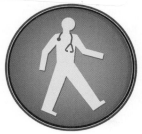

Resident Readiness™
Internal Medicine

Debra L. Klamen, MD, MHPE

Associate Dean for Education and Curriculum
Professor and Chair
Department of Medical Education
Southern Illinois University School of Medicine
Springfield, Illinois

Susan Thompson Hingle, MD

Professor of Medicine
Department of Internal Medicine
Southern Illinois University School of Medicine
Springfield, Illinois

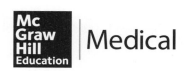

New York   Athens   Chicago   San Francisco   London   Madrid   Mexico City
Milan   New Delhi   San Juan   Singapore   Sydney   Toronto

1 2 3 4 5 6 7 8 9 0   DOC/DOC   18 17 16 15 14 13

ISBN 978-0-07-177318-8
MHID 0-07-177318-5

Notice

Medicine is an ever-changing science. As new research and clinical experience broaden our knowledge, changes in treatment and drug therapy are required. The authors and the publisher of this work have checked with sources believed to be reliable in their efforts to provide information that is complete and generally in accord with the standards accepted at the time of publication. However, in view of the possibility of human error or changes in medical sciences, neither the authors nor the publisher nor any other party who has been involved in the preparation or publication of this work warrants that the information contained herein is in every respect accurate or complete, and they disclaim all responsibility for any errors or omissions or for the results obtained from use of the information contained in this work. Readers are encouraged to confirm the information contained herein with other sources. For example and in particular, readers are advised to check the product information sheet included in the package of each drug they plan to administer to be certain that the information contained in this work is accurate and that changes have not been made in the recommended dose or in the contraindications for administration. This recommendation is of particular importance in connection with new or infrequently used drugs.

This book was set in Minion Pro by Thomson Digital.
The editors were Catherine A. Johnson and Cindy Yoo.
The production supervisor was Richard Ruzycka.
Project management was provided by Saloni Narang, Thomson Digital.
The designer was Eve Siegel; the cover designer was Anthony Landi.
RR Donnelley was the printer and binder.

This book is printed on acid-free paper.

Library of Congress Cataloging-in-Publication Data

Resident readiness. Internal medicine / [edited by] Debra L. Klamen, Susan Thompson Hingle.
    p. ; cm.
    Internal medicine
    Includes bibliographical references and index.
    ISBN 978-0-07-177318-8 (pbk. : alk. paper) — ISBN 0-07-177318-5 (pbk. : alk. paper)
    I. Klamen, Debra L., editor of compilation. II. Hingle, Susan Thompson, editor of compilation. III. Title: Internal medicine.
    [DNLM: 1. Diagnosis—Case Reports. 2. Internal Medicine—methods—Case Reports. 3. Therapeutics—Case Reports. WB 141]
    616.07′5—dc23

                                                            2012048773

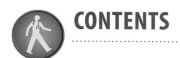

CONTENTS

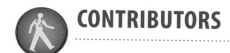

CONTRIBUTORS

Mohamad Alhosaini, MD
Assistant Professor of Clinical Medicine
Southern Illinois University School of Medicine
Springfield, Illinois
Chapters 2, 3, 4, 15

Muhammad Farooq Asghar, MD
Assistant Professor of Internal Medicine
Southern Illinois University School of Medicine
Springfield, Illinois
Chapters 8, 14

Edgard Cumpa, MD
Assistant Professor of Clinical Medicine
Southern Illinois University School of Medicine
Springfield, Illinois
Chapters 10, 24

Alan J. Deckard, MD, FACP
Associate Professor of Clinical Medicine
Chief, Division of General Internal Medicine
Department of Internal Medicine
Southern Illinois University School of Medicine
Springfield, Illinois
Chapter 20

Zak Gurnsey, MD, FACP
Assistant Professor/Hospitalist
Department of Internal Medicine
Southern Illinois University School of Medicine
Springfield, Illinois
Chapters 16, 18, 26

Se Young Han, MD
Division of General Internal Medicine
Southern Illinois University School of Medicine
Springfield, Illinois
Chapters 5, 7, 27

Susan Thompson Hingle, MD
Professor of Medicine
Department of Internal Medicine
Southern Illinois University School of Medicine
Springfield, Illinois
Chapters 6, 7, 27, 42

Sayeeda Azra Jabeen, MD, FACP
Assistant Professor of Clinical Medicine
Division of General Internal Medicine
Southern Illinois University School of Medicine
Springfield, Illinois
Chapters 1, 6, 13

Michael Jakoby, MD, MA
Associate Professor of Medicine
Chief, Division of Endocrinology and Metabolism
Southern Illinois University School of Medicine
Springfield, Illinois
Chapters 11, 12, 35, 38

Tiffany Leung, MD, MPH
Assistant Professor of Clinical Medicine
Division of General Internal Medicine
Southern Illinois University School of Medicine
Springfield, Illinois
Chapters 25, 34, 46, 47

Chaitanya K. Mamillapalli, MD
Assistant Professor
Division of Endocrinology and Metabolism
Southern Illinois University School of Medicine
Springfield, Illinois
Chapter 38

Owaise M. Y. Mansuri, MD
Fellow, Division of Endocrinology and Metabolism
Department of Internal Medicine
Southern Illinois University School of Medicine
Springfield, Illinois
Chapters 12, 35

Deepika Nallala, MD
Fellow, Division of Endocrinology
Department of Internal Medicine
Southern Illinois University School of Medicine
Springfield, Illinois
Chapter 11

Muralidhar Papireddy, MD
Academic Hospitalist
Assistant Professor of Clinical Medicine
Division of General Internal Medicine
Southern Illinois University School of Medicine
Springfield, Illinois
Chapters 7, 27, 42

Robert Robinson, MD, MS, FACP
Assistant Professor of Clinical Medicine
Department of Internal Medicine
Southern Illinois University School of Medicine
Springfield, Illinois
Chapters 21, 22, 29

J. Mark Ruscin, PharmD
Professor of Pharmacy Practice
Department of Pharmacy Practice
Southern Illinois University Edwardsville
School of Pharmacy
Edwardsville, Illinois
Chapter 46

Stacy Sattovia, MD, FACP
Associate Professor of Clinical Medicine/Hospitalist
Department of Internal Medicine
Director of Quality Improvement and Patient Safety
Southern Illinois University School of Medicine
Springfield, Illinois
Chapters 33, 48

Sheryll Mae C. Soriano, MD
Fellow, Division of Pulmonology
Southern Illinois University School of Medicine
Springfield, Illinois
Chapter 41

Vajeeha Tabassum, MD, FACP
Assistant Professor of Clinical Medicine
Division of General Internal Medicine
Southern Illinois University School of Medicine
Springfield, Illinois
Chapters 19, 28, 36

Thamilvani Thiruvasahar, MD
Rheumatology Fellow
Department of Medicine
Center of Excellence for Arthritic and Rheumatology
Shreveport, Louisiana
Chapter 17

Christine I. Todd, MD, FACP, FHM
Associate Professor of Internal Medicine
Division of General Internal Medicine
Southern Illinois University School of Medicine
Springfield, Illinois
Chapters 23, 43, 44, 45

Omar A. Vargas, MD, FACP
Assistant Professor of Internal Medicine
Division of Internal Medicine
Southern Illinois University School of Medicine
Springfield, Illinois
Chapters 31, 32, 39, 40

Siegfried W. B. Yu, MD, FACP
Associate Professor of Internal Medicine
Division of General Internal Medicine
Southern Illinois University School of Medicine
Springfield, Illinois
Chapters 9, 30, 37

ACKNOWLEDGMENTS

The resident readiness series evolved from ideas that a talented educator and surgeon, David Rogers, had about preparing senior students interested in going into surgery through a resident readiness course. This course was so successful at Southern Illinois University School of Medicine that it spread to other core clerkships, and resident readiness senior electives now exist throughout them. The idea for this book series was born by watching the success of these courses, and the interest the senior students have in them. It has been a great joy working with Susan Hingle, a singularly devoted physician who retains her humanity for others and passion for education, as well as with the other contributors to this book. We are grateful to the Dean, Dr. Kevin Dorsey, whose dedication to education and innovation allowed us to carve out time in our work to be creative. I (DLK) am greatly indebted to Catherine Johnson from McGraw-Hill, who helped me make the vision of a resident readiness series a reality. Her support and enthusiasm for the project have been unwavering. Likewise, the production editor on the internal medicine resident readiness book, Saloni Narang, has been completely dedicated to the task and is deserving of much thanks. We would also like to thank the many contributors to this book, whose commitment to medical education undoubtedly led to long nights writing and editing in its service. We would also like to thank our colleague dieticians, Gayle Jennings and Christina Rollins, for their expert contributions to the chapter on nutrition. Lastly, we appreciate our husbands' forbearance for the hours we spent in front of the computer at home; their patience and understanding are unparalleled.

Debra L. Klamen
Susan Thompson Hingle

INTRODUCTION

Facing the prospect of an internship is an exciting, and undoubtedly anxiety-provoking, prospect. Four years of medical school culminate in, after graduation, a rapid transition to someone calling you "Doctor" and asking you to give orders and perform procedures without, in many cases, a supervisor standing directly over your shoulder.

This book is organized to help senior medical students dip their toes safely in the water of responsibility and action from the safety of reading cases, without real patients, nurses, families, and supervisors expecting decisive action. The chapters are short, easy to read, and "to the point." Short vignettes pose an organizing context to valuable issues vital to the function of the new intern. Emphasis on the discussion of these cases is not on extensive basic science background or a review of the literature; it is on practical knowledge that the intern will need to function well in the hospital and "hit the ground running." Many of the cases include questions at the end of them to stimulate further thinking and clinical reasoning in the topic area discussed. References at the end of the cases are resources for further reading as desired.

HOW TO GET THE MOST OUT OF THIS BOOK

Each case is designed to simulate a patient encounter (or nurse request for a patient encounter in some instances) and is followed by a set of open-ended questions. Open-ended questions follow and are used purposely, since the cued nature of multiple choice questions will certainly not be available in a clinical setting with real patient involvement. Each case is divided into four parts.

Part 1

1. **Answers** to the questions posed. The student should try to answer the questions after the case vignette before going on to read the case review or other answers, in order to improve his or her clinical acumen, which, after all, is what resident readiness is all about.

2. A **Case Review:** A brief discussion of the case presented in the vignette will be presented, helping the student understand how an expert would think about, and handle, the specific issues at hand with the particular patient presented.

Part 2

Topic Title followed by **Diagnosis** and **Treatment** discussions: In this section, a more generalized, though still focused and brief, discussion of the general issues brought forward in the case presented will be given. For example, in the case of a patient presenting with coma and a significantly elevated glucose, the case review might discuss the exact treatment of the patient presented, while this part of the book will discuss, in general, the diagnosis and treatment of DKA. Of note, not all of the cases in the book will fit entirely into this model, so variations do occur as necessary. (For example, in the case of a patient in need of palliative care.)

Part 3

Tips to Remember: These are brief, bullet pointed notes that are reiterated as a summary of the text, allowing for easy and rapid review, such as when preparing a case presentation to the faculty in morning rounds.

Part 4

Comprehension Questions: Most cases have several multiple choice questions that follow at the very end. These serve to reinforce the material presented, and provide a self-assessment mechanism for the student.

Section I.
Inpatient Medicine

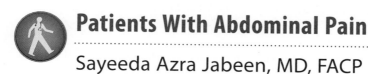

Patients With Abdominal Pain

Sayeeda Azra Jabeen, MD, FACP

A 75-year-old Man With Epigastric and Periumbilical Pain

Mr Jones is a 75-year-old gentleman admitted with a history of fever, cough, and shortness of breath. He was diagnosed with community-acquired pneumonia and started on levofloxacin. On admission his vitals were stable. The on-call intern gets a call at 2 AM by the nurse, stating Mr Jones has been complaining of excruciating constant abdominal pain (epigastric and periumbilical pain) radiating to the flank for the past 15 to 20 minutes. His pain is associated with nausea and vomiting but no fever or chills, hematuria, dysuria, or chest pain. He had a normal bowel movement today. Past medical history includes HTN, type 2 DM, and CAD; no h/o renal or gallstones. Social history is significant for smoking, and the patient reports no alcohol use. Medications include levofloxacin, hydrochlorothiazide, aspirin, metoprolol, and lovastatin; no NSAID use is noted. On physical examination, he looks to be in moderate distress.

Blood pressure lying down is 120/60, heart rate is 100, and the patient is afebrile. Heart and lung examinations are unremarkable. Abdominal examination reveals obese abdomen with moderate, diffuse tenderness without guarding or rigidity; bowel sounds are present but hypoactive. Pulses are diminished in the lower extremities. Rectal examination reveals Hemoccult-negative stool.

1. What should be included in your differential diagnosis (DDX)?

Answer

1. Pancreatitis

    Diverticular rupture (although pain would be expected more in the left lower quadrant [LLQ])

Peptic ulcer disease unless associated with perforation with signs of peritonitis (rebound tenderness and rigidity)

Ruptured abdominal aortic aneurysm (AAA)

CASE REVIEW: ABDOMINAL AORTIC ANEURYSM

The classic presentation of an AAA is a man with a history of HTN who has the triad of severe abdominal pain, a pulsatile abdominal mass, and hypotension. Physical examination is not sufficiently sensitive to rule out AAA. Although atherosclerosis is the most common cause for an AAA, there are a number of nonatherosclerotic causes, which include cystic medial necrosis, and infections such as syphilis and those caused by *Salmonella*. Aneurysms also occur with diseases such as Marfan syndrome or Ehlers-Danlos syndrome. Risk factors include smoking, male gender, family history, advanced age, and uncontrolled hypertension. Complications include aortic aneurysm rupture. Rates of rupture rise as the aneurysm increases in diameter size. Mortality with rupture is 70% to 90%. Bedside emergent ultrasound has been demonstrated to be highly accurate with a sensitivity of 96% to 100% and a specificity of 98% to 100%. For screening, ultrasound is preferred. Treatment may be surgical or medical. Urgent surgical management is used when the AAA has ruptured. For an asymptomatic AAA, repair is recommended when an aneurysm is greater than or equal to 5.5 cm, is tender, or has increased in size by more than 1 cm in 1 year. For smaller aneurysms that have not ruptured, medical management with smoking cessation, statin therapy, and blood pressure control is initiated.

Alternative diagnoses to consider include nephrolithiasis and diverticulitis.

Nephrolithiasis

The classic presentation is acute onset of severe back and flank pain that may radiate to the abdomen or groin. Pain may be associated with nausea, vomiting, or dysuria. Abdominal tenderness is unusual and, if present, should raise the possibility of other diagnoses.

Diverticulitis

A diverticulum is a sac-like protrusion of the colonic wall. A low-fiber diet and constipation are believed to cause diverticula to form by decreasing stool bulk, and increasing intraluminal pressure. Diverticulitis develops secondary to microscopic or frank perforation of the diverticula. Eighty-five percent to 90% develop in the sigmoid or descending colon. The classic presentation is gradually increasing LLQ pain. Fever is often present. Patients may present with diarrhea and/or constipation. Guarding and rigidity may be seen. Diverticulitis can be complicated with abscess formation, peritonitis, colonic obstruction, fistula formation, and sepsis. Computer tomography (CT) scanning of the abdomen with IV and oral contrast is the diagnostic test of choice. If the patient has no fever or elevated white blood cell count and is able to tolerate oral antibiotics, then start ciprofloxacin and metronidazole for 7 to 10 days. Encourage oral liquid intake. For moderate to severe attacks, broad-spectrum intravenous antibiotics should be started. Keep the patient NPO (nothing by mouth) and start intravenous fluids. If there is an abscess (5 cm or larger), obtain CT-guided drainage. Emergent surgery is indicated in cases of frank peritonitis, uncontrolled sepsis, clinical deterioration, obstruction, or large abscesses.

ABDOMINAL PAIN

Abdominal pain is one of the most common causes for hospital admission in the United States. It is caused by conditions that range from trivial to life-threatening.

Diagnosis

The first pivotal step in diagnosing abdominal pain is to identify the location of the pain. The DDX can then be narrowed to a subset of conditions that cause pain in that particular quadrant of the abdomen (see Figure 1-1).

There is overlap among the differential diagnoses in the various quadrants, and there are some different concerns based on age and gender.

History

The character and acuity of the pain are pivotal features that help prioritize the DDX. Other important historical points include factors that make the pain better or worse (eg, eating), radiation of the pain, duration of the pain, and associated symptoms (nausea, vomiting, poor appetite, inability to pass stool and gas, melena, hematochezia, fever, chills, weight loss, altered bowel habits, orthostatic symptoms, or urinary symptoms). Pulmonary symptoms or a cardiac history can be clues to pneumonia or myocardial infarction (MI) presenting as abdominal pain. In women, sexual and menstrual histories are very important. The patient should be asked about alcohol consumption as well.

Physical Examination

A few points about the physical examination are worth emphasizing. Vital signs such as hypotension, fever, tachypnea, and tachycardia are pivotal clinical clues that must not be overlooked. The HEENT examination should look for pallor or icterus. Careful heart and lung examinations can suggest pneumonia or other extra-abdominal causes of abdominal pain.

Right upper quadrant

Appendicitis (retrocecal)
Biliary colic
Cholangitis
Cholecystitis
Hepatitis
Hepatic abscess
Perforated duodenal ulcer
Pneumonia (right lower lobe)
Pulmonary embolism

Left upper quadrant

Gastric ulcer
Gastritis
Myocardial ischemia
Pancreatitis
Pneumonia (left lower lobe)
Pulmonary embolism
Splenic congestion or rupture

Right lower quadrant

Aortic aneurysm
Appendicitis
Crohn's disease
Diverticulitis (cecal)
Ectopic pregnancy
Endometriosis
Incarcerated inguinal hernia
Ischemic colitis
Ovarian cyst
Ovarian torsion
Pelvic inflammatory disease
Psoas abscess
Testicular torsion
Ureteral calculi

Left lower quadrant

Aortic aneurysm
Diverticulitis (sigmoid)
Ectopic pregnancy
Endometriosis
Incarcerated inguinal hernia
Ischemic colitis
Ovarian cyst
Ovarian torsion
Pelvic inflammatory disease
Psoas abscess
Testicular torsion
Ureteral calculi

Diffuse pain

Aortic aneurysm
Aortic dissection
Appendicitis (early)
Bowel obstruction
Gastroenteritis
Mesenteric ischemia
Metabolic disorders (Diabetic ketoacidosis, uremia)
Narcotic withdrawal
Pancreatitis
Perforated bowel
Peritonitis
Sickle cell crisis
Volvulus

Figure 1-1. DDX of abdominal pain.

Treatment

Acute abdominal pain frequently requires urgent investigation and management. Some patients require assessment of their airways, breathing, and circulation, followed by appropriate resuscitation. Many patients will require analgesics, which can be administered judiciously without compromising the physical assessment of peritoneal signs.

Patients with a suspected surgical abdomen must be transferred to an acute facility where surgical consultation and management are available.

Acute versus chronic pain: while an arbitrary interval, such as 12 weeks, can be used to separate acute from chronic abdominal pain, there is no strict time period. Pain in a sick or unstable patient should generally be managed as acute pain.

A 26-year-old Man With Diffuse Abdominal Pain for the Past 12 Hours

Mr Smith is a 26-year-old man with no significant past medical history who presents with diffuse abdominal pain that began 12 hours ago and is described as a pressure sensation, most intensely in the mid-abdomen. He has a decreased appetite but no nausea or vomiting. His last bowel movement was 2 days ago. He denies fevers and chills as well as hematuria, dysuria, and chest pain. The patient has no h/o gallstones, kidney stones, or abdominal surgeries. He takes no medications (no aspirin or NSAIDs) and reports occasional use of alcohol. Vitals are stable. Patient is afebrile. Cardiac and lung examinations are normal. Abdominal examination reveals a flat abdomen with hypoactive bowel sounds. There is mild, diffuse tenderness present. No guarding or rigidity is present. Rectal examination is normal. Stool is Hemoccult negative.

1. What should be included in your DDX?

Answer

1. Appendicitis (always to be considered in young adults)

   Peptic ulcer disease

   Pancreatitis (may present with epigastric or mid-abdominal pain)

   Early bowel obstruction

CASE REVIEW: APPENDICITIS

The classic presentation is diffuse abdominal pain that migrates to the right lower quadrant (RLQ) to McBurney point (1.5–2 in from the anterior superior iliac crest toward the umbilicus). The pain is associated with nausea, vomiting, fever, and anorexia. Appendicitis develops due to obstruction of the appendiceal orifice with secondary mucous accumulation, swelling, ischemia, necrosis, and perforation. Complications include perforation and abscess formation. The risk of perforation increases steadily with increasing age (50% in patients >75 years old). Fever, tenderness, guarding, and rebound may be absent in patients with appendicitis. Nonetheless, when present, they increase the likelihood of appendicitis. Eighty percent of patients with appendicitis have a WBC >10,000 with a left shift. Urinalysis may reveal pyuria and hematuria due to bladder inflammation from adjacent appendicitis. CT of abdomen and pelvis with IV and oral/rectal contrast is the test of choice. Although ultrasound is inferior to CT scan, it is the test of choice in pregnant patients. Frequent clinical observation is critical in patients with an unclear diagnosis. One should start intravenous fluids and broad-spectrum antibiotics and obtain a STAT surgical consult as urgent appendectomy is the treatment of choice.

Other diagnoses to consider in patients with RLQ pain include cecal diverticulitis, Meckel diverticulitis, acute ileitis, Crohn disease, and gynecologic conditions.

Cecal Diverticulitis

Cecal diverticulitis usually occurs in young adults and presents with signs and symptoms that are virtually identical to those of appendicitis.

Meckel Diverticulitis

A Meckel diverticulum is a congenital remnant of the omphalomesenteric duct. It contains all layers of the intestine and may have ectopic tissue present from either the pancreas or stomach. It is located on the small intestine 2 ft from the ileocecal valve, and is about 2 in in length. The small bowel may migrate into the RLQ and mimic the symptoms of appendicitis.

Acute Ileitis

Acute ileitis is due most commonly to an acute self-limited bacterial infection (Yersinia, Campylobacter, Salmonella, and others), and should be considered when diarrhea is a prominent symptom.

Crohn Disease

Crohn disease can present with symptoms similar to appendicitis. Fatigue, prolonged diarrhea with abdominal pain, weight loss, and fever, with or without gross bleeding, are the hallmarks of Crohn disease. Crohn disease should be suspected in patients who have persistent pain after surgery, especially if the appendix is histologically normal.

Gynecologic Conditions

A number of gynecologic conditions, most notably ectopic pregnancy and pelvic inflammatory disease (acute salpingitis), should be considered in the DDX. Always rule out pregnancy in women of childbearing age who complain of abdominal pain.

A 55-year-old Woman With Crampy Epigastric Pain

Ms Hampton is a 55-year-old female who presents to the emergency department with crampy epigastric pain that woke her up in the middle of the night. She has had similar attacks over the past several months that generally last for 3 to 4 hours. Heavy meals worsen the pain. She denies nausea and vomiting, has normal bowel movements, no fever or chills, and no hematuria, dysuria, or chest pain. Patient medical history is remarkable for type 2 DM, HTN, and lone atrial fibrillation. Medications include metoprolol, insulin, and aspirin; she occasionally takes acetaminophen for knee pain. She reports no alcohol use. On physical examination vitals are normal. The patient is afebrile. Sclera is nonicteric. Cardiac and lung examinations are normal except for the presence of an irregularly irregular cardiac rhythm. Abdominal examination shows a slightly obese abdomen. Bowel sounds are present. Abdomen is soft, with mild epigastric tenderness present. No guarding or rigidity is present. Murphy sign is negative. Rectal examination is normal. Stool is Hemoccult negative.

1. What should be included in your DDX?

Answer

1. Biliary colic
    Peptic ulcer disease
    Pancreatitis
    Irritable bowel syndrome (IBS)
    Mesenteric ischemia

CASE REVIEW: BILIARY COLIC

The classic presentation of biliary colic is a deep, sharp, severe, gnawing episodic pain that is localized to the right upper quadrant (RUQ) or the epigastrium. It may radiate to the back and be associated with nausea and vomiting. Patients are pain-free in between the episodes. Biliary colic occurs when a gallstone becomes lodged in the cystic duct and the gallbladder contracts against the obstruction, in response to a fatty meal. Complications include acute cholecystitis, pancreatitis, and ascending cholangitis. A RUQ ultrasound is the diagnostic test of choice due to its high sensitivity and specificity. Cholecystectomy is recommended. Dissolution therapies (eg, ursodiol) are reserved for nonsurgical candidates.

Alternative possible diagnoses include peptic ulcer disease (PUD), pancreatitis, IBS, ischemic bowel, mesenteric ischemia, and ischemic colitis.

Peptic Ulcer Disease

PUD presents with dull or hunger-like pain in the epigastrium that is either exacerbated or improved by food intake. Most ulcers are due to NSAID use, *Helicobacter pylori* infection, or both. Best predictors of PUD are a history of NSAID use and *H. pylori* infection. A significant number of patients with NSAID-induced ulcers do not experience pain. Anemia, GI bleeding, early satiety, or weight loss may be the only symptoms of PUD. Zollinger-Ellison syndrome is a rare cause of PUD. An esophagogastroduodenoscopy (EGD) should be considered with symptoms of significant bleeding, anemia, weight loss, early satiety, dysphagia, recurrent vomiting, a family history of GI cancer, or in patients who do not respond to initial therapy. Gastric ulcers always warrant biopsy to rule out adenocarcinoma. *H. pylori* testing should be done via the biopsied tissue.

One can also test for *H. pylori* with a urea breath test and *H. pylori* stool antigen in patients not undergoing EGD. A rapid urease test on biopsy and histology are preferred in patients undergoing EGD. Serology does not distinguish active from prior infection (avoid the use of serology on a routine basis). Active bleeding from PUD decreases the sensitivity of a rapid urease test. Patients with bleeding and a negative rapid urease test and negative histology should undergo a urea breath test several weeks after completing proton pump inhibitor (PPI) therapy.

Treatment goals include eradication of *H. pylori*, symptom alleviation, and ulcer healing. The regimen most commonly recommended for first-line treatment of *H. pylori* is triple therapy with a PPI (lansoprazole 30 mg twice daily, omeprazole 20 mg twice daily, pantoprazole 40 mg twice daily, rabeprazole 20 mg twice daily, or esomeprazole 40 mg once daily), amoxicillin (1 g twice daily), and clarithromycin (500 mg twice daily) for 10 to 14 days. Metronidazole (500 mg twice daily) can be substituted for amoxicillin, but only in penicillin-allergic individuals. An increased incidence of *H. pylori* resistance has led to the recommendation of posttreatment testing to confirm eradication. Appropriate testing includes stool antigen or urea breath test 4 to 6 weeks after completion of therapy. Don't forget to discontinue NSAIDs in these patients.

Pancreatitis

The classic presentation of pancreatitis is a constant, boring abdominal pain of moderate to severe intensity in the epigastrium that may radiate to the back. Pain is often associated with nausea, vomiting, low-grade fever, and abdominal distention. Alcohol abuse and choledocholithiasis cause 80% of acute pancreatitis cases. Other causes include idiopathic, post-endoscopic retrograde cholangiopancreatography (ERCP), and medications (hydrochlorothiazide, azathioprine, corticosteroids, sulfonamides, furosemide, etc). Less common causes are trauma, marked hypertriglyceridemia (>1000 mg/dL), hypercalcemia, and pancreatic divisum. Regardless of the inciting cause, trypsinogen is activated to trypsin that activates other pancreatic enzymes resulting in pancreatic autodigestion and inflammation. Patients with pancreatitis may develop psuedocysts, abscesses, or pancreatic necrosis. Systemic complications include hyperglycemia, hypocalcemia, acute respiratory distress syndrome, acute renal failure, and disseminated intravascular coagulation (DIC). Death may occur in patients with infected pancreatic necrosis and multiorgan system failure. Several predictive scores have been developed. These include Ranson criteria, the BISAP score, and the APACHE II score. The American Gastroenterology Association (AGA) recommends the use of the apache II system. Hemoconcentration (Hct ≥50%) on admission predicts severe pancreatitis. C-reactive protein >150 mg/dL at 48 hours can also predict severe pancreatitis. Diagnostic testing should include amylase and lipase. Transabdominal ultrasound is ideal to image the gallbladder and biliary tree to look for gallstones. CT scan is the test of choice to look for complications and assess severity.

Treatment is generally supportive care with IV fluids. It is recommended, after initial fluid resuscitation with 20 cm^3/kg IV fluids over 60 to 90 minutes, to give approximately 250 to 300 cm^3/h IV fluids for 48 hours if the patient's cardiac status permits. One should closely monitor vital signs, renal function, hematocrit, and fluid status. Patient should not eat and should be made NPO to rest the gut. Prophylactic antibiotics are controversial and not routinely indicated. It is reasonable to withhold antibiotics until there is clinical evidence of infection (fever, leukocytosis, or clinical deterioration). If there is necrotic tissue, then antibiotics should be started. ERCP and sphincterotomy can be therapeutic, but are invasive. They are only recommended in patients with gallstone pancreatitis with persistent obstruction or cholangitis.

Irritable Bowel Syndrome

IBS is characterized by intermittent abdominal pain accompanied by diarrhea, constipation, or both of years' long duration. The diarrhea is often associated with cramps relieved by defecation and passing flatus. Pain cannot be explained by structural or biochemical abnormalities. Symptoms of IBS are due to a combination of altered motility, visceral hypersensitivity, autonomic function, and psychological factors. Symptoms are often exacerbated by psychological or physical stress.

Diagnosis

The diagnosis is usually made by a combination of (1) fulfilling the Rome criteria, (2) the absence of alarm features, and (3) a limited workup to exclude other diseases.

1. Rome criteria: Recurrent abdominal pain or discomfort (of ≥6 months duration) at least 3 days per month for the past 3 months, associated with 2 or more of the following:

   A. Improvement with defecation

   B. Onset associated with a change in frequency of stool

   C. Onset associated with a change in form (appearance) of stool

2. Alarm symptoms suggest alternative diagnoses and necessitate evaluation

   A. Positive fecal occult blood test or rectal bleeding

   B. Anemia

   C. Weight loss >10 lb

   D. Fever

   E. Persistent diarrhea causing dehydration

   F. Sever constipation or fecal impaction

   G. Family history of colorectal cancer

   H. Onset of symptoms at age 50 years or older

   I. Major change in symptoms

   J. Nocturnal symptoms

   K. Recent antibiotic use

3. Workup

   A. Common recommendations for patients fulfilling Rome criteria without alarm symptoms include the following:

      - CBC.

      - Test stool for occult blood.

      - Serologic tests for celiac sprue (eg, IgA tissue transglutaminase or IgA EMA) in patients with diarrhea as the predominant symptom.

      - Routine chemistries are recommended by some experts.

   B. Colonoscopy with biopsy (to rule out microscopic colitis) is recommended in patients with alarm symptoms, in patients aged ≥50 years, and in patients with a marked change in symptoms.

C. There is no evidence that flexible sigmoidoscopy or colonoscopy is necessary in young patients without alarm symptoms.

D. In addition to the above testing, the following should be evaluated in patients with alarm symptoms:
- Thyroid function levels
- Basic chemistries
- Stool for *Clostridium difficile* toxin and presence of ova and parasites

A variety of serum and fecal markers, including ASCA, p-ANCA, fecal calprotectin, and fecal lactoferrin, are useful in selected patients and can suggest bowel inflammation or inflammatory bowel disease (IBD).

Treatment

Treatment of IBS includes avoiding certain foods (milk products, caffeine, alcohol, fatty foods, gas-producing vegetables, etc) that may worsen symptoms. Specific therapy is based on predominant symptoms. When abdominal pain is a predominant symptom, medications such as anticholinergics (dicyclomine or hyoscyamine) and/or smooth muscle relaxants may be beneficial. Cognitive behavioral therapy is also useful. When diarrhea is the predominant symptom, medications such as loperamide, diphenoxylate, and cholestyramine may be useful. Alosetron, a 5-HT3 receptor antagonist, is also useful with diarrhea, but is generally only prescribed by gastroenterologists, as serious complications such as bowel obstruction and ischemic colitis may occur with its use. When constipation is the predominant symptom, a change to a high-fiber diet and osmotic laxatives such as lactulose and polyethylene glycol are used.

Ischemic Bowel

There are 3 distinct subtypes of ischemic bowel, including chronic mesenteric ischemia (chronic small bowel ischemia), acute mesenteric ischemia (acute ischemia of small bowel), and ischemic colitis (ischemia of the large bowel).

Mesenteric ischemia

This is a life-threatening condition that virtually always presents with the abrupt onset of acute, severe abdominal pain that is typically out of proportion to a relativity benign physical examination. It may be associated with nausea, vomiting, and abdominal pain. This ischemia usually occurs due to a superior mesenteric artery embolism (50%) that is frequently due to a dislodged thrombosis from the left atrium, left ventricle, or cardiac valves. Mesenteric arterial thrombosis (15%–25%) occurs due to progressive atherosclerotic stenosis of the involved artery. Mesenteric venous thrombosis occurs often due to portal hypertension, hypercoagulable states, and intra-abdominal inflammation.

Nonobstructive mesenteric ischemia (NOMI) (20%–30%) often occurs in elderly patients with atherosclerotic disease and superimposed hypotension (MI, heart failure, cardiopulmonary bypass, dialysis, or sepsis). Mortality is high at 30% to 65%. Complications include bowel infarction and peritonitis. Lactic acid level is typically elevated. Although CT angiography and magnetic resonance angiography have been used, direct mesenteric angiography is the gold standard diagnostic test.

Treatment consists of emergent revascularization via thromboembolectomy, thrombolysis, vascular bypass or angioplasty, and surgical resection of necrotic bowel. Broad-spectrum IV antibiotics, volume resuscitation, and preoperative and postoperative anticoagulation to prevent thrombosis propagation are also essential. Intra-arterial papaverine has been used to block reactive mesenteric arteriolar vasoconstriction and improve blood flow.

Ischemic colitis

Ischemic colitis presents with left-sided abdominal pain that is frequently associated with bloody or maroon-colored stools and/or diarrhea. It occurs due to a nonocclusive decrease in colonic perfusion (hypotension, MI, sepsis, CHF, etc). It typically involves the watershed area of the colon, most commonly the splenic flexure, descending colon, and rectosigmoid junction. Lactic acid level is elevated. Colonoscopy is the preferred diagnostic test. CT scan may demonstrate segmental circumferential wall thickening (when nonspecific) or appear normal. Treatment is generally supportive with bed rest, IV fluids, and broad-spectrum antibiotics. Colonic infarction occurs in a small percentage of patients and requires surgical intervention.

A 55-year-old Woman With a Diagnosis of Biliary Colic, Now Presenting With Constant RUQ Pain, Fever, and Chills

Mrs Hampton's history suggests biliary colic. A RUQ ultrasound reveals multiple small gallstones. CBC is normal. Serum lipase and liver enzymes were normal. Urea breath test for *H. pylori* was negative. After surgical consultation, cholecystectomy was planned in the next few weeks. Unfortunately, Mrs Hampton returned to the emergency department prior to scheduled surgery with constant pain in her RUQ associated with fever and chills. She looks in acute distress. She reports dark urine. Vitals are stable except for the presence of fever at 38.3°C. Sclera was anicteric. Abdominal examination reveals RUQ tenderness with positive Murphy sign.

1. What should be included in your DDX?

Answer

1. Common bile duct (CBD) obstruction (also known as choledocholithiasis)
   Ascending cholangitis
   Acute cholecystitis
   Hepatitis

CASE REVIEW: CHOLEDOCHOLITHIASIS AND ASCENDING CHOLANGITIS

The classic presentation is RUQ pain, fever, and jaundice, also known as Charcot triad. This occurs due to CBD obstruction, most commonly from a gallstone. Complications include obstruction, jaundice, fever, leukocytosis, sepsis, and pancreatitis. ERCP is both diagnostic and therapeutic. It is the preferred test of choice in patients with a high pretest probability of CBD stone with obstruction. It allows direct cannulation of CBD and relieves obstruction via simultaneous stone extraction and sphincterotomy. In patients who are less likely to have a CBD stone, a less invasive test such as magnetic resonance cholangiopancreatography (MRCP) or endoscopic ultrasound (EUS) would be appropriate as an initial study. Treatment includes IV hydration, IV broad-spectrum antibiotics, decompression of the biliary system (via ERCP in patients with persistent pain, hypotension, altered mental status, persistent high fever, WBC ≥20,000, bilirubin >10 mg/dL) and electively in more stable patients, and/or cholecystectomy.

Alternative diagnoses to consider include acute cholecystitis and acute hepatitis.

Acute Cholecystitis

Acute cholecystitis presents as persistent RUQ or epigastric pain associated with fever, nausea, and vomiting. Murphy sign may be present (sensitivity 65% and specificity 87%). Acute cholecystitis is caused by persistent obstruction of the cystic duct with stones resulting in gallbladder inflammation and pain. It may be complicated with necrosis, infection, and gangrene. The test of choice is a RUQ ultrasound. Cholescinitigraphy (HIDA scan) is useful when the pretest probability is high and ultrasound is nondiagnostic. Nonvisualization of the gallbladder suggests cystic duct obstruction and is highly specific for acute cholecystitis. Treatment includes IV hydration and IV antibiotics.

Acute Hepatitis

Viral or alcoholic hepatitis should be considered in a patient presenting with abdominal pain, jaundice, anorexia, nausea, malaise, hepatomegaly, or hepatic tenderness. Liver enzymes are very high in acute hepatitis. If suspected, appropriate serologies should be ordered.

A 70-year-old Man With Crampy Mid-abdominal Pain

Mr Lantern is a 70-year-old man with a history of hypertension, type 2 DM, and coronary artery disease who presents with intermittent, crampy, mid-abdominal pain that started 2 days ago and is associated with nausea, vomiting, constipation, and an unintentional weight loss of 10 lb over the past 2 months. No fever or chills, hematuria, dysuria, or chest pain is noted. The patient has no history of gallstones, kidney stones, or abdominal surgeries. Medications: lisinopril, aspirin, metoprolol, simvastatin, and insulin. He reports no alcohol use. On physical examination the patient looks moderately distressed. Vitals are significant for orthostasis with the heart rate increasing by 20 beats/min and blood pressure dropping by 20 mm Hg when the patient sits up. The patient is afebrile. Sclera are nonicteric. Cardiac and lung examinations are normal except for an irregularly irregular rhythm. Abdominal examination reveals a distended abdomen with hyperactive bowel sounds. Rectal examination is normal. Stool is Hemoccult positive.

1. What should be included in your DDX?

Answer

1. Large bowel obstruction (LBO)

   Small bowel obstruction (SBO)

CASE REVIEW

Large Bowel Obstruction

LBO typically presents with severe, diffuse, crampy abdominal pain that appears in waves associated with vomiting. Abdominal pain and the absence of bowel movements or flatus suggest bowel obstruction. Initially, patients may have several bowel movements as the bowel distal to the obstruction is emptied. Obstruction can be due to cancer, volvulus, diverticular disease, or external compression from metastatic cancer, etc. LBO may be complicated by bowel infarction, perforation, peritonitis, and sepsis. Plain x-rays of the abdomen may show air-fluid levels and distension of large bowel (>6 cm) and also free air under the diaphragm in the case of perforation. CT scan of the abdomen and pelvis is also accurate in the diagnosis of LBO (91% sensitive and 91% specific). Hypaque enema (water-soluble enema) is 96% sensitive and 98% specific and is highly accurate for larger bowel obstruction. It can be both diagnostic and therapeutic. It can also exclude acute colonic pseudo-obstruction (Ogilvie syndrome, distension of the cecum and colon without mechanical obstruction). Colonoscopy can decompress pseudo-obstruction and prevent cecal perforation. Treatment of LBO includes aggressive hydration, broad-spectrum antibiotics, and a surgical consultation. Emergent surgical indications include perforation or ischemia. Nonemergent indications include increasing abdominal distension and failure to resolve with conservative management.

Small Bowel Obstruction

SBO presents similarly to LBO, except that the patient typically has a history of prior abdominal surgeries. It is usually caused by adhesions, malignant obstruction, hernias, IBD strictures, or radiation-induced strictures. SBO complications include bowel infarction, perforation, peritonitis, and sepsis. Plain x-rays of the abdomen may show 2 or more air-fluid levels or dilated loops of bowel proximal to the obstruction (>2.5 cm diameter of small bowel). Complete obstruction is unlikely if air is seen in the rectum or in the colon. CT scan of the abdomen is the diagnostic test of choice. It may delineate the etiology of the obstruction as well. Obstruction is suggested by a transition point between bowel proximal to the obstruction, which is dilated, and bowel distal to the obstruction, which is collapsed. A small bowel series may be useful when CT is nondiagnostic. SBO treatment includes aggressive IV hydration, keeping the patient NPO with a nasogastric tube to suction, careful frequent observation, repeated physical examinations over the first 12 to 24 hours, and frequent plain radiographs. Broad-spectrum IV antibiotics are typically initiated. Surgical indications include signs of ischemia, infarction on CT scan, and obstruction due to hernia.

TIPS TO REMEMBER

- DDX of abdominal pain may be very expansive.
- History is the most important element in developing and refining your list of diagnostic possibilities.
- Localizing the pain to a quadrant helps to refine and narrow your DDX.
- Not all abdominal pain is of gastrointestinal origin.
- Workup should be targeted based on the history and physical examination.

SUGGESTED READINGS

Fishman M, Aronson M. Differential diagnosis of abdominal pain in adults. In: Fletcher R, Sokol N, eds. *UpToDate*. 2011.

Mohler E, Fairman R. Natural history and management of abdominal aortic aneurysm. In: Eidt J, Mills J, Collins K, eds. *UpToDate*. 2011.

Panner R, Majumdar S. Diagnostic approach to abdominal pain in adults. In: Edit J, Mills J, Collins K, eds. *UpToDate*. 2012.

Stern S, Cifu A, Altkorn D. Abdominal pain. In: Benoit J, Stein S, eds. *Symptom to Diagnosis: An Evidence Based Guide*. 2nd ed. New York: McGraw Hill (Lange Clinical Medicine); 2010.

Yamada T. *Approach to the Patient with Abdominal Pain. Handbook of Gastroenterology*. Philadelphia: Lippincott Williams & Wilkins; 1998:49–58.

Yamada T. *Approach to the Patient with Acute Abdomen. Handbook of Gastroenterology*. Philadelphia: Lippincott Williams & Wilkins; 1998:59–67.

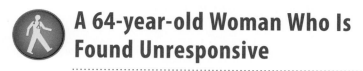

A 64-year-old Woman Who Is Found Unresponsive

Mohamad Alhosaini, MD

A 64-year-old female with a history of COPD and obstructive sleep apnea was admitted to the hospital for suspected methicillin-resistant *Staphylococcus aureus* cellulitis. The patient was started on intravenous vancomycin. She refused to use the hospital CPAP machine during the night. At 6:00 AM the phlebotomist found the patient unresponsive and the rapid response team was called. The patient had a Glasgow coma score of 5. Her vital signs were normal except for an O_2 saturation of 85% on room air. ABG showed: pH of 7.01, Po_2 of 55, $P\check{c}o_2$ of 90, and HCO_3 of 30.

1. What is the acid-base abnormality?
2. What is the cause of this abnormality?
3. What would you do for the patient?

Answers

1. The patient has acute noncompensated respiratory acidosis.

2. The patient had acute hypercapnic respiratory failure secondary to worsening apnea most likely secondary to not using the CPAP machine.

3. The patient needs emergent intubation. Noninvasive ventilation is not appropriate in this case because of her poor mental status and severe acidosis.

METABOLIC ACIDOSIS

High Anion Gap Metabolic Acidosis

Diagnosis
High anion gap metabolic acidosis (HAGMA) is simply caused by adding acid to the serum. The excessive hydrogen ions will be buffered by bicarbonate, so bicarbonate concentration will decrease. Chloride concentration will stay the same because the loss of bicarbonate will be replaced by the negatively charged anion part of the added acid. The low bicarbonate and the normal chloride concentrations will result in a high anion gap.

The most clinically important acids that cause HAGMA and their etiologies are shown in Table 2-1. A simplified algorithm to HAGMA is shown in Figure 2-1.

Advanced chronic kidney disease (CKD) is commonly associated with HAGMA when GFR decreases to less than 20 mL/min. Metabolic acidosis promotes protein catabolism and worsens bone disease in this group. Acidosis is

Table 2-1. Etiologies of HAGMA

Lactic acid → shock, drugs (metformin, salicylates, INH, methanol, ethylene glycol, propofol, linezolide, stavudine, didanosine), seizure, liver failure, malignancy, cyanide poisoning, and carbon monoxide poisoning
Ketones → diabetes, starvation, ethanol
Salicylates → salicylate toxicities
Glycolic and oxalic acids → ethylene glycol toxicity
Formic acid → methanol toxicity
Pyroglutamic acid → acetaminophen
Phosphoric acid, sulfuric acid, and other acids → advanced chronic kidney disease
D-Lactic acidosis → after small bowel resection
Iron intoxication

effectively corrected by hemodialysis. Patients not on hemodialysis may need sodium bicarbonate to keep serum bicarbonate above 20 mEq/L. The starting dose is usually 650 mg 3 times a day. Loop diuretics are frequently added to avoid volume overload.

Treatment
Lactic acidosis treatment should be directed at the underlying cause. Bicarbonate should be avoided because it may have an adverse effect on cardiac function and may even worsen the acidosis. When the pH is less than 7.1, bicarbonate may be used. The goal is to get the pH above 7.1 and not to the normal range.

Ketoacidosis is caused by diabetes, starvation, or ethanol. Diabetic keto-acidosis is treated with fluids and insulin. Starvation and alcohol ketoacidosis should be treated with glucose administration (inducing insulin release will decrease lipolysis in adipose tissue as well as keto acid production from liver). Again, bicarbonate should be used only if the pH is less than 7.1.

Ethanol dehydrogenase is responsible for producing formic, oxalic, and formic acids from ethylene glycol and methanol. Inhibition of ethanol dehydrogenase by intravenous fomepizole or intravenous ethanol is an essential part of treatment. In contrast to lactic acidosis and ketoacidosis, intravenous bicarbonate should be used in HAGMA secondary to ethylene glycol or methanol intoxication (a higher pH makes these toxins water soluble and unable to cross the blood-brain barrier). Emergent hemodialysis should be done if the ethylene glycol or methanol intoxication is confirmed, and the patient has acute kidney injury (AKI), metabolic acidosis, or very high serum toxin levels (>50 mg/dL of methanol or >8.1 mmol/L of ethylene glycol).

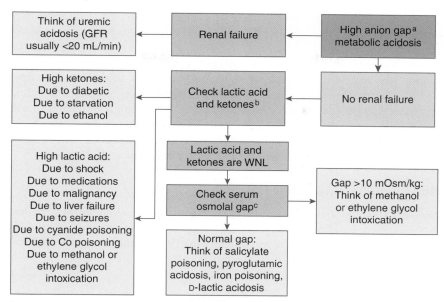

^aPatients with hypoalbuminemia may have lower normal anion gap than the regular normal gap (which is 10–12 mEq/L in most laboratories). If your patient has hypoalbuminemia, the normal anion gap will be lower by 2.5 for each 1 g/L decrease in serum albumin. Forgetting to correct the anion gap in hypoalbuminemia states may result in falsely diagnosing normal anion gap metabolic acidosis instead of high anion gap metabolic acidosis.

^bAcetone and acetoacetate are detected in urine or blood. Negative acetone or acetoacetate doesn't rule out ketones because they can be converted to beta-hydroxybutyrate in cases of excessive NADH/NAH ratio. If you have high suspicion for ketones, add beta-hydroxybutarate to your order list.

^cSerum Osmolal gap = measured serum osmolality – calculated osmolality
(calculated osmolality = $2 \times$ [Na] + [glucose]/18 + [urea]/2.8 + ETOH/4.6). Normal gap is 10 mOsm/kg.

Figure 2-1. Approach to high anion gap matabolic acidosis.

Salicylate poisoning should be treated by increasing blood and brain pH. Intravenous bicarbonate will increase the negatively charged fraction of salicylic acid. This ionized fraction will have less ability to cross the blood-brain barrier and higher solubility in the urine. The end result will be less CNS toxicity and higher urinary excretion. When the serum concentration is above 80 mg/dL, hemodialysis may be tried.

D-Lactic acidosis is a rare cause of metabolic acidosis. It is seen in patients who have a history of small intestine resection. If such a patient ate a large carbohydrate meal, more carbohydrate will reach the colon. In the colon, bacteria will produce D-lactic acid from carbohydrate metabolism. The typical presentation is confusion, ataxia, and acidosis after a meal rich in carbohydrate. The symptoms and the acidosis improve after discontinuation of the meal. The serum lactic acid test is normal in this condition because the test detects only the more common L-lactic acid. If you have a suspicion of D-lactic acidosis, ask the lab to check it specifically. Low-carbohydrate meals and antibiotic use to decrease bacterial overgrowth in the colon are the main measures used to prevent the acidosis episodes.

Another uncommon cause of HAGMA is pyroglutamic acidosis. This is usually seen in critically ill patients who have been ill for a long period of time and who are on acetaminophen. Both chronic critical illness and acetaminophen (even at therapeutic levels) decrease glutathione. The low glutathione in turn will cause the accumulation of pyroglutamic acid. Diagnosis is confirmed by checking urine pyroglutamic acid levels. Acetaminophen should be stopped in these patients. N-Acetylcystine may be used to increase glutathione production.

Non-anion Gap Metabolic Acidosis

Non-anion gap metabolic acidosis (NAGMA) is caused either by bicarbonate loss (diarrhea, renal tubular acidosis [RTA] type II) or by inability of the kidney to excrete hydrogen (RTA type I, RTA type IV, and mild-to-moderate renal failure).

Diagnosis

Most of the time, a history and simple workup will be sufficient to learn the etiology. If you are still not sure of the etiology, urine anion gap (UAG) will help narrow the differential diagnosis. UAG is calculated by the following formula: UAG = urine [Na] + urine [K] - urine [Cl]. Positive UAG is found in renal etiologies (AKI, RTA), and negative UAG is found in extrarenal etiologies (such as diarrhea). The UAG will be positive if the urine [Cl] is low and will be negative if the urine [Cl] is high. Lower urine [Cl] is associated with lower urine ammonium (NH_4). Urine ammonium reflects the kidney's ability to acidify the urine, so low urine ammonium in the setting of acidosis indicates an inappropriate response of the kidney to the acidosis (so the kidney is the cause of the acidosis). Higher urine [Cl] is associated with higher urine ammonium, and indicates appropriate response of the kidney to the acidosis (so the kidney is not the etiology of the acidosis). The major characteristics of the different RTA types are summarized in Table 2-2.

Treatment

Acidosis secondary to diarrhea is corrected by treating the diarrhea. If that is not possible or the acidosis is severe, alkali may be used. Potassium should always be replaced, as alkali treatment will worsen hypokalemia.

Renal failure–related acidosis should be treated with oral bicarbonate (see above). RTA type II may be treated with a thiazide diuretic. The volume contraction induced by thiazide will increase the bicarbonate threshold loss in the proximal tubule. RTA type I is treated by alkali administration. Potassium citrate is preferred because of the associated hypokalemia in RTA type I. RTA type IV treatment is mainly directed toward hyperkalemia. Achieving normal potassium

Table 2-2. Comparison of Major Types of RTA

	Type I	Type II	Type IV
Hyperchloremic acidosis	Yes	Yes	Yes
Minimum urine pH	>5.5	<5.5 (but usually >5.5 before the acidosis becomes established)	<5.5
Plasma potassium	Low-normal	Low-normal	**High**
Renal stones	**Yes**	No	No
Defect	Reduced H^+ excretion in distal tubule	Impaired HCO_3 reabsorption in proximal tubule	Impaired cation exchange in distal tubule

levels will help in controlling the acidosis. Low-potassium diet and loop diuretics are usually first tried. If there is no response, fludrocortisone can be tried to induce urinary potassium secretion.

Intravenous Bicarbonate Replacement in Metabolic Acidosis

Isotonic bicarbonate solution can be made by adding 3 ampules of sodium bicarbonate (50 mEq each) to 1 L of D5W.

A bicarbonate deficit can be calculated by the following formula:

$$\text{Deficit } HCO_3 = (0.5 \times \text{lean body weight [kg]}) \times (24 - \text{current } HCO_3 \text{ levels})$$

Keep in mind that the above formula underestimates the deficit if there is edema or if the HCO_3 level is less than 5 mmol/L. The first part in parentheses on the right-hand side of the formula may need to be increased in situations like this.

Only half of the bicarbonate deficit should be corrected over the first 24 hours. After 24 hours, bicarbonate level and the patient condition should be evaluated again before any further bicarbonate treatment.

METABOLIC ALKALOSIS

Diagnosis

Chloride depletion metabolic alkalosis is seen in more than 90% of metabolic alkalosis cases. Pendrin, which is an HCO_3–Cl exchanger protein on the apical membrane of the distal tubule, plays a major role in chloride depletion alkalosis. This protein reabsorbs chloride and excretes bicarbonate. In chloride depletion states, there will be less chloride in the tubule and thus pendrin will be suppressed. Bicarbonate will not be secreted and alkalosis will occur. Chloride depletion also induces hydrogen and potassium urinary excretion in the collecting tubule. The resultant hypokalemia will worsen the alkalosis by further induction of urinary hydrogen loss. The major causes of chloride depletion metabolic alkalosis are vomiting, nasogastric tube suctioning, and loop or thiazide diuretic use in edematous patients.

Metabolic alkalosis rarely has clinically significant adverse effects. If serum bicarbonate is increased to more than 50 mmol/L, serious complications may occur. Seizures and delirium can be caused by alkali-induced hypocalcemia. Hypoxia may occur secondary to hypoventilation (lung compensation to metabolic alkalosis). Serious cardiac arrhythmia may occur secondary to hypokalemia.

Treatment

Replacing the chloride with intravenous normal saline will treat the alkalosis in most patients with vomiting or nasogastric tube suctioning. Rarely, normal saline will not be enough and hydrogen chloride solution is needed.

Holding loop or thiazide diuretics can be enough to treat diuretic-induced alkalosis. If this is not successful, increasing the bicarbonate clearance by acetazolamide may be tried. Another advantage of acetazolamide is its ability to treat the edema in these patients.

Hypokalemia should always be looked for and treated in all metabolic alkalosis patients. Potassium chloride is the treatment of choice.

In a minority of cases, there will be no evidence of gastric fluid loss or diuretic use from a history and physical examination. Checking a random urine chloride may help narrow the differential diagnosis (see Figure 2-2).

RESPIRATORY ALKALOSIS

Diagnosis

Respiratory alkalosis results from hypocapnia. Hyperventilation is the underlying mechanism of hypocapnia. It is induced by signals from the lungs, the peripheral ventilation chemoreceptors, or the central ventilation chemoreceptors. Maladjusted mechanical ventilation is another common cause of respiratory alkalosis. See Table 2-3 for etiologies of respiratory alkalosis.

The clinical manifestations of respiratory alkalosis usually start when the P_{CO_2} drops to less than half the normal range. Usual symptoms include light-headedness, circumoral numbness, chest discomfort, and paresthesia of the extremities.

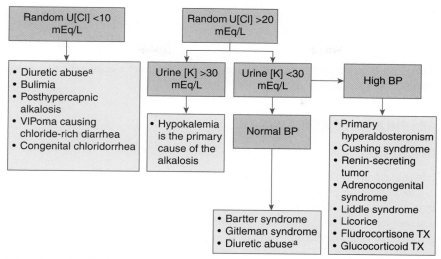

aUrine chloride will be high during the diuretic abuse and low after the use.

Figure 2-2. Differential diagnosis of metabolic alkalosis based on urine chloride.

Hypocapnia causes cerebral vasoconstriction that can have serious neurological complications in patients with a history of traumatic brain injury or acute stroke. Respiratory alkalosis can cause cardiac arrhythmia as well.

Table 2-3. Respiratory Alkalosis Etiologies

Hyperventilation secondary to stimulated chest receptors:

Pneumonia, asthma, pneumothorax, flail chest, acute respiratory distress syndrome, pulmonary edema, pulmonary embolism, pulmonary fibrosis

Hyperventilation secondary to severe hypoxia stimulating the peripheral chemoreceptors:

Pulmonary pathologies, high altitude, laryngospasm, drowning, severe anemia, left shift deviation of HbO_2 curve

Hyperventilation secondary to stimulating central chemoreceptors:

Pain, anxiety, psychosis, voluntary, sabarachnoid hemorrhage, CVA, meningoencephalitis, trauma, drugs (progesterone, salicylates, xanthenes, epinephrine, norepinephrine), fever, sepsis, exercise, pregnancy, hepatic failure

Data from Floege J, Johnson RJ, Feehally J. *Comprehensive Clinical Nephrology.* 4th ed. Philadelphia: Mosby; 2007.

Treatment

Hypocapnia is not a benign finding and can cause long-term brain injury. Therefore, respiratory alkalosis should always be taken seriously and treated. Treatment should be directed to the underlying etiology. When arterial pH rises to more than 7.55, acetazolamide may be used.

RESPIRATORY ACIDOSIS

Diagnosis

Lungs are responsible for keeping the P_{CO_2} within the normal range by exhaling it. The exhalation process increases or decreases depending on the production of P_{CO_2} by the body. Hypoventilation occurs when the lung fails to exhale the normal production of CO_2 or fails to increase this process in response to higher CO_2 generation. Hypoventilation will cause an increase in the P_{CO_2} and respiratory acidosis may develop. Causes of this failure may be divided into central nervous system–related etiologies, neuromuscular-related etiologies, and lung etiologies illustrated in Table 2-4.

Most hypercapnic symptoms are related to the CNS. Confusion is common, and in untreated cases, coma may occur. Tremor, myoclonic jerks, or seizures may occur. The hypercapnia-induced CNS vasodilation can be severe and cause increased intracranial pressure. Less commonly, the cardiovascular system can be affected with arrhythmia, decreased cardiac output, and labile blood pressure.

Table 2-4. Respiratory Acidosis Etiologies

CNS etiologies:
   Depressed level of consciousness secondary to drugs or encephalopathy of any etiology causing decreased respiratory drive, hypothyroidism[a]

Neuromuscular etiologies:
   Myasthenia gravis, Guillain–Barré syndrome, muscular dystrophy, amyotrophic lateral sclerosis, botulism, dermatomyositis/polymyositis, Lambert–Eaton syndrome, hypermagnesemia, hypothyroidism[a]

Lung etiologies:
   COPD, asthma, obstructive or central sleep apnea, hypoventilation syndrome, thoracic skeletal deformities, advanced pulmonary fibrosis

[a]Hypothyroidism causes decreased hypoxic and hypercapnic ventilation drives and muscle weakness.

Treatment

Inappropriate use of oxygen is common and is an easily preventable precipitator of respiratory acidosis. In patients with chronic CO_2 retention status, correcting hypoxia to a normal range will further increase the Pco_2 by 3 mechanisms. First, O_2 will reverse the hypoxia-induced pulmonary vasoconstriction, which in turn will increase the perfusion to the lung areas that have minimum ventilation and thus the dead space ventilation will increase. Second, O_2 will increase Pco_2 release from red blood cells by decreasing hemoglobin's affinity to CO_2. Third, respiratory drive in chronic CO_2 retainers depends on hypoxia and O_2 administration will suppress this drive.

Another preventable cause of respiratory acidosis in hospitals is discontinuing the use of CPAP or BiPAP machines. Very often, sleep apnea patients don't tolerate the hospital machines and prefer to use their home machines. Patients should always be encouraged to bring their home machines to the hospital as soon as possible. If that is not possible, try machines with lower pressure, autotitrated pressure, or a nasal-only mask. This may make it easier for patients to use the hospital machine.

If respiratory acidosis develops, management largely depends on the Po_2 level and the patient's mental status. If the Po_2 is more than 60 mm Hg and the patient is alert, careful observation is recommended. If Po_2 is less than 55 mm Hg and the patient is alert, you may try a small dose of oxygen till you get the Po_2 more than 60 mm Hg (don't try to get saturation more than 90%–92%). If the patient respirator status does not improve, noninvasive positive pressure ventilation may be tried. Arterial blood gases should be drawn 2 hours after starting noninvasive ventilation. If there is no improvement in the Pco_2 levels, intubation should not be delayed. Any time a patient starts to become confused, intubation should be considered. Noninvasive ventilation in confused patients is a relative contraindication because of the higher risk for aspiration.

TIPS TO REMEMBER

- Lactic acidosis, ketoacidosis, and advanced renal failure are the most common etiologies of HAGMA.

- Intravenous bicarbonate should not be used in lactic acidosis or ketoacidosis unless the arterial pH is less than 7.1.

- The most common causes of NAGMA are diarrhea and renal failure.

- Chloride-deficient metabolic alkalosis is the most common cause of metabolic alkalosis. Treatment is based on intravenous normal saline and holding the diuretics if they are being used.

- Respiratory alkalosis causing hypocapnia is not benign and should always be reversed.

- Oxygen should be used very carefully in patients with chronic CO_2 retention in order to decrease the risk of respiratory acidosis.
- Respiratory acidosis can be treated with noninvasive ventilation if it is not severe and the patient is awake enough to cooperate with the machine.

COMPREHENSION QUESTIONS

1. A medical consult was called for persistent elevated bicarbonate and hypokalemia in a 63-year-old male. The patient underwent emergent partial gastrectomy 2 weeks ago for a perforated gastric ulcer. His hospital course was complicated by early wound infection and gastrocutaneous fistula. He completed a 7-day course of intravenous piperacillin and tazobactam. For the last 3 days the patient has received several intravenous potassium supplements because of persistent hypokalemia. He is on a clear liquid diet and on normal saline fluid at a rate of 150 cm^3/h. Today, the patient is hemodynamically stable. His physical examination is significant only for a 10 cm-midline epigastric incision. The incision is healed except for the lower 0.5 cm that is open with wet dressing around it.
Laboratory findings:

      ABG: pH of 7.47, Po_2 of 85, and Pco_2 of 48
      Sodium: 138
      Potassium: 2.8
      Chloride: 88
      Bicarbonate: 39
      BUN: 15
      Creatinine: 0.8
      Glucose: 120
      Calcium: 8.5
      Albumin: 3.0

Which of the following is the best to do next?
      A. Acetazolamide
      B. Potassium citrate
      C. Potassium chloride
      D. Decrease intravenous fluid rate

2. A 50-year-old female patient with a history of AIDS and type 1 DM presents to the ER with nausea, epigastric discomfort, and generalized weakness of 2 days duration. The patient reported intermittent diarrhea for the last 3 months after she was started on a new HAART regimen.
Laboratory findings:
      Sodium: 136
      Potassium: 5.4
      Chloride: 109

Bicarbonate: 15
BUN: 25
Creatinine: 0.9
Glucose: 300
Calcium: 7.3
Albumin: 2.0
ABG: pH of 7.25, Po_2 of 95, and Pco_2 of 31

What is most likely etiology of this patient's acid-base abnormality?
   A. Diarrhea
   B. Diabetic ketoacidosis
   C. Acute kidney injury
   D. Renal tubular acidosis type IV

Answers

1. **C.** This patient's metabolic alkalosis is most likely secondary to chloride depletion through the fistula. Potassium replacement is essential not only to prevent arrhythmia but also to treat the patient's metabolic alkalosis. Potassium chloride is the best choice here. Potassium citrate is alkali treatment and it will worsen the alkalosis. The patient is losing fluids through the fistula and is on only a clear liquid diet, so he is at risk for hypovolemia; therefore, using acetazolamide or decreasing the intravenous fluid rate is not appropriate here.

2. **B.** The patient's anion gap is 12 mEq/L. Because her albumin is only 2.0, her expected normal anion gap should be lowered by 5 mEq/L more than the usual normal range (usual normal anion gap is 10–12 mEq/L; this patient's expected normal anion gap is around 5–7 mEq/L). After correcting the anion gap, it is clear that this patient has a HAGMA. The only listed etiology that can cause HAGMA is diabetic ketoacidosis. AKI will cause NAGMA most of the time. Severe AKI may cause a high anion gap acidosis, but there is no evidence that this patient has severe AKI.

SUGGESTED READING

Floege J, Johnson RJ, Feehally J. *Comprehensive Clinical Nephrology*. 4th ed. Philadelphia: Mosby; 2007.

A 65-year-old Woman With Chest Pain

Mohamad Alhosaini, MD

A 65-year-old female with a history of hypertension and DM type 2 was admitted to the general medical floor with fever and cough for 3 days. The patient was diagnosed with community-acquired pneumonia and was started on levofloxacin. She improved and her fever resolved. On hospital day 3, the patient complained of severe pressure-like substernal chest pain with radiation to the left shoulder of 20 minutes duration. The pain was associated with sweating and nausea. The on-call internal medicine resident was paged. The patient was sitting on the edge of the bed and looked very distressed. Her vital signs showed temperature of 36.5°C, heart rate of 88 bpm, blood pressure of 160/95, respiratory rate of 24/min, and blood oxygen saturation of 98% on room air.

The patient has a history of poorly controlled diabetes mellitus type 2, hypertension, and hypercholesterolemia. She is a heavy ex-smoker. Physical examination is significant only for crackles over the right lower lung base.

The nurse had already done an ECG before the resident arrived (Figure 3-1).

1. What do you think is wrong with this patient?

2. What should you do next?

Answers

1. This is a 65-year-old female patient with several risk factors for coronary artery disease who is presenting with cardiac chest pain. Her ECG showed deep T-wave inversion in the anterior leads, which is consistent with ischemia.

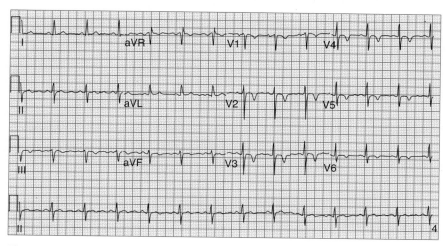

Figure 3-1. Patient's EKG.

31

2. The patient is having an acute coronary syndrome (ACS), and needs emergent diagnostic and therapeutic plans. Sublingual nitroglycerine (NTG) should be given for pain. The patient should chew 2 tablets of 81 mg aspirin (ASA). A high dose of clopidogrel and an intravenous beta-blocker should be given as soon as possible.

You should check cardiac enzymes, complete blood count, coagulation profile, basic metabolic panel, and magnesium levels stat. The patient should be moved to a telemetry floor with frequent vital sign checks and closer nursing observation. A cardiologist should be contacted immediately. Discussion with the cardiologist should focus on the decision of medical versus early invasive therapy, and the best anticoagulation to be given.

ACUTE CORONARY SYNDROME

Diagnosis

You will frequently face patients presenting with ACS during training. Fast and accurate management is crucial in improving patient outcomes. This review will summarize the most important elements of ACS management.

ACS can be divided into unstable angina, NSTEMI, and ST elevation MI (STEMI) (Table 3-1). The algorithm for unstable angina and NSTEMI management is the same. The initial management of all ACSs is the same; however, it differs significantly subsequently. The review will be arranged in the same way (initial acute management, unstable angina/NSTEMI management, and STEMI management). The last 2 sections review the MI complications and a summary of an effective discharge process.

Treatment (Initial Acute Management)

The adverse outcomes of ACS, such as lethal arrhythmia, heart failure, and recurrent ischemia, can be reduced if anti-ischemic, antiplatelet, and

Table 3-1. Acute Coronary Syndromes

Unstable angina: acute cardiac chest pain that comes and goes without relation to exertion along with ST segment depression or T-wave inversions. Cardiac enzymes are normal
NSTEMI: elevated cardiac enzymes with acute cardiac chest pain or/and ECG changes (ST segment depression or T-wave inversion)
STEMI: acute cardiac chest pain, ST segment elevations, and elevated cardiac enzymes

Table 3-2. Initial Acute Management

The 7 early treatment measures in ACS:
1. Oxygen
2. Nitroglycerine
3. Morphine
4. Beta-blocker
5. Aspirin
6. Clopidogrel
7. Anticoagulation
Initial workup plan:
Move to a telemetry unit
Check cardiac enzymes, CBC, CMP, Mg, PT, PTT
Contact cardiology immediately

anticoagulation medications are administered early. These early therapies should come to your mind once you have diagnosed a patient with ACS (Table 3-2). You must be able to order these measures for appropriate patients within a few minutes.

Patients with respiratory distress or O_2 saturation of less than 90% should be started on oxygen to keep saturation within a normal range. Starting oxygen in patients with normal oxygen saturation possibly causes direct vasoconstriction on coronary arteries, so the routine use of oxygen in all patients is discouraged.

Pain associated with ACS is usually severe and contributes to the ischemia by inducing further sympathetic output. Treating the pain is an essential part of early ACS treatment and should be started immediately. NTG 0.4 mg sublingual can be administered if the systolic blood pressure is more than 90 mm Hg. This usually works within a few minutes. The same dose can be repeated 2 more times in 5-minute intervals as needed. Make sure the patient has not received any phosphodiesterase inhibitor-5 during the last 24 hours before giving NTG. If pain persists, 2 to 4 mg of morphine sulfate should be tried. Sometimes, pain is refractory to sublingual NTG and morphine. In such circumstances, an intravenous NTG drip can be started if there is no concern about right ventricle infarction (to avoid excessive preload reduction and precipitating cardiac shock in these patients).

Beta-blockers decrease early complications and improve long-term mortality in patients with ACS. If blood pressure allows, all patients should receive a beta-blocker as soon as possible. Cardioselective beta-blockers such as atenolol or metoprolol are preferred. Five milligrams of intravenous metoprolol every 2 minutes for a total of 3 doses, and then 50 mg orally 15 minutes after the last intravenous dose can be given. The patient should be on 50 mg every 6 hours for the first 48 hours, and then he or she can be switched to a maintenance twice-daily dose or a once-daily long-acting form. Even if the patient does not tolerate the intravenous dose, you can try a small dose of oral metoprolol (such as 12.5–25 mg) and follow the patient closely.

Platelet aggregation plays an important role in ACS. Current evidence supports the early use of dual antiplatelet agents. If there is no contraindication, patients should chew aspirin at a dose of 162 to 325 mg. In addition to aspirin, a loading dose (300 mg) of clopidogrel should be administered. Some cardiologists prefer a 600 mg dose of clopidogrel, and you should familiarize yourself with your institution's practice. If a patient has a history of gastrointestinal bleeding, a proton pump inhibitor can be added.

Thrombosis from plaque disruption is one of the main causes of coronary artery obstruction. Thrombus-related events are preventable by anticoagulation. Heparins and direct thrombin inhibitors block the ongoing coagulation and reduce the death rate after MI. Table 3-3 shows the different anticoagulants used for MI. There is no definitive evidence to support the use of any of these medications over the other. Discussion with the treating cardiologist is important to choose the best anticoagulation in each case.

All patients with ACS should be moved to a telemetry bed for continuous monitoring and closer observation. Cardiac enzymes, complete blood count, coagulation profile, basic metabolic panel, and magnesium levels should be obtained stat. Platelet counts and the coagulation profile can affect the antiplatelet and anticoagulation choices. Creatinine level is important for adjustment of medication doses and allows for contrast nephropathy prophylaxis measures to be ordered if the patient has chronic kidney disease. Potassium and magnesium should be kept above 4.0 and 2.0 mEq/L, respectively, as this may decrease the risk of tachyarrhythmias. The cardiology team should be involved in the care of ACS patients as early as possible.

Table 3-3. Anticoagulation Medications Used in MI

Anticoagulation Drug	Mechanism of Action
Unfractionated heparin	Activates antithrombin III that inactivates IIa and Xa
Enoxaparin	Activates antithrombin III that inactivates IIa and Xa
Fondaparinux	Antithrombin III–selective inhibition of Xa
Bivalirudin	Direct thrombin inhibitor

Table 3-4. The TIMI Risk Score for Unstable Angina/NSTEMI

Age ≥65 years?	Yes: +1
≥3 risk factors for CAD?	Yes: +1
Known coronary artery disease?	Yes: +1
ASA use in past 7 days?	Yes: +1
Severe angina (≥2 episodes within 24 h)?	Yes: +1
ST changes ≥0.5 mm?	Yes: +1
Positive cardiac marker?	Yes: +1

Treatment Measures Specific to Unstable Angina/Non-ST Elevation Myocardial Infarction

The main decision to be taken in this group is whether to treat them with early invasive intervention or more conservatively. Thrombolysis in Myocardial Infarction (TIMI) score (Table 3-4) is a well-studied and validated score that is used to help make this decision. The TIMI score can be calculated in a few seconds from any smart phone or online. Like any other scoring system, TIMI score is an assistant tool for physicians and can't replace clinical judgment in controversial cases.

Patients with TIMI score between 0 and 2 usually have a lower mortality compared with those with higher scores. This group of patients can be treated conservatively with aspirin, clopidogrel, beta-blockers, statins, and an anticoagulation agent. The patient should be observed closely in a telemetry unit. Any sign of further chest pain, heart failure, or arrhythmia warrants reevaluation for possible switching to more invasive treatment. After stabilizing the patient, further testing with echocardiography and a stress test should be done to reassess the risk. Based on the ejection fraction (EF) and the stress test results, cardiologists can decide if the patient needs PCI or medical treatment alone.

Patients with higher TIMI scores (3 or more) usually have a more critical coronary artery blockage, and urgent PCI for possible revascularization should be done within 24 hours. If you are caring for such a patient, you should discuss with cardiology the need for anti-glycoprotein IIb/IIIa receptors prior to catheterization as this has shown to be beneficial.

Treatment Measures Specific to ST Elevation MI

Managing patients with STEMI is more straightforward than managing those with NSTEMI. The main goal of treatment is emergent reperfusion with either primary PCI or fibrinolytic therapy.

Table 3-5. Absolute Contraindications to Fibrinolytics

History of hemorrhagic stroke

History of ischemic stroke during the last year

Intracranial neoplasm

Active internal bleeding

Suspected aortic dissection

Primary PCI is superior to fibrinolytic therapy in patients with STEMI if it is done within 12 hours of the chest pain onset as it shows more patent infarct-related arteries. Because of that, PCI is always considered first. In hospitals that are not prepared to have emergent PCI, patients should be transferred to another hospital if it can be done within 2 hours. While the patient is on the way to the cardiology laboratory, you should continue all the early treatment measures (Table 3-2) along with anti-GP IIb/IIIa inhibitors.

Because of its serious bleeding side effects, fibrinolytics should be administered with great caution in a critical care setting and only in well-selected patients. Most hospitals have certain protocols that have to be filled before administration. You should be familiar with this protocol in your institution (Table 3-5).

Twelve hours after chest pain onset, infarction is less likely to be reversed. Therefore, fibrinolytic therapy is not indicated and PCI is less likely to help. Patients should be treated medically. However, if there is continuous chest pain, pulmonary edema, or recurrent arrhythmias, PCI is conducted by some cardiologists.

Complications of MI

In the era of PCI, complications of MI are less common than before. The most common complications of MI will be reviewed, as well as the role of an internist in managing them.

Right ventricular infarction

Infarction of the small right ventricle can easily affect the left ventricle preload and causes cardiogenic shock. Prognosis of MI is worse when it is complicated with right ventricular infarction.

Right ventricular infarction is associated with inferior MI and right coronary artery occlusion. The triad of jugular vein distention, normal chest examination, and hypotension should raise the suspicion of right ventricular infarction.

Whenever you suspect a right ventricular infarction, try to avoid preload reducing agents. In hypotensive patients, try normal saline to support the blood pressure and improve the right ventricular perfusion. Dobutamine may be used if the patient didn't improve with fluids.

Tachyarrhythmia

Ischemia triggers tachyarrhythmia in both atria and ventricles. Ventricular fibrillation (VF) and sustained ventricular tachycardia (VT) have the worst prognosis.

Any tachyarrhythmia with shock should be treated with electrical cardioversion. If the patient is hemodynamically stable, treatment will depend on the type of arrhythmia. A general rule in any tachyarrhythmia is that stat K^+ and Mg^{2+} should be ordered and kept above 4.0 and 2.0, respectively.

VT can be divided into sustained and nonsustained. Sustained VT lasts more than 30 seconds and can be symptomatic or asymptomatic. Amiodarone is the drug of choice for asymptomatic patients. It can be given as a drip or as boluses every 10 to 15 minutes. Nonsustained VT lasts less than 30 seconds and is not symptomatic in most patients. There is no need for anything more than observation and keeping the electrolytes above the recommended range.

Atrial fibrillation (A fib) can occur secondary to ischemia and can worsen any heart failure symptoms. The main goal is to control the heart rate to less than 110 in order to prevent pulmonary edema or further tachycardia-induced ischemia. The first line of treatment is a beta-blocker. A calcium channel blocker with or without digoxin can be tried next. A fib after ischemia is usually reversible within 48 hours and long-term anticoagulation is not needed as long as it is not recurrent or persistent after that.

Bradyarrhythmia

ACS can affect the cardiac conduction system. The effect can be transient or permanent depending on the severity and extent of the infarction. Small inferior MIs are commonly associated with bradyarrhythmia, and this is usually transient. On the other hand, an anterior MI is less likely to be associated with bradyarrhythmia, and if it is, the infarct is large and it is associated with both higher mortality and the need for a higher rate of permanent pacing.

The decision as to placement of a permanent pacemaker is beyond the scope of the internist. However, you are expected to be able to do the first-line treatment of bradyarrhythmia if needed before definite treatment is done by cardiology.

Asymptomatic bradycardia or Mobitz type I second-degree AV block can be treated with observation only. If it becomes symptomatic, try intravenous atropine. If there is no response, you can place the patient on an external pacer while waiting for cardiology to place a temporary transvenous pacemaker.

Mobitz type II AV block and third-degree AV block should be treated with temporary transvenous pacemakers even if the patient is asymptomatic. Other indications for a temporary transvenous pacemaker include asystole, alternating bilateral fascicular block of any age, or new and fixed bilateral fascicular block.

Mechanical Complications After STEMI

There are 3 complications after STEMI that have a very poor prognosis. Think of them when you have a patient with sudden-onset cardiogenic shock between days 3 and 7 post-STEMI. These complications include papillary muscle rupture, ventricular septal defect, and free wall rupture of the left ventricle.

Papillary muscle rupture

This complication usually takes place after inferior MI. It causes either acute tricuspid or mitral valve regurgitation with shock and pulmonary edema. You may or may not hear a short early systolic murmur, but the diagnostic modality of choice is emergent echocardiography. The patient should be sent to the OR, but the prognosis is poor.

Ventricular septal defect

This usually takes place after an anteroseptal MI. It also causes sudden-onset cardiogenic shock with a diffuse holosystolic murmur. Diagnosis is with echocardiography and the next step is emergent surgery.

Free wall rupture

Large anterior MIs are associated with this complication. It causes acute pericardial tamponade with sudden shock and syncope. Prognosis is grave.

Discharging the Patient After ACS

Mortality after ACS is closely related to the continuity of treatment in the outpatient setting. When you discharge such patients, you must write accurate discharge instructions and a complete medications list. Counseling and educating the patient is also very important.

All patients should be discharged on aspirin and clopidogrel. Aspirin should be taken for the rest of the patient's life. The duration of clopidogrel is less clear. Medically treated patients and those who received a bare metal stent have to take it for at least 1 month and up to 1 year. Drug-eluting stent patients should take clopidogrel for at least 1 year, and some cardiologists prefer to have these patients on clopidogrel lifelong. Educate patients with a drug-eluting stent very well that failure to take clopidogrel even for a few days can cause thrombosis at the stent site and life-threatening STEMI.

Another mandatory medication is a cardioselective beta-blocker. Even if the patient did not receive a beta-blocker in the first few days after admission, it should be tried and an effort should be made to send the patient home on it. Beta-blockers should be taken for life.

Statin should be initiated in all patients with ACS before discharge, and all patients who were on statins before admission should continue taking it. Statin benefits are not restricted to lowering low-density lipoprotein (LDL), but they also stabilize atherosclerotic plaques. There is evidence that high-dose atorvastatin

(80 mg once a day) is superior to other statins, and it is recommended for use as early as possible. Although a lipid panel is checked in all patients, it is important to remember that LDL can be falsely lower in the ACS setting and it should be repeated in 2 months after discharge. The LDL goal in this group of patients is less than 100.

Echocardiography is part of the workup in all patients with ACS. EF and motion motility has therapeutic and prognostic values. If the EF is 40% or less, give angiotensin-converting enzyme inhibitors or angiotensin receptor blockers before discharge even if there is no sign of heart failure. Patients with an EF of less than 35% are qualified to have a defibrillator placed for primary prevention of sudden cardiac death.

Patients with a history of smoking should be counseled prior to discharge to stop. Dietary counseling is also important before discharge. A diet rich in vegetables, fruits, fibers, low salt, and white meat is associated with better outcomes.

Exercise should be avoided in the first few days after ACS, but after that patients should be educated about the importance of exercise and its positive effect on delaying mortality. It is recommended to have at least 150 minutes a week of moderate-intensity aerobic exercise or 75 minutes a week of vigorous aerobic exercise. If the patient has A fib or aortic stenosis, it would be safer to begin exercise in a supervised setting.

Finally, make sure you get an appointment for your patient with the primary care doctor and the cardiologist soon after discharge. Involve the patient care facilitator early on admission if the patient needs a new primary care doctor. This will shorten the time spent waiting before a patient can see a physician after discharge.

Table 3-6 provides a checklist that may help you remember the essential medications and recommendations when you discharge ACS patients.

Table 3-6. Discharge Checklist

- ASA
- Clopidogrel
- Cardioselective beta-blocker
- Atorvastatin
- ACEi or ARB in patients with EF less than 40%
- Defibrillator in patients with EF less than 35%
- Smoking cessation counseling
- Diet and exercise counseling
- Appointment with the PCP and the cardiologist

TIPS TO REMEMBER

- Oxygen, nitroglycerin, morphine, aspirin, clopidogrel, cardioselective beta-blockers, and anticoagulation are the mainstays of initial treatments that you should start on patients diagnosed with ACS.

- Unstable angina/NSTEMI patients with a TIMI score of 2 or less should be treated medically and observed closely.

- Unstable angina/NSTEMI patients with a TIMI score of 3 or more should be treated with early invasive therapy.

- STEMI patients should be treated with PCI if presented within 12 hours after chest pain onset. When PCI is not available in the hospital, patients should be transferred to a hospital that can do emergent PCI as long as it can be done within 2 hours of transfer.

- When PCI is not possible, patients with STEMI should be treated with fibrinolytic therapy if there are no contraindications.

- After ACS, patients should be discharged on aspirin, clopidogrel, beta-blockers, and a statin. ACE inhibitor (ACEi) or ARB should be added to patients with EF of 40% or less.

COMPREHENSION QUESTIONS

1. A 70-year-old male patient presents to the ER with confusion of 5 hours duration. Physical examination is significant only for bilateral leg edema. The patient's BP is 90/45, heart rate is 100 bpm, oxygen saturation is within the normal range, and temperature is 36.8°C. Past medical history is significant for hypertension and congestive heart failure. ECG showed ST segment depression in the inferior leads. Troponin was 2.8 (normal is less than 0.01); brain natriuretic peptide (BNP) was 800 (normal is less than 100). CBC and BMP are within normal limits.

What is the most appropriate next step for this patient?

2. A 60-year-old male was admitted to your hospital for STEMI. The patient had PCI done successfully with 1 drug-eluting stent placed in the left anterior artery. Echocardiography done prior to discharge showed an EF of 40%. Lipid panel showed LDL of 60, HDL of 30, and TG of 150. The patient is doing fine without any chest pain or shortness of breath. His physical examination is completely normal. His past medical history is significant for hypertension and gout only. He used to take amlodipine. The patient is ready for discharge. His vital signs now are: BP 135/85, HR 80 bpm, RR 20/min, and temperature 37°C.

What medication should be included on the discharge medication list?

Answers

1. The patient is presenting with confusion and hypotension. He has ST depression in the inferior leads and significantly elevated troponin. Because of the normal CBC and the absence of fever, sepsis is less likely. The most likely diagnosis in this patient is inferior NSTEMI with cardiogenic shock. Delirium is one of the atypical presenting signs of MI. This patient needs intravenous fluid to support preload and enhance coronary perfusion.

Even though the patient has a history of CHF, there is no evidence of pulmonary edema on physical examination in this patient. MI can cause the elevated BNP, and there is evidence that the degree of elevated BNP is related to the prognosis. Giving furosemide to this patient may worsen the cardiogenic shock and should be avoided.

Dobutamine is a beta-agonist medication that improves myocardial contractility and improves cardiogenic shock. It also causes arrhythmias and increases the risk of ischemia. Starting this patient on dobutamine is a premature step, and intravenous fluids should be tried first.

Metoprolol is an essential treatment in ACS. However, in this patient, a beta-blocker may worsen the cardiogenic shock, so it is better to wait till the blood pressure improves before starting it.

2. Atorvastatin is recommended for all patients with ACS. Statins improve mortality not only by lowering the LDL but also by a direct mechanism on coronary arteries. The normal LDL in this patient could be affected by the ACS he had and should be repeated in 1 to 2 months to evaluate the effect of atorvastatin.

Niacin can lower the LDL and increase the HDL; however, statins are always a first-line treatment for patients after MI and there is no evidence to support the use of niacin in that setting. You can add niacin if the LDL is still elevated after treatment with a statin for a sufficiently long period of time.

Even though the patient has a low EF, he doesn't have any symptoms or signs of CHF. Asymptomatic CHF should be treated with beta-blockers and ACEi or ARBs. However, diuretics are not indicated if there is no dyspnea or edema.

Blood pressure control is important after MI. The BP goal is less than 140/90. The patient will be started on a beta-blocker and ACEi because of his MI and his low EF. Continuing amlodipine with the ACEi and beta-blocker in this patient is not indicated because his blood pressure is acceptable at this point. Remember that the blood pressure measurement is always more accurate in the outpatient setting. If this patient's BP is still elevated in the outpatient setting, his PCP should start him on a third antihypertensive such as amlodipine.

SUGGESTED READINGS

Kushner FG, Hand M, Smith SC Jr, et al. 2009 focused updates: ACC/AHA guidelines for the management of patients with ST-elevation myocardial infarction (updating the 2004 guideline and 2007 focused update) and ACC/AHA/SCAI guidelines on percutaneous coronary intervention (updating the 2005 guideline and 2007 focused update) a report of the American College of Cardiology Foundation/American Heart Association Task Force on Practice Guidelines. *J Am Coll Cardiol.* 2009;54:2205–2241. doi:10.1016/j.jacc.2009.10.015.

Wright RS, Anderson JL, Adams CD, et al. 2011 ACCF/AHA focused update incorporated into the ACC/AHA 2007 guidelines for the management of patients with unstable angina/non-ST-elevation myocardial infarction: a report of the American College of Cardiology Foundation/American Heart Association Task Force on Practice Guidelines developed in collaboration with the American Academy of Family Physicians, Society for Cardiovascular Angiography and Interventions, and the Society of Thoracic Surgeons. *J Am Coll Cardiol.* 2011;57:e215–e367. doi:10.1016/j.jacc.2011.02.011.

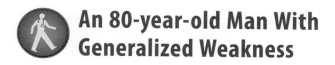

An 80-year-old Man With Generalized Weakness

Mohamad Alhosaini, MD

An 80-year-old male was transferred from his nursing home to the emergency room for generalized weakness of 3 days duration. His weakness got worse to the extent that he found it difficult to go to the bathroom. He also mentioned worsening dysuria and difficulty passing urine for the last week. There was no chest pain, fever, cough, abdominal pain, back pain, hematuria, diarrhea, melena, or rash.

The patient has a history of dementia, benign prostatic hypertrophy (BPH), congestive heart failure (CHF) with an ejection fraction of 40% as measured 6 months ago, chronic kidney disease (CKD) stage III, diabetes mellitus type 2, and hypertension. He takes donepezil, memantine, tamsulosin, finasteride, lisinopril, metoprolol, amlodipine, torsemide, and metformin. The patient is a widower who has lived at the nursing home for the last 4 years. He has never smoked or drunk alcohol.

Vital signs in the ER: blood pressure of 100/60, heart rate of 100, and respiratory rate of 20. He had a normal temperature and oxygen saturation on room air. The patient was closing his eyes during the physical examination and trying to sleep. His mucosa looked dry. Neck, heart, and lung examinations were unremarkable. There was mild abdominal tenderness in the hypogastric area with dullness to percussion. There was a +1 bilateral pitting edema. Neurological examination was within normal limits. Void collector on the bedside contained 30 cm^3 of dark yellow urine.

Initial workup:

WBC: 9000 with normal differential

Hemoglobin: 10

Platelets: 200,000

Sodium: 130

Potassium: 5.1

Chloride: 103

Bicarbonate: 16

Blood urea nitrogen: 95

Creatinine: 8.5 (patient's baseline is 1.8; last check was 1 month ago)

Glucose: 220

CXR: mild bilateral interstitial infiltrates and cardiomegaly

ECG showed sinus tachycardia with peaked T waves in the anterior leads

1. What is the most important next step?

2. How would you work up the patient's acute kidney injury (AKI)?

Answers

This is a case of an elderly patient with a history of CKD, CHF, and benign prostatic hypertrophy (BPH) who is presenting with weakness and difficulty passing urine. He had poor oral intake for a week prior to admission. On examination, he has hypogastric tenderness and dullness to percussion over that area. His heart rate is 100 and his blood pressure is 100/60. Labs showed severe AKI, severe hyperkalemia, and low bicarbonate.

1. The patient needs an immediate therapeutic and diagnostic plan. Foley catheter should be inserted to help in getting an accurate urine output (UOP) and to relieve any obstruction at the prostate level. Because of the decreased oral intake, tachycardia, and mild hypotension, intravenous normal saline should be started. Continuous oximeter and serial lung examinations are important in such patients with low ejection fraction. The unknown UOP is being treated with fluids. Metformin, ACE inhibitors, and diuretics should be held. Insulin is the hypoglycemic agent of choice in this case to treat the hyperglycemia.

2. The low bicarbonate raises the suspicion of metabolic acidosis and an arterial blood gas will help assess this possibility. Urinalysis, urine osmolality, urine protein, urine urea, urine creatinine, and renal ultrasound should be obtained as soon as possible. The patient's input and output must be strictly documented.

ACUTE KIDNEY INJURY (ACUTE RENAL FAILURE)

Diagnosis

AKI is very common in the inpatient setting (range from 0.5%–13%). The wide incidence range can be explained by the different definitions of AKI among different authors and physicians.

Because of its reversibility in the early stages and its impact on morbidity and mortality, we suggest having a low threshold to diagnose AKI. An increase in serum creatinine of 0.3 mg/dL or by 1.5 times the baseline should raise your suspicion of AKI. A more important, but not widely used, criterion is the decrease in UOP to less than 0.5 mL/kg/h for at least a 6-hour duration. The decrease in UOP actually precedes the decrease in glomerular filtration rate (GFR) and the increases in serum creatinine. UOP criteria are more practical in the intensive care unit where more accurate UOP measurement is conducted. There is ongoing research to evaluate urinary biomarkers that can detect AKI at much earlier stages. None of these biomarkers is used in practice yet.

Commonly, baseline creatinine will not be available for comparison. In situations like this, it becomes hard to differentiate between CKD and AKI when faced with elevated creatinine. Anemia, hypocalcemia, and hyperphosphatemia are abnormalities seen in CKD, and their presence makes CKD more likely than AKI. Small kidney size and thinning of the cortex on renal ultrasound are the

Table 4-1. Acute Kidney Injury Etiologies

Prerenal (Hypoperfusion of the Kidney)	Renal (Tubular or Glomerular Injury)	Postrenal (Obstruction of the Urinary Tract)
Volume depletion (diarrhea, vomiting, bleeding, burns, pancreatitis, hyperglycemia, excessive diuresis, sepsis)	Acute tubular necrosis	Urinary retention
	Vascular causes (Wagner's, polyarteritis nodosa, Churg–Strauss, hemolytic uremic syndrome, thrombotic thrombocytopenic purpura, cholesterol emboli)	Urological malignancies
Decreased intravascular effective circulation (CHF, cirrhosis)		Pelvic masses
		Obstructing nephrolithiasis
Renal artery thrombosis	Glomerulonephritis	
Renal artery dissection	Acute interstitial nephritis	
	Cast nephropathy	
	Contrast nephropathy	
	Myoglobin nephropathy	
	Tumor lysis syndrome	

most accurate markers that can differentiate CKD from AKI. Keep in mind that the kidney size is normal in diabetic nephropathy, amyloidosis, and polycystic kidney disease.

The easiest way to approach AKI is by dividing the etiologies into 3 categories: prerenal, renal, and postrenal (Table 4-1). It is important to remember that overlap among different etiologies is a common scenario.

Detailed history and careful physical examination is an essential part of the diagnosis process. Mild-to-moderate AKI secondary to volume depletion, or secondary to decreased intravascular effective circulation, is a very common scenario in the inpatient setting. In situations like this, volume status assessment is crucial. Unfortunately, physicians commonly fail to accurately classify the volume status because of the ongoing loss of physical examination skills and the limited predictive values of these signs (Table 4-2).

Simple urine tests and renal imaging will often identify the etiology of the AKI. In the majority of cases, they are the only needed workup. Biopsy is rarely done.

Urine tests

Urinalysis is an inexpensive and valuable test that can help narrow the differential diagnosis of AKI. Urine tests should include the following: dipstick test, microscopic and sediment evaluations, osmolality, fractional excretion of sodium (FeNa) (or urea), and urine creatinine to serum creatinine ratio.

Table 4-2. Volume Status Signs

Heart rate and blood pressure	Tachycardia is more sensitive for hypovolemic states than for hypotension, but both are sometimes absent in hypovolemic patients
	Patients on beta-blocker may not have reflex tachycardia when they are hypovolemic
	Tachycardia is not specific for hypovolemia (it can be seen in euvolemic and hypervolemic states)
Orthostatic hypotension	Good specificity for hypovolumia (>90%) but low sensitivity (22%)
	Common mistakes when checking for orthostatic hypotension are: not having the patient stand up long enough (at least 2 min) and not counting the heart rate
Dry mucosa and diminished skin turgor	Both these signs don't necessary mean hypovolemia in the elderly. Mouth breathing, a common problem in the elderly, can cause dry mouth regardless of the volume status. Skin turgor diminishes in the elderly
CVP	Low CVP has a modest positive predictive value (47%) in detecting volume-responsive patients
Jugular venous distention (JVD)	Good specificity for hypervolemia but low sensitivity
	JVD in pure right heart failure can be seen even if the patient is hypovolemic
	Carotid pulsation should not be mistaken for JVD; carotid pulsation is faster and brisker than JVD. It has only 1 phase, while JVD has multiple phases. Carotid pulsation is synchronized with the radial pulsation
Third heart sound	Good specificity for hypervolemic state (80%–90%) but low sensitivity (30%–40%)
Bilateral pitting edema	Peripheral edema is seen in hypervolemic states. But it is also seen in low albumin states and venous stasis states regardless of the volume status
Rales	Elderly can have fine crackles in the lower parts of the lung fields regardless of the volume status (age-related crackles)

Dipstick and microscopic tests should be reviewed carefully. In acute tubular necrosis (ATN), the kidneys' acidification function can be impaired, and urine pH of more than 6.5 is seen sometimes in these patients. Hematuria is seen in obstructive AKI—like prostate pathology, nephrolithiasis, or urological malignancy.

A positive blood dipstick with only a few red blood cells should raise the suspicion of myoglobinuria.

Proteinuria is common in AKI. The protein to creatinine ratio in a random urine spot is a quick and easy test that can give you an idea about the 24-hour protein urine. Trace to mild proteinuria is seen in prerenal etiologies. Moderate proteinuria (to less than 1 g in 24 hours) is seen with ATN. Proteinuria that is more than 1 g in 24 hours should make one think of a nephritic syndrome or cast nephropathy, and it is more helpful in narrowing the differential diagnosis than just mild-to-moderate proteinuria.

Identification of casts is also a very important part of urinalysis. Hyaline casts can be seen in normal persons, so their presence or absence is of little value. Muddy brown casts and cellular debris are seen in ATN; however, their absence doesn't rule it out. Red blood cell casts are pathognomonic for glomerulonephritis (GN). White blood cell casts are seen with acute interstitial nephritis (AIN). Again, the absence of red blood cell casts or white blood cell casts doesn't rule out GN or AIN, respectively. Cast identification needs good skills and practice. Experienced nephrologists examine the urine themselves looking for casts. We encourage residents to learn this important skill during their nephrology elective.

Urine osmolality can help differentiate between prerenal AKI and ATN. Osmolality of more than 500 mOsm/kg is more consistent with prerenal etiologies. Urine osmolality of less than 400 mOsm/kg is seen with ATN. Keep in mind that elderly, CKD patients, and patients on diuretics have impaired water reabsorption, so they have low urine osmolality even when they are volume depleted. Having high osmolality in these groups indicates a severe volume contraction state.

FeNa is another useful test that helps differentiate prerenal from renal AKI. In volume depletion states, the FeNa will be less than 1% due to the excessive sodium reabsorption. An FeNa of more than 2% is consistent with intrarenal injury. However, a number of intrarenal AKI etiologies are associated with an FeNa of less than 1% (contrast nephropathy, myoglobin nephropathy, GN, and early stages of ATN*). On the other hand, high FeNa is seen in prerenal AKI secondary to excessive vomiting. This is because the consequent bicarbonaturia is associated with excessive urinary sodium loss.

The high urine sodium seen in patients taking diuretics makes FeNa less helpful. In this situation, the fractional excretion of urea (FeUrea) is the best alternative. An FeUrea of less than 35% is suggestive of prerenal etiologies, while values more than 50% suggest ATN.

---

*In nonoliguric ATN, the intact tubules will face large loads of water and sodium and they will try to preserve the body's sodium by excessive reabsorption. In this situation the overall result will be a low FeNa. In oliguric ATN, the intact tubules will face small loads of water and sodium. To avoid significant sodium retention, the intact tubules will reabsorb less sodium and the FeNa will be high. The take-home message is that FeNa is most likely to be useful in oliguric AKI.

Imaging

Renal ultrasound is a helpful tool when you suspect obstructive AKI or when you are not sure of the diagnosis. Pelvicalyceal dilatation is a very sensitive sign for obstruction. During early obstruction, dilatation may not appear. Also, in some malignancies, there will be ureteral encasement and retroperitoneal fibrosis, and dilatation will not appear. Because of that, in cases of high suspicion for obstruction with negative ultrasound or CT scan, retrograde or anterograde pyelography is recommended due to its improved accuracy.

Biopsy

Renal biopsy is rarely needed for diagnosis. Think about it when you suspect GN, vasculitis, or AIN. It can also be done in cases of persistent elevated creatinine when prerenal and postrenal etiologies have been ruled out and the etiology of the intrinsic AKI is still unclear.

Treatment

General management

After an AKI diagnosis, avoidance of further injury is a main goal for all patients. Contrast materials, kidney insulting medications, and hypotension should be avoided as much as possible.

Most patients with volume depletion–induced AKI improve with hydration or/and blood transfusion if it is caught early. If there is no improvement after fluid administration, reevaluate the patient for ATN or other diagnoses.

In CHF patients, the differentiation between AKI caused by acute exacerbation of CHF and AKI caused by excessive diuresis is sometimes tough. The best strategy is a diuretic trial. Diuretics will improve the renal function if the injury is caused by a CHF exacerbation, and will make it worse if excessive diuresis is the cause. In the latter case, diuretics should be stopped and a small fluid challenge should be tried. Remember to look at the patient as a whole; the decision of holding diuretics and giving fluid to improve the renal function should be weighed against worsening of the cardiac condition. Thorough discussion with the cardiology service is important in such cases.

The balance between fluid administration and diuresis is more complicated in intensive care unit patients. As mentioned earlier, volume status assessment is a challenging task especially in the ICU. Echocardiogram is probably the most accurate tool available now to help in making the decision of giving or restricting fluids. If the cardiac output of a patient is expected to increase with fluids, the patient is called volume responsive (organ perfusion will increase by fluids). If the cardiac output of a patient is expected to be the same after fluid administration, the patient is called volume nonresponsive (organ perfusion will not increase by fluids) and fluid restriction or diuretics will be beneficial if the patient has poor cardiac function. Echocardiogram helps estimate the cardiac output by measuring the stroke volume. In patients who are not on a ventilator, the change in stroke volume is measured when the patient is flat and after the patient raises the legs 45°. Raising the legs will increase the venous return and the preload to the heart, an effect that is similar to fluid bolus. If the cardiac input variation is more than 15% with this maneuver, the patient is considered volume responsive.

Echocardiogram is also useful in ventilated patients. During mechanical ventilation, the positive pressure with inspiration will increase the pressure in the chest. This will decrease the venous return to the right ventricle. The venous return will increase during expiration. This variation of the venous return will cause variation of the stroke volume, and hence the cardiac input. By using the echocardiogram, this variation can be estimated. Respiratory variation of more than 20% in the stroke volume predicts positive response to fluid expansion.

Hepatorenal syndrome, GN, AIN, and cast nephropathy managements are beyond the internist level and a nephrology consult is recommended anytime you suspect these diagnoses.

Benign prostate hypertrophy–induced urinary retention and AKI is a common scenario. Relieving the obstruction by Foley catheter should be done as soon as possible and it is usually enough to treat the AKI. Other causes of obstruction should be managed in coordination with emergency help from a urologist.

Dietary modification should always be considered in AKI patients. In oliguric AKI, water and sodium excretion is limited and restriction of both is important to prevent any pulmonary edema. Potassium and phosphorus dietary restriction is also recommended because of impaired excretion in AKI. The potassium level should always be observed to prevent any cardiac complications from hyperkalemia. In the polyuric phase of AKI, potassium and phosphorus depletion may occur. Close monitoring and replacement is required. Patient with AKI are at risk for protein-energy malnutrition and should be on at least 1.5 g/kg of protein everyday.

Renal recovery after AKI usually takes place during the first 2 weeks after diagnosis. Renal recovery after ATN and in CKD patients is a long and incomplete process. Even after creatinine normalization, it is better to avoid any nephrotoxic medication whenever this is possible. If there is no improvement after 8 weeks of onset, end-stage renal disease becomes very likely.

Management of complications

AKI complications are life threatening and need quick intervention. A nephrology consult is a must anytime you suspect the patient needs dialysis or specialist management.

Fluid overload Patients with oliguric AKI are at high risk for pulmonary edema. Mild-to-moderate pulmonary edema can be treated with loop diuretics. Oxygen, morphine, and nitroglycerine can be helpful too. Patients with severe pulmonary edema or those who don't respond to diuretics may need to have emergent hemodialysis. Remember the ABC rule, and consider intubation before diuresis or hemodialysis when indicated.

Hyperkalemia Hyperkalemia has a major effect on the cardiac conduction system and includes bradycardia and asystole. Once hyperkalemia is discovered, immediate medical treatment should be started. Unresponsive and persistent hyperkalemia should be treated with hemodialysis.

Acid-base abnormalities Metabolic acidosis is the most common acid-base complication of AKI. Contributing factors are: decreased bicarbonate regeneration, decreased ammonium excretion, and accumulation of other unmeasured anions. Anion gap stays normal in 50% of acidosis cases.

Bicarbonate may be replaced when it is lower than 15 mmol/L or the pH is less than 7.20 (see Chapter 2 to learn bicarbonate replacement principles). Keep in mind that sodium bicarbonate administration can induce volume overload. Refractory acidosis should be treated with hemodialysis.

TIPS TO REMEMBER

- AKI has a significant effect on the morbidity and mortality of the inpatient population.
- A decrease in UOP to less than 0.5 mL/kg for 6 hours and 0.3 mg/dL change in serum creatinine are the 2 main criteria to diagnose AKI.
- Urinalysis, urine osmolality, random protein to creatinine ratio, FeNa, and renal ultrasound are enough to diagnose the etiology of AKI in most cases.
- Volume depletion–induced AKI is reversible with early volume resuscitation.
- AKI secondary to an acute exacerbation of CHF improves with diuretics.
- Obstructive AKI warrants an early urology consult.
- Pulmonary edema resistant to diuretics, refractory hyperkalemia or metabolic acidosis, and symptomatic uremia are indications for hemodialysis in AKI.

COMPREHENSION QUESTIONS

1. A 75-year-old female presents to the emergency department with vomiting, high-grade fever, and left flank pain of 2 days duration. Prior to that, the patient started having dysuria a week ago and her primary care doctor started her on ciprofloxacin. The dysuria did not improve.

The patient has a history of CHF with an ejection fraction of 35% (measured 1 month ago), and coronary artery disease status post–coronary bypass surgery 5 years ago. Home medications include: aspirin, carvedilol, lisinopril, ciprofloxacin, furosemide, and spironolactone. The patient mentioned a CT of the chest was done 10 days prior to this presentation for follow-up of a pulmonary nodule found incidentally on CXR 6 months ago.

On examination, the patient is lying on the bed and sweating. Vital signs: temperature 39°C, blood pressure 100/60, heart rate 110 bpm, respiratory rate 22/min, and oxygen saturation 97% on room air. Positive findings on clinical examination include: bilateral fine crackles in both lung bases, a systolic ejection murmur at the heart base rated 3/6 with radiation to the carotids, and left costophrenic tenderness.

CXR showed an enlarged cardiac silhouette and a 3 cm nodule in the right middle lobe. Initial labs—WBC: 18,000 with 15% bands, Hg: 12, HCT: 36, platelets: 250,000, Na: 131, K: 3.7, Cl: 99, HCO_3: 28, BUN: 80, Cr: 2.8 (last Cr was 0.7 ten days ago), glucose: 95, Ca: 8.0, BNP: 300, and lactic acid: 3.0 (normal is up to 2.0). Urinalysis showed elevated white blood cells, trace protein and blood, bacteriuria, and many hyaline casts. Urine sodium was 8 mmol/L. FeNa was <1%.

What is the most likely cause of the patient's AKI?

A. Contrast nephropathy

B. AIN

C. AKI secondary to volume depletion

D. AKI secondary to CHF

E. ATN

2. An 80-year-old female with a history of advanced CHF is admitted to the hospital with acute on chronic systolic heart failure. The patient was started on a high dose of intravenous furosemide twice a day. The next day, she made a good amount of urine and her shortness of breath improved slightly. Her creatinine increased to 2.1 (baseline is 1.5). On hospital day 3, the patient's creatinine increased to 2.4. Her respiratory rate is 24/min and her saturation is 92% on 6 L by nasal cannula. On examination, her estimated jugular venous pressure is 15 and she has bilateral fine crackles heard diffusely in both lung fields. Her input in the last 24 hours was 1500 cm^3, and her UOP was 2700 cm^3.

What would you do next?

A. Hold furosemide and repeat BMP the next day.

B. Continue IV furosemide.

C. Switch to oral furosemide.

D. Hold furosemide, give 250 cm^3 of normal saline, and repeat BMP.

E. Call nephrology for hemodialysis.

Answers

1. C. The patient's presentation is consistent with severe sepsis and pyelonephritis. She was vomiting for 2 days. She is tachycardic and sweating. Her lactic acid is elevated. This indicates that the patient is in a hypovolemic state. Urine sodium concentration is low even though the patient is on furosemide and spironolactone, which means the kidney is reabsorbing a higher fraction of urine sodium because of the severe prerenal state.

Patients with AKI secondary to CHF are usually in a significant exacerbation, which is not the case here. It is not uncommon to see mild edema in the lower extremities and fine crackles in the lungs of elderly patients with stable CHF

(New York Heart Association Functional Class I). BNP of 300 is not so high as to indicate a hypervolemic state, and, more importantly, BNP should be interpreted very carefully in low GFR states (serum BNP level will be high with poor kidney function). The CXR did not show any pulmonary edema.

After contrast administration, the vast majority of contrast nephropathy patients will have an elevated creatinine within the first 72 hours, and it usually comes back to normal in 5 to 7 days. This patient had contrast given 10 days ago, which makes contrast nephropathy a very unlikely cause of her AKI.

The patient was started on ciprofloxacin a few days ago, and this definitely put her at risk for AIN. Fifty percent to 60% of AIN patients have proteinuria (less than 1 g in 24 hours urine), pyuria, and hematuria. Leukocyte casts are also seen with AIN. However, because it is a much less common etiology of AKI than prerenal causes, AIN is usually a diagnosis of exclusion. This patient has only trace protein-uria and hematuria. More importantly, the patient's presentation and initial workup is very consistent with prerenal AKI. If the renal function doesn't improve after fluid resuscitation, the patient should be evaluated for other etiologies including AIN.

ATN is an important differential diagnosis in this case. Prolonged dehydra-tion and sepsis are risk factors for ischemia and subsequent ATN. The low FeNa in this case does not rule out ATN. That is because FeNa is less than 1% during the early stages of nonoliguric ATN. The only way to differentiate between the 2 conditions is by fluid challenge. If there is no improvement, ATN becomes more likely. Because prerenal AKI is more common than ATN, choice C is the right answer at this stage of the patient's presentation.

2. **B.** The patient's kidney function got worse with an intravenous diuretic. How-ever, she is still in acute heart failure (saturation is 92% on 6 L of oxygen, high JVP, diffuse crackles on chest auscultation). IV furosemide should be continued at this point in order to improve the cardiac function. The UOP and creatinine should be followed very closely. Later on, the diuretics can be switched to oral, and the kidney function will most likely improve after that.

Holding the furosemide with or without fluid bolus at this stage may improve the kidney function, but the patient's acute heart failure will get worse. If this occurs, the patient will be at a higher risk for acute respiratory failure that has a higher mortality than mild-to-moderate AKI.

Before switching from intravenous to oral diuretics, patients should be back to their baseline volume status and with minimal or no symptoms of heart failure. It is still premature to switch this patient to oral diuretics.

Some CHF patients will be resistant to diuretics. In situations like this, increas-ing the dose or adding a thiazide diuretic should be tried. If this doesn't work and the kidney function worsens with low UOP, hemodialysis should be considered. In this patient, intravenous furosemide improved her symptoms slightly and she is still making a good amount of urine. Continuing the intravenous furosemide will most likely improve her volume status.

SUGGESTED READINGS

McPhee S, Papadakis M. *Current Medical Diagnosis & Treatment*. New York, NY: McGraw-Hill Companies; 2011:869–878.

Szerlip H. Acute kidney injury. In: *Internal Medicine Essentials for Students*. Philadelphia: American College of Physicians and RR Donnelly Publishing; 2011:231–235.

A 48-year-old Man With Restlessness, Tremulousness, and Hypertension

Se Young Han, MD

A 48-year-old man is admitted to a hospital because of pneumonia. Two days after the hospitalization, the patient becomes agitated and restless with tachycardia and hypertension. On physical examination, the patient is noted to be alert, but anxious, tremulous, and disoriented to place and time. And these findings differ from those on examination at admission. His alcohol history is significant (eg, drinking 3 or more vodkas a day for years; most recent alcohol intake occurred 2 days before coming to the hospital), but no history of liver diseases or alcohol withdrawal is evident. Subsequent physical examinations reveal no specific changes from the admission assessment except disorientation and anxiety. His respiratory status appears stable, and repeated CXR does not show any progression compared with the admission assessment. Routine laboratory workups including CBC, CMP, EKG, and blood glucose are stable. Since he has a history of alcohol dependence, alcohol withdrawal is considered.

1. **What is the next step to determine the treatment? Once you start medications, how do you adjust the dose of them? And before deciding how to give them, what should you consider first?**

Answer

1. Patients may develop autonomic instability within 48 hours of admission, given significant alcohol use. Therefore, under the suspicion of alcohol withdrawal, it is necessary to calculate Clinical Institute Withdrawal Assessment for Alcohol scale (revised) (CIWA-Ar; see below) score to determine the use of benzodiazepine. If the score is more than 20, pharmacologic treatment is indicated. Since dose of benzodiazepine needs to be adjusted according to patient's symptom report, you should make sure that the patient is able to communicate his symptoms before implementing the protocol.

CASE REVIEW

Given his history of alcohol abuse and symptoms, he is at high risk for alcohol withdrawal and possibly delirium tremens (DTs).

APPROACH TO ALCOHOL WITHDRAWAL PROBLEMS

Screen a patient at risk of alcohol abuse, and assess the necessity of initiating withdrawal protocol.

Alcohol-related problems are estimated in up to 20% of patients in community teaching hospitals. We are frequently asked to manage these problems in a patient who was admitted to the hospital for other medical or surgical illnesses. Although DTs had a mortality rate as high as 20% in the untreated, early recognition of a patient at risk and initiation of appropriate treatment can lower the mortality significantly.

The easiest method to screen a patient at risk of alcohol withdrawal is the CAGE mnemonic (cut–annoyed–guilty–eye opener). More than 2 positive responses correlate highly with severe alcohol abuse and should raise concerns as to whether the patient will experience alcohol withdrawal.

Diagnosis

Currently, CIWA-Ar is recommended for determining the need to treat alcohol withdrawal. In general, a score of less than 10 requires no pharmacologic treatment; a score of 10 to 20 requires at least later assessment, if not treatment; and a score of more than 20 usually merits pharmacologic treatment or a gradual increase to a higher dosage for a person receiving treatment.

CLINICAL INSTITUTE WITHDRAWAL ASSESSMENT FOR ALCOHOL SCALE

Scoring

The cumulative score provides the basis for treatment of patients undergoing alcohol withdrawal (Table 5-1).

Assessment Tool

Nausea and vomiting
Ask: "Do you feel sick to your stomach? Have you vomited?" (See Table 5-2.)

Table 5-1. CIWA Scoring Interpretation

Cumulative Score	
0–8	No medication is necessary
9–14	Medication is optional for patients with a score of 8–14
15–20	A score of ≥15 requires treatment with medication
>20	A score of >20 poses a strong risk of delirium tremens
67	Maximum possible cumulative score

Table 5-2. Nausea Scoring

Score	
0	No nausea and no vomiting
1	Mild nausea with no vomiting
2	
3	
4	Intermittent nausea with dry heaves
5	
6	
7	Constant nausea, frequent dry heaves, and vomiting

Tremor
Arms extended and fingers spread apart (Table 5-3).

Paroxysmal sweats
See Table 5-4.

Anxiety
Ask: "Do you feel nervous?" (See Table 5-5.)

Agitation
See Table 5-6.

Tactile disturbances
Ask: "Have you any itching, pins and needles sensations, burning sensations, or numbness, or do you feel bugs crawling on or under your skin?" (See Table 5-7.)

Table 5-3. Tremor Scoring

Score	
0	No tremor
1	Not visible, but can be felt fingertip to fingertip
2	
3	
4	Moderate, with patient's arms extended
5	
6	
7	Severe, even with arms not extended

Table 5-4. Sweating Scoring

Score	
0	No sweat visible
1	Barely perceptible sweating, palms moist
2	
3	
4	Beads of sweat obvious on forehead
5	
6	
7	Drenching sweats

Table 5-5. Anxiety Scoring

Score	
0	No anxiety, at ease
1	Mildly anxious
2	
3	
4	Moderately anxious, or guarded, so anxiety is inferred
5	
6	
7	Equivalent to acute panic states as seen in severe delirium or acute schizophrenic reactions

Table 5-6. Activity Scoring

Score	
0	Normal activity
1	Somewhat more than normal activity
2	
3	
4	Moderately fidgety and restless
5	
6	
7	Paces back and forth during most of the interview, or constantly thrashes about

Table 5-7. Neurologic Scoring

Score	
0	None
1	Very mild itching, pins and needles, burning, or numbness
2	Mild itching, pins and needles, burning, or numbness
3	Moderate itching, pins and needles, burning, or numbness
4	Moderately severe hallucinations
5	Severe hallucinations
6	Extremely severe hallucinations
7	Continuous hallucinations

Auditory disturbances

Ask: "Are you more aware of sounds around you? Are they harsh? Do they frighten you? Are you hearing anything that is disturbing to you? Are you hearing things you know are not there?" (See Table 5-8.)

Visual disturbances

Ask: "Does the light appear to be too bright? Is its color different? Does it hurt your eyes? Are you seeing anything that is disturbing to you? Are you seeing things you know are not there?" (See Table 5-9.)

Headache, fullness in head

Ask: "Does your head feel different? Does it feel as if there is a band around your head?" Do not rate for dizziness or light-headedness. Otherwise, rate severity (Table 5-10).

Table 5-8. Auditory Disturbance Scoring

Score	
0	Not present
1	Very mild harshness or ability to frighten
2	Mild harshness or ability to frighten
3	Moderate harshness or ability to frighten
4	Moderately severe hallucinations
5	Severe hallucinations
6	Extremely severe hallucinations
7	Continuous hallucinations

Table 5-9. Visual Disturbance Scoring

Score	
0	Not present
1	Very mild sensitivity
2	Mild sensitivity
3	Moderate sensitivity
4	Moderately severe hallucinations
5	Severe hallucinations
6	Extremely severe hallucinations
7	Continuous hallucinations

Orientation and clouding of sensorium

Ask: "What day is this? Where are you? Who am I?" (See Table 5-11.)

Besides patient's history on alcohol, what clues may help us figure out to define possible alcohol use and risk of developing withdrawal symptoms?

Physical examinations may give you clues about alcohol abuse: mild fluctuation hypertension, repeated infections such as pneumonia, particularly aspiration pneumonia, and otherwise unexplained cardiac arrhythmias such as atrial fibrillation (so-called "holiday heart syndrome").

If a patient has severe alcoholism enough to produce liver damage, changes in liver function tests such as an AST:ALT ratio >2:1 may be seen. Among other laboratory tests, elevated carbohydrate-free transferrin (>20 U/L) and gamma-GT (>35 U) are the most sensitive and specific (>70%) to make a diagnosis of alcohol

Table 5-10. Headache Scoring

Score	
0	Not present
1	Very mild
2	Mild
3	Moderate
4	Moderately severe
5	Severe
6	Very severe
7	Extremely severe

Table 5-11. Orientation Scoring

Score	
0	Oriented and can do serial additions
1	Cannot do serial additions or is uncertain about date
2	Disoriented for date by no more than 2 calendar days
3	Disoriented for date by more than 2 calendar days
4	Disoriented for place and/or person

abuse; the combination of the 2 is likely to be more accurate than either alone. These tests are also useful in monitoring abstinence as well. Other than the afore-mentioned tests, a high MCV (>91 μm³) and serum uric acid (>7 mg/dL) can be useful in identifying heavy drinkers.

Once alcoholism is confirmed through either history or laboratory tests, we should start some interventions to prevent alcohol withdrawal syndromes.

The primary effect of alcohol on the CNS is depression of excitability and conduction, so patients with alcoholism seem to have compensated for the depressant effect because the brain has been exposed repeatedly to high doses of alcohol. When alcohol intake is terminated or the alcohol level in the CNS decreases, withdrawal symptoms occur. Since withdrawal is a form of rebound overactivations from the suppression, many of these withdrawal symptoms are the opposite of those produced by intoxication. That is, symptoms of increased CNS activity, particularly agitation, and autonomic hyperactivity such as an increase in heart rate, respiratory rate, and temperature are seen. Patients may develop various withdrawal signs and symptoms depending on the time from the last alcohol use.

Alcohol psychosis develops 12 to 24 hours after discontinuing alcohol use. Patients typically have distinctive visual hallucination without autonomic instability. This is in contrast to the tactile hallucination with autonomic instability in DTs.

Alcohol withdrawal seizures (typically a single generalized seizure) may occur within 48 hours after stopping alcohol, and usually do not require prophylactic antiseizure medications.

DTs refers to delirium associated with a tremor and autonomic hyperactivity, and generally occurs 2 to 7 days after stopping alcohol. This is seen in <5% of alcohol-dependent individuals. The chance of DTs during any single withdrawal is <1%. DTs is most likely to develop in patients with concomitant severe medical disorders. However, in case of very severe alcoholism, patients may have DTs earlier than the typical time frame. In this case, they may have positive blood alcohol in spite of the presence of DTs, which means that their brains have been chronically and severely depressed by higher alcohol. Consequently, their hospital courses and detoxifications may take much longer and be more likely complicated.

Treatment

The goals of treatment are amelioration of symptoms and prevention of complications.

Mild symptoms can be managed supportively. If a patient progresses symptomatically despite supportive measures, pharmacologic treatment should be instituted. Most withdrawal symptoms are caused by the rapid removal of a CNS depressant (in this case, alcohol). The symptoms can be controlled by administering any CNS depressant in doses that decrease agitation, and gradually tapering the dose over 3 to 5 days.

High-dose benzodiazepine is a drug of choice if pharmacologic treatment is required.

Among CNS depressants, benzodiazepines have the highest margin of safety and lowest cost and are, therefore, the preferred class of drugs. All benzodiazepines are effective in the treatment of alcohol withdrawal symptoms. Benzodiazepines with a short half-life are especially useful for patients with serious liver impairment or preexisting encephalopathy. However, short-acting benzodiazepines such as lorazepam can produce rapidly changing drug blood levels and must be given every 4 hours to avoid abrupt fluctuations that may increase the risk of seizures. Therefore, most clinicians use drugs with longer half-lives, such as diazepam or chlordiazepoxide.

Dosage can be adjusted by a symptom.

A key point in treating alcohol withdrawal is to begin with a larger dose of benzodiazepines than usual, which are prescribed for anxiety. The patient's response should be observed, and the dosage needs to be adjusted accordingly. Previously, fixed-dose schedules were used for the treatment, but multiple studies have shown that a symptom-triggered approach may be as efficacious as the fixed one and result in less drug use.

Prerequisite to start CIWA-Ar protocol.

Before implementing a symptom-triggered protocol, 2 factors should be considered: first, is the patient at risk of developing alcohol withdrawal syndrome? (A remote history of alcoholism does not increase the risk of symptom development and therefore doesn't need a treatment protocol.) Second, does the patient have intact verbal communication? Since this protocol is a symptom-triggered treatment, it is ineffective if the patient is not able to communicate symptoms.

In addition to alcohol withdrawal syndrome, there are other medical problems complicating the treatment of patients with alcohol withdrawal, especially nutritional deficiencies:

1. Thiamine deficiency:

   A. Wet beriberi (aka beriberi syndrome) is characterized by high output heart failure (alcoholism is 1 of the reversible causes of dilated cardiomyopathy).

   B. Dry beriberi (either Wernicke syndrome or Korsakoff psychosis).

In Wernicke syndrome, patients typically manifest ataxia, ophthalmoplegia (diplopia with nystagmus due to lateral gaze palsy, often affecting VI cranial nerve, abducens nerve), and confusion.

In Korsakoff psychosis, patients may develop a combination of anterograde and retrograde amnesia, confabulation, or spur cell on peripheral blood smear. It is associated with a poor prognosis.

Management: give thiamine first before replacing glucose in patients with alcoholism. Thiamine is a vital cofactor for glucose metabolism; therefore, giving glucose prior to thiamine would worsen the status of the patient.

2. Refeeding syndrome (phosphate deficiency): Patients who chronically use alcohol are phosphate-depleted as well. If they are fed a high-carbohydrate diet without correcting hypophosphatemia, it will lead to the depletion of more phosphate because it will be used to make ATP and phosphate-bound glucose in the liver and muscles. Consequently, patients may develop hemolysis, muscle breakdown, and respiratory distress.

3. Vitamin B_{12} and folate deficiency: Clinically, vitamin B_{12} results in both hematologic and neurologic sequelae while folate deficiency causes only hematologic problems.

Biochemically, the level of vitamin B_{12} and folate can be measured directly. However, the folate level can be affected by even 1 folate-rich diet, making it appear normal. Moreover, vitamin B_{12} levels are often borderline low (250–500). If these levels are normal but clinical suspicion is high, measure the indirect metabolites of vitamin B_{12} and folate: MMA and homocysteine. If both are elevated, there is a vitamin B_{12} deficiency, and if only homocysteine is high, a folate deficiency is likely present.

In vitamin B_{12} deficiency, neurologic complications come first before hematologic manifestations such as megaloblastic anemia (MCV is often higher than 110). Therefore, even without hematologic findings, dementia or gait problem such as a "high stepping gait" in a clinical context may be a symptom of vitamin B_{12} deficiency.

4. Miscellaneous: hyponatremia (beer potomania), magnesium deficiency, and calcium deficiency.

TIPS TO REMEMBER

- Alcohol-related problems are common in the hospital. Early recognition of a patient at risk and initiation of appropriate treatment can lower the mortality significantly.

- CIWA-Ar is recommended for determining the need to treat alcohol withdrawal.

- Many of alcohol withdrawal symptoms seen are due to increased CNS activity, particularly agitation and autonomic hyperactivity such as an increase in heart rate, respiratory rate, and temperature.

- DTs refers to delirium associated with a tremor and autonomic hyperactivity, and generally occurs 2 to 7 days after stopping the use of alcohol.

- Benzodiazepines are the preferred class of drugs to treat the alcohol withdrawal syndrome.

COMPREHENSION QUESTION

1. A 42-year-old man was admitted for vomiting blood. On admission, his examinations including vital signs were unremarkable. Initial laboratory tests showed mild macrocytic anemia on CBC, normal LFT, and a negative alcohol level. The next day, he started to see "spiders hanging from the ceiling." Examination revealed temperature 97.8°F, heart rate 74/min, respiratory rate 12/min, and blood pressure 130/80 mm Hg. There was mild tremulousness. His past medical history was significant for alcohol abuse. CIWA-Ar protocol was started.

   What is the most likely diagnosis?
   A. DTs
   B. Minor withdrawal symptoms
   C. Acute withdrawal seizure
   D. Alcohol hallucinosis
   E. Korsakoff psychosis

Answer

1. A. Lack of autonomic hyperactivity in addition to atypical time course (onset less than 48 hours from last drinking) makes DTs highly unlikely. Patients with DTs typically show disorientation and their hallucinations are tactile other than visual. Patients may develop minor withdrawal symptoms such as tremulousness, mild anxiety, and nausea usually within 6 hours of cessation of drinking. Alcohol withdrawal seizure, often a single generalized seizure, may occur within 48 hours after stopping alcohol. Based on the development of distinctive visual hallucination without autonomic instability, the patient with withdrawal symptoms is diagnosed with alcoholic hallucination, which happens in 12 to 24 hours after discontinuing alcohol. This patient does not have features of Korsakoff psychosis.

SUGGESTED READINGS

Fauci AS, Braunwald E, Kasper DL, et al. Alcohol and alcoholism. In: *Harrison's Principles of Internal Medicine*. 17th ed. New York, NY: McGraw-Hill Professional; 2008:2725–2728 [chapter 387].

Hecksel KA, Bostwick JM, Jaeger TM, Cha SS. Inappropriate use of symptom-triggered therapy for alcohol withdrawal in the general hospital. *Mayo Clin Proc.* 2008;83(3):274–279.

Lohr R. Treatment of alcohol withdrawal in hospitalized patients. *Mayo Clin Proc.* 1995;70(8):777–782.

Arrhythmias

Sayeeda Azra Jabeen, MD, FACP and
Susan Thompson Hingle, MD

A 55-year-old Man With Fatigue and Decreased Exercise Tolerance

A 55-year-old male with a past medical history of hypertension, hyperlipidemia, and obesity presents to the outpatient internal medicine clinic with a 3-day history of fatigue and decreased exercise tolerance. He used to be able to walk 2 blocks without shortness of breath, but now he gets winded even walking in from the parking garage. He feels as though his heart is beating fast but denies palpitations. He has no chest pain, dizziness, visual changes, edema, or orthopnea. His medications include chlorthalidone, lovastatin, and aspirin.

On physical examination, his blood pressure is 120/60 mm Hg, pulse is 100 bpm, respiratory rate is 16/min, and pulse oximetry is 96% on room air. He is alert and answers questions appropriately. His lungs are clear to auscultation. His cardiac examination reveals an irregularly irregular rhythm that is tachycardic. Extremities reveal no edema. EKG is shown in Figure 6-1.

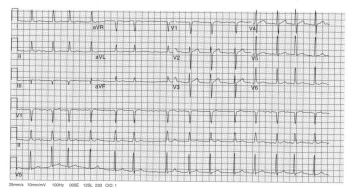

Figure 6-1. Patient's EKG.

1. What is your diagnosis?

Answer

1. Atrial fibrillation, a form of supraventricular tachycardia (SVT).

ARRHYTHMIAS

A thorough clinical history and physical examination, as in any other case, are very important. Clinically significant tachyarrhythmias may produce symptoms of palpitations, lightheadedness, syncope, or dyspnea. Look for any triggering factors such as infection, inflammation, myocardial ischemia, drug toxicity, excess use of caffeine, tobacco, excessive alcohol intake, thyroid abnormalities, catecholamine excess, or electrolyte imbalances as potential causes.

A reasonable way to organize arrhythmias is into the following categories: supraventricular tachyarrhythmias, ventricular tachyarrhythmias, bradyarrhythmias, and conduction blocks.

A 30-year-old Woman With Palpitations and Anxiety

A 30-year-old female is admitted with fever, elevated WBC, diarrhea, and abdominal pain and found to have *C. difficile* colitis. The patient complains of palpitations associated with anxiety. The nurse reports the patient's BP is 130/70 with a heart rate of 150 bpm. The EKG is shown in Figure 6-2.

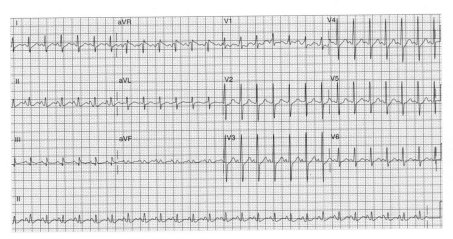

Figure 6-2. Patient's EKG.

1. What is the best next step?

Answer

1. The EKG reveals SVT with a HR of 150 bpm. The best step to perform next is carotid sinus massage. If there is no response, try intravenous adenosine. Continue to treat the underlying infection as well.

SUPRAVENTRICULAR ARRHYTHMIAS

Supraventricular Tachycardia

Diagnosis

SVT refers to paroxysmal tachyarrhythmias that involve the atria, the atrioventricular (AV) junction, or both. It should be noted that while all of the above terms are technically causes of SVT, clinicians should use the specific diagnosis, when possible, such as atrial flutter and atrial fibrillation with rapid ventricular response.

Most SVTs have a narrow QRS complex on ECG, but SVT with aberrant conduction can produce a wide complex tachycardia that may mimic ventricular tachycardia (VT). These tachycardias commonly occur as a result of a precipitating illness or drug interaction.

Treatment

Managing SVT is relatively straightforward. If the patient is hemodynamically unstable, proceed to cardioversion. If the patient is hemodynamically stable, treatment includes carotid massage, IV adenosine, beta-blockers, and/or calcium channel blockers.

A 69-year-old Man With Tachycardia and Wheezing

A 69-year-old gentleman is admitted with pneumonia and COPD exacerbation. The nurse calls you saying the patient has developed tachycardia and active wheezing, and his rhythm is irregular. She is worried and wants you to look at the EKG (Figure 6-3). The nurse shows you the following 12-lead EKG from the patient:

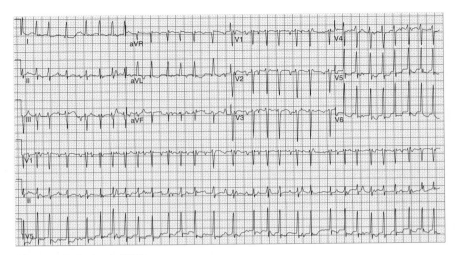

Figure 6-3. Patient's EKG.

1. What is your diagnosis and treatment plan?

Answer

1. The EKG shows multifocal atrial tachycardia (MAT). The patient's underlying lung disease must have precipitated MAT. Treating the COPD exacerbation with beta-2-adrenergic agonist inhalation is the treatment of choice. Make sure to correct hypomagnesemia or hypokalemia if present.

Multifocal Atrial Tachycardia

Diagnosis

MAT is an irregular SVT with a heart rate of more than 100 bpm distinguished by at least 3 p-wave morphologies (Figure 6-4). It is often associated with COPD and congestive heart failure. Therapy in patients with MAT should be aimed at treating the underlying disease.

Treatment

Medical therapy for the tachyarrhythmia is indicated only if MAT causes a sustained rapid ventricular response that causes or worsens myocardial ischemia, heart failure, peripheral perfusion, or oxygenation. For patients with symptomatic MAT requiring ventricular rate control, we recommend therapy with verapamil or a beta-blocker.

Wandering Atrial Pacemaker

This disorder is similar to MAT in that there are 3 morphologically distinct p-waves but the heart rate is less than 100 bpm (Figure 6-5).

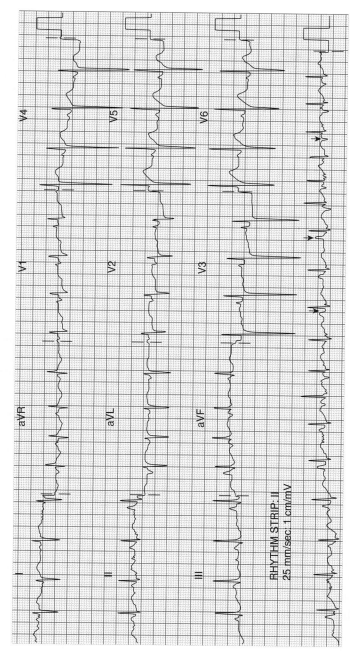

Figure 6-4. MAT with an irregular rhythm and with at least 3 different morphological p-waves and tachycardia.

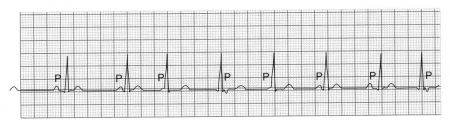

Figure 6-5. *Note*: Irregular rhythm with 3 morphologically distinct p-waves with a heart rate of less than 100 bpm.

Atrial Fibrillation

Diagnosis

Atrial fibrillation is characterized by the absence of discrete p-waves (Figure 6-6). Rapid atrial activity can be seen as fibrillatory f waves at a rate that is generally between 350 and 600 bpm; the f waves vary in amplitude, morphology, and intervals. The RR interval shows no repetitive pattern, and is thus labeled as "irregularly irregular." The ventricular rate usually ranges from 90 to 170 bpm.

Treatment

Studies have shown that rhythm control and rate control result in similar mortality and stroke rates, even in patients with underlying heart failure. Quality of life should be considered when deciding upon treatment. Therapy should be directed at rate control with a goal of less than 100 bpm. Rate control is generally achieved with beta-blockers, a calcium channel blocker, or digoxin. Digoxin is less effective in controlling ventricular response during activity and in paroxysmal atrial fibrillation. It is useful in patients with decreased LV function. Anticoagulation should be started in patients at high risk for stroke as determined by the CHADS2 scoring system. (See scoring system below.)

CHADS2 system:

Congestive heart failure (current or any previous history) gets 1 point.

Hypertension (current or any prior history) gets 1 point.

Age ≥75 years gets 1 point.

Diabetes mellitus gets 1 point.

Stroke. Patients with a history of a systemic embolic event get 2 points. Secondary prevention in patients with a prior ischemic stroke or a transient ischemic attack is of utmost importance.

If the patient scores 2 or more points, then anticoagulation is indicated to prevent stroke.

If the patient scores less than 2 points, only aspirin is indicated.

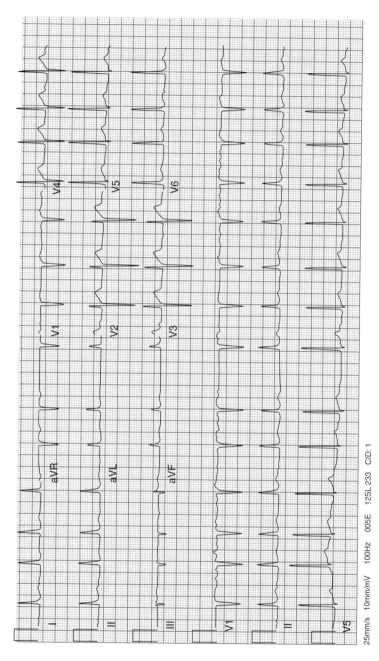

25mm/s   10mm/mV   100Hz   005E   005E   12SL 233   CID: 1

Figure 6-6. Atrial fibrillation with an irregularly irregular rhythm with no p-waves. Note the fibrillatory or f waves.

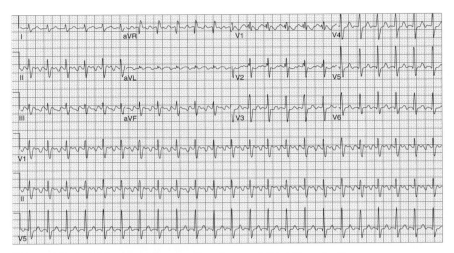

Figure 6-7. Atrial flutter with sawtooth pattern and 2:1 AV conduction.

Atrial Flutter

Diagnosis
Atrial flutter results from a single reentrant circuit around a functional or structural barrier to conduction within the atria (Figure 6-7). The 12-lead EKG has a characteristic "sawtooth" pattern with an effective atrial rate of 250 to 350 bpm. There is typically 2:1 (flutter waves:QRS response) conduction across the AV node. As a result, the ventricular rate is usually one half the flutter rate in the absence of AV node dysfunction.

Treatment
The clinical presentation and treatment strategies are similar to atrial fibrillation, which include rate control and anticoagulation. There is a high rate of success with radio-frequency ablation for typical atrial flutter.

A 75-year-old Man With Sudden Shortness of Breath and Weakness

A 75-year-old male with a past medical history significant for hypertension, diabetes, and coronary artery disease presents to the emergency department with a 1-hour history of sudden shortness of breath and generalized weakness.

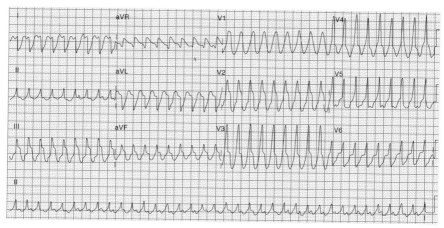

Figure 6-8. Patient's EKG.

On examination, he is noted to have a blood pressure of 90/58. He is clammy and diaphoretic. His lungs are clear to auscultation. His heart examination reveals tachycardia.

His EKG is shown in Figure 6-8.

1. What is your diagnosis?

Answer

1. VT.

VENTRICULAR ARRHYTHMIAS

Ventricular Tachycardia

Diagnosis

VT is the most frequently encountered life-threatening arrhythmia. It is defined as a series of 3 or more ventricular complexes that occur at a rate of 100 to 250 bpm. Typically, the QRS complex is wide (usually >120 milliseconds). In the setting of significant structural heart disease, sustained VT (defined as an episode longer than 30 seconds) predicts a poor prognosis. This is a potentially life-threatening arrhythmia because it may lead to ventricular fibrillation (VF), asystole, and sudden death.

Treatment

Patients suffering from pulseless VT or unstable VT are hemodynamically compromised and require immediate cardioversion. For patients who are hemodynamically stable, antiarrythmic agents such as amiodarone, lidocaine, procainamide, or sotolol should be used.

A 75-year-old Man Status Post–Myocardial Infarction With Stent Placement

A 75-year-old male with HTN, DM2, ESRD, PVD, and CAD with a CABG in the past is admitted with an acute ST elevation myocardial infarction status post–cardiac stent placement. He has a BP of 90/50, and a heart rate of 110 bpm early in the morning. You are at the nurses' station and the telemetry monitor goes off showing the rhythm in Figure 6-9.

1. What do you do next?

Answer

1. Call a code blue, followed by cardioversion and IV amiodarone.

Ventricular Fibrillation

Diagnosis

VF is the most frequent mechanism of sudden cardiac death (SCD). It is a rapid, disorganized ventricular arrhythmia resulting in no uniform ventricular contraction, no cardiac output, and no recordable blood pressure. The electrocardiogram in VF shows rapid (300–400 bpm), irregular, shapeless QRST complexes with variable amplitude, morphology, and intervals. Over time, these waveforms decrease in amplitude. Ultimately, asystole occurs.

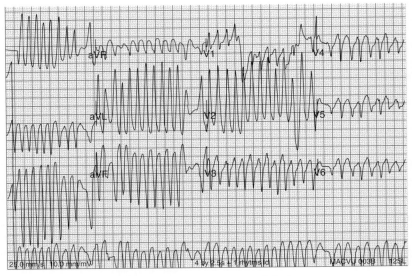

Figure 6-9. Ventricular fibrillation with disorganized rhythm.

Treatment

Immediate unsynchronized cardioversion is the treatment of choice, followed by intravenous antiarrythmics such as amiodarone.

A 65-year-old Woman With Syncopal Episodes

A 65-year-old woman comes in for her Welcome to Medicare examination. She has a history of hypertension and diabetes mellitus type 2. On questioning, she says she has had 2 syncopal episodes in the past week. On physical examination, her blood pressure is 138/78 mm Hg, her pulse is 80 bpm, and her respiratory rate is 14/min. Lungs are clear to auscultation. Cardiovascular examination reveals a regular rate and rhythm with no murmurs, gallops, or rubs. Her extremities have no edema.

Her EKG is shown in Figure 6-10.

1. What is your diagnosis?

Answer

1. Mobitz type II AV block.

HEART BLOCKS

First-degree AV Block

Diagnosis

First-degree AV block usually results from a conduction delay within the AV node in which the PR interval is lengthened beyond 200 milliseconds. The most

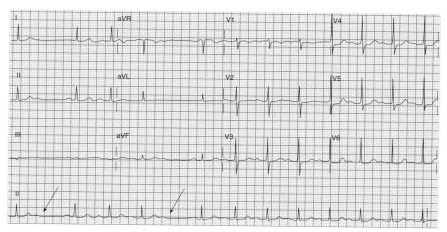

Figure 6-10. First degree AV block.

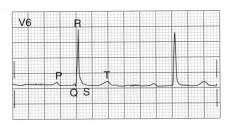

Figure 6-11. First degree AV block.

common causes include increased vagal tone (athletes), drug effect, electrolyte abnormalities, ischemia, and conduction system disease.

Treatment

Asymptomatic patients require no therapy. Stop or decrease the dose of AV node blocking medications such as beta-blockers or calcium channel blockers if these are being used (Figure 6-11).

Second-degree AV Block

Diagnosis

There are 2 types of second-degree AV blocks. These are recognized based on their pattern of impulse conduction, and the distinction between type I and type II is important, as the 2 types carry different prognostic implications.

Mobitz Type I (Wenckebach) Block

Mobitz type I heart block is characterized by the progressive prolongation of the PR interval on consecutive beats followed by a blocked p-wave (Figure 6-12). This

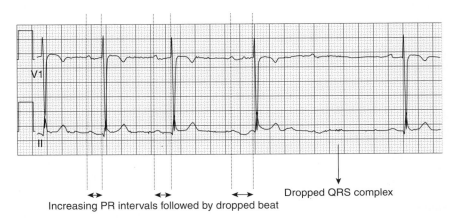

Dropped QRS complex

Increasing PR intervals followed by dropped beat

Figure 6-12. Mobitz type I block.

is recognized as a dropped QRS complex. After the dropped QRS complex, the PR interval resets and the cycle repeats. The RR interval progressively shortens before a blocked p-wave.

Treatment

Prior to initiating treatment for Mobitz type I AV block, reversible causes of slowed conduction such as myocardial ischemia, increased vagal tone, and medications should be excluded. If no reversible causes are present, and the patient is asymptomatic, no specific therapy is required. Atropine can be used emergently, and for persistent symptomatic bradycardia a permanently implanted pacemaker is indicated.

Mobitz Type II Block

Diagnosis

Mobitz type II block is characterized by an abrupt AV conduction block without evidence of conduction delay in preceding conducted impulses (Figure 6-13). The ECG demonstrates no change in the PR interval preceding conducted impulses. This type of AV block may progress rapidly to complete heart block, in which no escape rhythm may emerge. In this case, the person may experience a Stokes-Adams attack, cardiac arrest, or SCD.

Treatment

The definitive treatment for this form of AV block is an implantable pacemaker.

Third-degree (Complete) AV Block

Diagnosis

Complete heart block occurs when all of the atrial impulses fail to conduct to the ventricle and the prevailing ventricular escape rhythm is slower than the atrial rhythm (Figure 6-14). The PR interval will be variable, and the hallmark of complete heart block is no apparent relationship between p-waves and QRS complexes.

Treatment

Therapy for complete heart block begins by looking for and correcting reversible causes such as myocardial ischemia, increased vagal tone, and drugs that depress AV conduction. If no reversible causes are present, treatment is a permanent pacemaker for most patients.

TIPS TO REMEMBER

- Quick recognition of arrhythmias is important and comes with practice and experience.
- Anticoagulation with warfarin has significant risks, so should be reserved for patients with high CHADS2 scores.
- Mortality outcomes are similar for patients with atrial fibrillation who are treated with rhythm control compared with those treated with rate control.

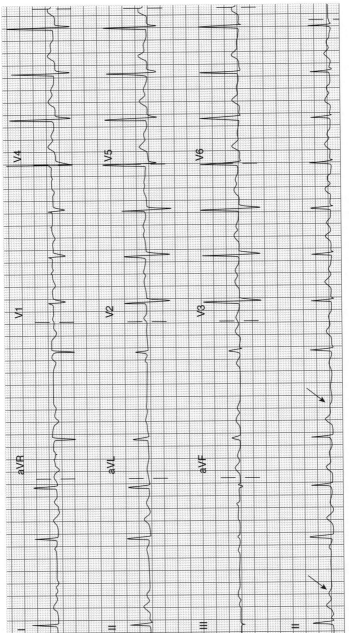

Figure 6-13. Mobitz type II with consistent PR interval and an unpredictable blocked p-wave.

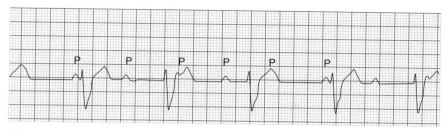

Figure 6-14. Third-degree heart block. Note p-waves marching through and QRS complexes without a correlating p-wave.

SUGGESTED READINGS

Ahya SN, Flood K, Paranjothi S. *Cardiac Arrhythmias. The Washington Manual of Medical Therapeutics*. 30th ed. Philadelphia: Lippincott Williams & Wilkins; 2001:153–167.

Cheng A, Kumar K. Overview of atrial fibrillation. In: Zimetbaum P, Saperia G, eds. *UpToDate*. 2012.

Phang R. Overview of the evaluation and management of atrial flutter. In: Zimetbaum P, Saperia G, eds. *UpToDate*. 2012.

A 40-year-old Man With Chest Pain

Muralidhar Papireddy, MD, Se Young Han, MD, and Susan Thompson Hingle, MD

A 40-year-old man presented to emergency department with a 2-day history of chest pain. He also has a 1-week history of sore throat, runny nose, dry cough, and generalized body aches. Yesterday, he woke up with chest pain, which he describes as a severe, sharp, substernal chest pain that is aggravated by cough, deep breathing, and lying down. No dyspnea, orthopnea, paroxysmal nocturnal dyspnea, palpitations, or syncope. He is physically active and is training for a 20-mile marathon. He has a history of hypertension, diabetes type 2, and dyslipidemia. No medication allergies. He drinks 1 glass of red wine on most nights. No history of tobacco or illicit drug use. He is on hydrochlorothiazide, metformin, and lovastatin. On examination, he appears to be in moderate distress from the chest pain. Vitals signs are within normal limits. Cardiac examination shows normal heart sounds with a pericardial rub. The remainder of the physical examination is unremarkable. Complete blood count is normal; basic metabolic profile is within normal range. Cardiac enzymes are normal. Electrocardiogram done in the emergency room shows diffuse ST segment elevation without reciprocal changes and PR segment depression in the limb leads. Chest radiograph is within normal limits.

1. What is the diagnosis and treatment of this condition?

Answer

1. Acute pericarditis.

CASE REVIEW

His symptoms and signs are typical for acute pericarditis. Patient had chest pain for 2 days, which is sharp, constant, and worsened by position and deep breathing. Electrocardiogram shows diffuse ST elevation without reciprocal changes that helps to differentiate it from myocardial infarction where you will find reciprocal ST depression with evolution of Q waves. Most cases of pericarditis are idiopathic or viral in etiology. Treatment is to begin nonsteroidal anti-inflammatory medication.

APPROACH TO CHEST PAIN

One of the most common presenting complaints in the emergency department, clinics, and even in hospital inpatients is chest pain. Several conditions can present as chest pain, and the challenge is in identifying the life-threatening causes from benign conditions.

In patients with chest pain who are not having a myocardial infarction, 50% to 60% of them have musculoskeletal and gastroesophageal disorders as the etiology of their chest pain. Unknown causes and psychiatric condition account for another 8% to 35% of the cases. Realizing this, it is also important to recognize that chest pain is a symptom of some life-threatening conditions that require further investigation and management. Patients who are discharged with a diagnosis of noncardiac chest pain of unknown origin have survival rates of 94% at 10 years and 88% at 20 years.

A thorough history and physical examination can identify the etiology of the chest pain in most cases. In some cases, though, we may need additional testing to confirm or refute a clinical diagnosis.

History

Characteristics of the pain tell a lot about the underlying process. Every detail may have significance. Classical teaching with pneumonic, OLD-CA^{2}R^{2}T (*o*nset, *l*ocation, *d*uration, *c*haracter, *a*ggravating factors/*a*ssociated symptoms, *r*adiation/*r*elieving factors, *t*iming of the pain), can be applied.

Onset: Information on onset of the pain may provide a great deal of information in the evaluation of the patients with chest pain. With aortic dissection, pneumothorax, and pulmonary embolism, the onset of the pain is sudden. Myocardial ischemia is usually gradual in onset.

Location: If a patient points with a finger to the apex or sternal border of the heart, the etiology of the pain is probably musculoskeletal. Describing the pain with a closed fist or palm suggests ischemia.

Duration: Pain that is constant and lasts weeks or a few seconds; pain is probably not from myocardial ischemia. Stable angina generally lasts 2 to 10 minutes, unstable angina (UA) 10 to 20 minutes, and myocardial infarction >30 minutes.

Character: Pain is described as sharp in pneumothorax, aortic dissection, pleurisy, and pericarditis. Pain in myocardial ischemia is described as a discomfort, a pressure, tightness, heaviness, or squeezing. Burning pain is most likely from esophageal reflux.

Aggravating factors: Exertion, cold weather, or stress aggravation suggests ischemia. Cough and deep breathing aggravation suggest pleurisy. In esophageal reflux and pericarditis, the pain worsens with lying down. Movement and rotation worsen chest pain in patients with musculoskeletal pain. Swallowing worsens pain in esophageal disorders, but with postprandial pain, do not forget to think about myocardial ischemia as a possibility.

Associated symptoms: Chest pain with dyspnea suggests pulmonary embolism, pneumonia, myocardial ischemia, pneumothorax, or eroding lung tumors. Nausea, vomiting, and diaphoresis may be associated with myocardial ischemia. Cough may be present with a pulmonary process or

GERD. Syncope may occur concomitantly with aortic dissection, massive PE, or critical aortic stenosis.

Radiation: If the chest pain radiates to the neck, jaw, shoulders, back, or arms, this may suggest myocardial ischemia or aortic dissection. In pain that radiates down the neck and then causes chest pain, one should think about cervical radiculopathy. Pericarditis pain radiates to trapezius area.

Relieving factors: Leaning forwards improves pain in pericarditis. Sitting up improves the pain in esophageal reflux disease. Resting improves chest pain in myocardial ischemia from stable angina. Improvement with antacids and eating suggests gastroesophageal problems. Pain relieved by nitroglycerin does not rule out acute coronary syndrome (ACS).

Timing of the pain: Early morning pain may occur in myocardial ischemia. If chest pain occurs at night while sleeping, think about gastroesophageal reflux or myocardial ischemia. Chest pain that happens after heavy exercise, weight lifting, or moving furniture suggests cardiac ischemia or musculoskeletal sources. Chest pain after recurrent retching or vomiting should make you think about esophageal rupture. If the pain occurs while swallowing, think esophagitis or spasm.

Also important is gathering information on the risk factors for different conditions in consideration on your differential diagnostic hypothesis list. Knowledge of the risk factors may give you pertinent information regarding disease likelihood. But it is also important to remember that having no cardiac risk factors in patients presenting with acute chest pain does not rule out ACS.

Physical Examination

Examination should focus on palpation of the upper and lower extremity pulses, bilateral upper extremity blood pressure measurements, a thorough cardiac and respiratory examination, an abdominal examination, and, last but not the least, examination of the musculoskeletal system.

EKG and Chest Radiograph

An EKG should be ordered as a part of an acute evaluation of chest pain. A chest radiograph may be helpful in evaluating nonischemic causes of chest pain.

Rapid Evaluation

A rapid evaluation should be carried out on presentation to identify the patients who may be having 1 of the life-threatening conditions (see Table 7-1). These conditions may result in death, if ignored. Once we know that the chest pain is not from 1 of these life-threatening conditions, the next question to ask is the following: does this patient need admission to the hospital for further management or

Table 7-1. Life-threatening Causes of Chest Pain

Acute coronary syndrome
Pulmonary embolism
Pneumothorax
Aortic dissection
Esophageal rupture

can the patient be managed as an outpatient? The algorithm in Figure 7-1 can help us make decisions regarding further care. We will discuss life-threatening causes of the chest pain and end with discussion of the common causes of chest pain.

Acute coronary syndrome

UA, non–ST elevation myocardial infarction (NSTEMI), and ST elevation myocardial infarction (STEMI) are all considered to be ACSs. For the convenience of the readers, UA and NSTEMI are discussed together as they are closely related conditions with similar management strategy.

UA is defined as an ischemic pain occurring at rest that lasts for more than 10 to 20 minutes, new-onset chest pain, or increasing angina that is more frequent, lasts longer, or occurs at a lower threshold, with negative cardiac enzymes and EKG showing ST depression or T-wave inversion. In myocardial infarction pain, the pain lasts longer than 30 minutes and is more intense. It is classified as STEMI or NSTEMI based on presence or absence of ST segment elevation, respectively.

Symptoms and signs Chest pain is often described as a pressure-like pain, chest tightness, squeezing, heaviness, indigestion, or chest discomfort that radiates to the jaw, neck, arms, or shoulder. If a patient has had a myocardial infarction in the past, he or she may relate the pain to the previous episode. Cardiac ischemia is often associated with dyspnea, diaphoresis, weakness, nausea, or vomiting. Patients often show the painful area by placing a palm or a closed fist over the chest. Obtaining a history of comorbid conditions such as hyperthyroidism, gastrointestinal bleeding, and renal and pulmonary diseases may be important too. On physical examination, attention should be paid to general appearance, vitals, pulses, cardiac, lung examination, musculoskeletal examination, signs of heart failure, and fluid overload.

Chest pain that is pleuritic, lasts only a few seconds, radiates to the lower extremities, and is reproduced with movement or palpation of the chest is not an ischemic pain. Also if the pain is constant and lasts for hours, with negative EKG and cardiac enzymes, then chest pain is probably from some cause other than cardiac ischemia. A word of caution is that patients with ACS may have pleuritic chest (13%) or reproducible chest pain on palpation (7%).

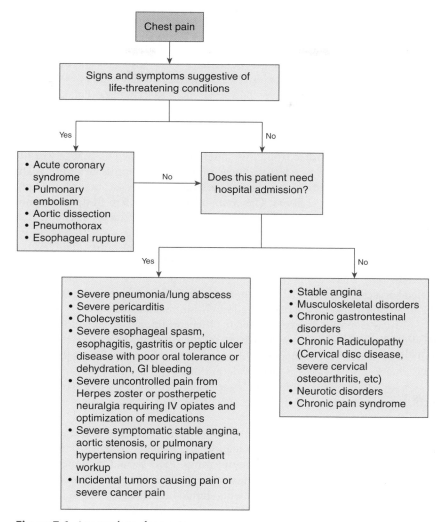

Figure 7-1. Approach to chest pain.

In patients with classic symptoms of ACS, traditional risk factors for CAD are less important than the symptoms, EKG findings, and the cardiac enzymes. In other words, risk factors may have no role in diagnosing ACS. Elderly patients, women, and diabetic patients may present with dyspnea alone in ACS. Relief of angina with nitroglycerin does not rule out ACS. Also relief of chest pain with a GI cocktail (mixture of viscous lidocaine, antacids, and an anticholinergic) does not rule out ACS.

EKG It as an important tool to risk stratify patients on presentation. ST elevation seen on an EKG needs emergent cardiology consultation for immediate reperfusion therapy. ST depression of more than 0.5 mm and symmetric T-wave inversions during symptoms suggest ischemia. Patients with ST segment deviation of less than or equal to 0.5 mm are at increased risk of death and new MI at 1 year compared with isolated T-wave changes or no EKG changes. Patients with a normal ECG on presentation with chest pain may have ACS. One percent to 6% of chest pain patients go on to develop MI, and 4% have UA.

Cardiac biomarkers Cardiac troponins should be determined as part of work for ACS. If they are negative, serial enzymes should be done for up to 12 hours after the symptom onset. Cardiac troponins are elevated as early as 2 hours and may be delayed for up to 8 to 12 hours. They remain elevated for 5 to 14 days. Troponin levels provide prognosis beyond what is known from EKG and predischarge stress test. There is a quantitative relationship with risk of death.

CK-MB is not as sensitive or specific for myocardial injury. The levels of CK-MB become elevated at the same time as cardiac troponins but remain elevated for only 1 to 2 days because of a short half-life. They may be elevated with skeletal muscle injury. CK-MB may be useful to assist in knowing the extension of the infarct or to diagnose a periprocedural MI in the hospital.

Cardiac troponin may be elevated in other conditions too. Therefore, in making the diagnosis of myocardial infarction, there should be a characteristic rise and fall of cardiac troponin along with ischemic description of chest pain and/or EKG changes. See Chapter 3 for new definition of MI.

Brain natriuretic peptide and C-reactive protein have no role in diagnosing ACS, but may have prognostic value.

Initial risk stratification Early risk stratification is the most important step in the management of ACS. This helps to identify the patients at high risk for cardiac events to intervene early to improve outcomes. EKG should be done as part of rapid assessment while performing history and physical examination. If the EKG shows there is ST elevation, then patients should be treated as STEMI.

For patients with UA and NSTEMI, we need to identify the patients who are at extremely high risk (as shown in Table 7-2), since this group of patients should go for urgent coronary intervention. If there is no urgent indication for coronary intervention, these patients should be risk stratified using one of the risk stratification models. The TIMI risk score is the most often used, because it is easy to remember and apply. Within the first 2 weeks, the risk of death, myocardial infarction, and severe recurrent ischemia requiring intervention increases with increasing TIMI score. Zero to 2 is low risk, 3 to 4 intermediate risk, and 5 to 7 high risk.

Once risk stratified, very-high-risk patients need to go for an urgent coronary angiography and revascularization. High- and intermediate-risk patients on TIMI score benefit from early intervention (<24 hours).

Table 7-2. Unstable Angina/NSTEMI Early Risk Stratification

Extremely high-risk features requiring urgent coronary angiography and revascularization
Ongoing chest pain despite optimal medical management
Hemodynamic instability/shock
Electrical instability (sustained ventricular tachycardia)
Pulmonary edema/new-onset or worsening heart failure/severe ventricular dysfunction
New or worsening mitral regurgitation
TIMI risk score: 7 variables
Age >65
>2 episodes of chest pain in the last 24 h
>3 risk factors (hypertension, diabetes, dyslipidemia, smoker, and significant family history of early MI)
Known coronary artery disease with >50% stenosis
ST segment deviation on admission EKG
Positive cardiac biomarkers
On ASA for the preceding 7 days

For STEMI, the time from first medical contact to percutaneous coronary intervention (PCI) should be less than 90 minutes (also known as door to balloon time). If the patient is transferred from a non-PCI center, the time to PCI should be no more than 120 minutes. If PCI center is not accessible, then fibrinolytics should be given within 30 minutes of arrival and can be given within 12 hours of the symptom onset.

In patients with symptoms suspicious for ACS, but not confirmed based on negative initial EKG and cardiac troponin, the patient needs to be admitted to a chest pain unit or a monitored bed to obtain serial EKGs and cardiac enzymes. Remember that cardiac troponin may take up to 8 to 12 hours to rise. Low-risk patients should undergo a stress test within 72 hours.

Detailed management is discussed in Chapter 3.

Pulmonary embolism
The incidence of pulmonary embolism is rising presumably due to improved quality of imaging and widespread availability of CT scanners. Not all pulmonary embolisms are life-threatening, but proximal ones may pose significant risk of death and morbidity.

Symptoms and signs Pulmonary embolism without infarction may present with dyspnea at rest or exertion. Pleuritic chest pain suggests pulmonary infarction from pulmonary embolism. Patients may complain of cough, wheezing, and calf or thigh pain. Examination may be significant for respiratory distress, sinus tachycardia, and an S3. Massive PE may present with right-sided heart failure.

Diagnosis Prior to ordering imaging, pretest probability should be assessed to avoid unnecessary investigations and cost burden. The Wells score is a well-validated prediction model. A modified Wells criterion provides a pretest probability for PE. Based on the score, patients are categorized into (1) PE likely (score >4) or (2) PE unlikely (score of 4 or less).

For the PE unlikely category, if the D-dimer is negative, PE is essentially ruled out. For the PE likely category and the PE unlikely category with positive D-dimers, CT pulmonary angiogram (CT-PA) should be ordered, unless contraindicated. If CT-PA is negative, it should be followed up with lower extremity ultrasound to rule out DVT, if there is clinical suspicion.

If the CT is contraindicated, V/Q scan should be ordered. The traditional Wells score should be used in conjunction with V/Q scan results to confirm or refute the diagnosis of PE. Normal V/Q scan with any clinical probability rules out PE. With a low clinical probability and low probability V/Q scan, PE is ruled out. High clinical probability and high probability V/Q scan confirms PE. Any other combination should be followed up with traditional pulmonary angiogram or serial lower extremity Doppler to rule out DVT.

EKG may show S1Q3T3, anterior T-wave inversion, or right bundle branch pattern, but the most common EKG finding is simply sinus tachycardia. S1Q3T3 is not common, but, if present, it suggests that there may be a massive PE and/or severe pulmonary hypertension.

Treatment Thrombolysis is considered if there is a massive PE. Massive PE is defined as proximal PE with associated hypotension (SBP <90 mm Hg or a drop in SBP of more than 40 mm Hg from baseline for more than 15 minutes). Embolectomy may be considered for similar reasons, if there is contraindication to thrombolytic therapy. Anticoagulation is the mainstay of treatment for PE. It should be continued for 3 to 6 months. IVC filter is placed in patients who have ongoing bleeding or have contraindications for anticoagulation. It is not a definitive therapy but a palliative measure.

Pulmonary embolism is discussed in Chapter 29.

Aortic dissection

Aortic dissection is another life-threatening condition that requires prompt diagnosis and urgent intervention. It starts as an intimal tear or as a hematoma within the wall and may extend both proximally and distally. Trauma, instrumentation, uncontrolled hypertension, coarctation of aorta, cystic medial degeneration in connective tissue disorders, and pregnancy are some of the etiological causes for aortic dissection. Anatomically, aortic dissection is divided into Stanford type A and type B. Type A involves ascending aorta and type B elsewhere.

Symptoms and signs Aortic dissection presents with severe sharp tearing anterior chest pain (in ascending aortic dissection) and similar posterior chest and back pain (in descending aortic dissection). Thirteen percent of the cases with ascending aortic dissection may have associated syncope. In the International Registry of Acute Aortic Dissection, 73% reported chest pain and out of these 85% had an abrupt onset and 91% described it as worst pain ever. Patients present in severe distress with diaphoresis. A pulse deficit is more common in ascending dissections than the descending dissections and may be found in up to 15% to 30% of the cases. Aortic insufficiency murmurs may be noted in up to 32% of these patients.

Diagnosis Chest radiograph is relatively insensitive but may show widened mediastinum in up to 62% of the cases. EKG may be normal in one third of the cases. Negative D-dimer can rule out aortic dissection in low-risk patients, but if the suspicion is high, further investigation should be carried out. If the patient is stable, CT scan with aortic dissection protocol or MRI is a good screening test in the ED. If unstable, patients need emergent transesophageal echocardiography (TEE).

Treatment Ascending dissections are managed surgically and descending dissections medically.

Pneumothorax

Pneumothoraces are classified as primary spontaneous pneumothorax (PSP) and secondary spontaneous pneumothorax (SSP). PSP is without underlying lung disease, and SSP is secondary due to underlying lung disease. Pneumothoraces most often occur at rest.

Symptoms and signs Pneumothorax presents as an acute onset of pleuritic chest pain and dyspnea. Physical examination findings are decreased chest excursion on the side of pneumothorax, absent breath sounds, hyperresonance on percussion, and reduced tactile vocal fremitus. If the pneumothorax is large, patients may be in distress with labored breathing, tachycardia, and hypotension.

Diagnosis Chest radiograph is adequate to diagnose pneumothorax. The pneumothorax appears as a dark area with no vascular markings with a white pleural border.

Treatment Small pneumothoraces (<3 cm for PSP and <1 cm for SSP) are managed conservatively with supplemental oxygen and follow-up chest radiographs. If patients present with a tension pneumothorax with mediastinal tracheal shift and hemodynamic compromise, a quick bedside needle decompression (passing a long angiocatheter or spinal needle in the second or third intercostal space in the midclavicular line) improves mortality outcomes. If stable, a chest tube insertion followed by pleurodesis is the recommended treatment.

Esophageal rupture

Esophageal rupture is a potentially fatal condition that needs urgent intervention. It was first described by Boerhaave, so is called Boerhaave syndrome. Boerhaave syndrome is when a patient presents with esophageal rupture following severe retching or vomiting. Risk factors for the rupture include recent endoscopic procedures, esophagitis from infections, medications or caustic ingestion, Barrett esophagus, and esophageal cancers.

Symptoms and signs Esophageal rupture presents with a sudden severe excruciating retrosternal chest pain occurring after severe retching or vomiting. Patients may have dyspnea, odynophagia, or fevers. Physical examination will likely be significant for tachycardia, tachypnea, diaphoresis, and possible subcutaneous emphysema. If the patient presents late in the course, he or she may have fever and shock due to mediastinitis.

Diagnosis Chest radiograph may show pneumomediastinum and pleural effusion. Computed tomography provides more information, including the abscess or fluid collections. Gastrografin esophagogram is another way to diagnose this. Performing an esophagogastroduodenoscopy (EGD) is controversial.

Treatment In a healthy patient with no history of esophageal cancer, an urgent reconstruction surgery should be performed within 24 hours. If the perforation is contained, conservative management may be a reasonable approach. This includes continuous NG suction, antibiotics, and parenteral nutrition. For patients with esophageal cancers, palliative stenting is an option.

Other causes of chest pain

Other causes of chest pain are discussed in the following table with symptoms, signs, and further enquire to understand the etiology of the chest pain better in Table 7-3. Once we know that the cause of the chest pain is not life-threatening or 1 of the causes that need inpatient workup, patients may be discharged with outpatient management and follow-up.

TIPS TO REMEMBER

- The most important step in the management of chest pain is the initial rapid assessment to rule out the causes that may cause death (MI, PE, pneumothorax, aortic dissection, esophageal rupture).
- History and physical examination are crucial in the evaluation of chest pain, and then followed by EKG and chest radiograph.
- Do not miss ST segment elevation on the EKG.
- Risk factors for coronary artery disease predict long-term risk of ACS, but they have limited role in identifying ACS with ongoing symptoms. The absence of risk factors will not exclude ACS.

Table 7-3. Other Causes of Chest Pain

Condition	Symptom	Signs	Further Enquire
Musculoskeletal	Aching pain, worsened by movement, sometimes respirophasic. Tender to touch	May have chest wall erythema/swelling. Light and deep palpation may reproduce the symptoms	Recent weight lifting, heavy exercise, trauma, slept in an abnormal posture/new bed
Esophageal disorders	Esophageal spasm presents as tightness or burning or squeezing pain. Esophagitis may present similarly, but burning pain is the common complain	Pharyngeal erythema from reflux	New medications, caustic ingestion, and similar problems in the past
Reflux disease	Burning or tightness. Sensation of warmth/discomfort traveling up the retrosternum with sour taste in the mouth and sometimes ends with coughing Worse on lying down and more symptomatic at night after a late or large meal at night	Pharyngeal erythema. Epigastric tenderness if associated with gastritis or peptic ulcer disease	New medications, eating patterns, positions worsening the symptoms
Peptic ulcer disease/gastritis	Epigastric pain and retrosternal pain described as burning sensation	Epigastric tenderness	New medications, smoking, alcohol history, and stress and feeding habits. Other family members being affected for infectious gastritis

(continued)

Table 7-3. Other Causes of Chest Pain (*Continued*)

Condition	Symptom	Signs	Further Enquire
Stable angina	Exertional central chest discomfort that is described as a pressure, heaviness, tightness, crushing, indigestion, or discomfort that radiates to neck, jaw, arms, or shoulders. Usually lasts 2 to 10 min. Relieved by rest or nitroglycerine	Ejection systolic murmur if the cause is aortic stenosis. Pulmonic heave in pulmonary hypertension. Pallor in anemia	Exacerbating factors such as bleeding, stress, and cold exposure. Other conditions such as aortic stenosis or pulmonary hypertension can present with angina
Pneumonia	Pleuritic chest pain with cough, fevers, and dyspnea	Pleural rub along with other signs of pneumonia	Ask to show the area of pain, as patients often develop musculoskeletal pain from recurrent coughing and the respirophasic pain may not be a pleuritic pain
Herpes zoster/ postherpetic neuralgia	Acute sharp pain in a dermatomal distribution	Acute infection can present with vesicular rash. Postherpetic neuralgia patients may have a faint healed rash	History of dermatomal zoster rash in the past if this was not due to active zoster
Stress/mental health issues	Fleeting pain lasting seconds or days	May have precordial tenderness	Palpate other areas of the body as patients with neurotic disorders or fibromyalgia have tenderness in most other sites of the body

- ECG is the easiest and simplest tool for diagnosis of ACS, but due to its low sensitivity, serial ECGs should be performed in a patient with ongoing chest pain. If there is ST deviation or T-wave inversion during the periods of symptoms, this suggests ischemia.

- All patients with suspected ACS should undergo serial cardiac biomarker sampling. If baseline data are negative, further sampling should be obtained 6 to 8 hours later depending on symptom onset.

- Early risk stratification is a crucial step in the management of ACS.

- A serial rise and fall in troponin associated with ACS may help distinguish ACS from non-ACS conditions.

- Patients who are not in the early invasive strategy for ACS should have a stress test done within 72 hours to risk stratify.

- For STEMI, door to balloon time for primary PCI should be 90 minutes. If transferred from a non-PCI center, it is 120 minutes.

- Thrombolysis for STEMI can be done for up to 12 hours after symptom onset. There is no benefit beyond that period.

- Aortic dissection is a difficult diagnosis to make, and high levels of vigilance are required. Chest radiograph may show widened mediastinum, but the test is not very sensitive.

- Using clinical pretest probability scores such as Wells score can help categorize the patients into PE likely or PE unlikely category. For PE unlikely group, negative D-dimer rules out PE.

- If the clinical suspicion for PE is high, do not wait for the image confirmation; start therapeutic anticoagulation if there is no obvious contraindication.

- Pneumothorax is a clinical diagnosis supported by chest radiograph. Do not wait for chest tube insertion; if there is tension pneumothorax, proceed with needle decompression.

- Esophageal rupture in the hospital is more often secondary to the procedures. Have a low suspicion if patients had any upper GI procedures recently or have known esophageal pathology to cause the rupture.

- Gastroesophageal disorders and musculoskeletal problems are the most common causes of chest pain in the emergency department and the outpatient clinic.

COMPREHENSION QUESTION

1. A 38-year-old woman with no significant past medical history presents to the emergency department with left-sided pleuritic chest pain, shortness of breath, and dizziness for a day. She became short of breath while watching television. When she tried to get up, she felt light-headed, so she went back to bed. She

awoke this morning with severe chest pain that worsened with cough and deep breathing. She is physically active and runs 5 miles at least 4 times per week. There is no history of trauma, fever, chills, or rigors. She has had no similar episodes in the past. She does not smoke. She drinks a glass of wine occasionally. She is not married and has never been pregnant. She takes oral contraceptive pills but no other medications. She works for a pharmaceutical company and travels to most parts of the world. She just returned from Australia 2 days ago. Examination significant for moderate distress, respiratory rate of 28/min, heart rate of 124/min, blood pressure 110/68 mm Hg, temperature of 100.3°F, and saturating 87% on room air. Routine labs are normal except a white cell count of 12,000 cells/mm^3 with a left shift. Troponin is mildly elevated at 0.104 ng/mL (normal high <0.034). EKG shows sinus tachycardia but otherwise normal. Chest radiograph shows left upper lobe infiltrate. Wells score is 4, and the D-dimer is elevated at 2.8 µg/mL. Pulmonary embolism is considered as the cause of her symptoms.

What do we do next?

A. Get lower extremity Doppler to rule out DVT.

B. Get V/Q scan.

C. Get CT-PA.

D. Start weight-based enoxaparin 1 mg/kg and order a CT-PA.

E. Start antibiotics for community-acquired pneumonia and discharge home.

Answer

1. **D.** She has pulmonary embolism until proved otherwise. CT angiogram is the next investigation of choice, but we should not waste time to confirm the diagnosis. The earlier the anticoagulation is started, the better the outcomes will be as the anticoagulation will help prevent further clot extension. Troponins can be elevated in up to 50% of the patients with large thromboembolic clot burden. Troponin level normalizes within 40 hours in PE. This is compared with the troponin elevation after myocardial infarction that may remain elevated for 5 to 14 days. Elevated troponins carry a poorer prognosis compared with negative troponins in patients with PE.

SUGGESTED READINGS

Bense L, Wiman LG, Hedenstierna G. Onset of symptoms in spontaneous pneumothorax: correlations to physical activity. *Eur J Respir Dis.* 1987;71(3):181–186.

Fruergaard P, Launbjerg J, Hesse B, et al. The diagnoses of patients admitted with acute chest pain but without myocardial infarction. *Eur Heart J.* 1996;17(7):1028–1034.

Hagan PG, Nienaber CA, Isselbacher EM, et al. The International Registry of Acute Aortic Dissection (IRAD): new insights into an old disease. *JAMA.* 2000;283(7):897–903.

Henrikson CA, Howell EE, Bush DE, et al. Chest pain relief by nitroglycerin does not predict active coronary artery disease. *Ann Intern Med.* 2003;139:979–986.

Klinkman MS, Stevens D, Gorenflo DW. Episodes of care for chest pain: a preliminary report from MIRNET. Michigan Research Network. *J Fam Pract.* 1994;38(4):345–352.

Kontos MC, Diercks DB, Kirk JD. Emergency department and office-based evaluation of patients with chest pain. *Mayo Clin Proc.* 2010;85(3):284–299.

Leise MD, Locke GR 3rd, Dierkhising RA, Zinsmeister AR, Reeder GS, Talley NJ. Patients dismissed from the hospital with a diagnosis of noncardiac chest pain: cardiac outcomes and health care utilization. *Mayo Clin Proc.* 2010;85(4):323–330.

Pasricha PJ, Fleischer DE, Kalloo AN. Endoscopic perforations of the upper digestive tract: a review of their pathogenesis, prevention, and management. *Gastroenterology.* 1994;106(3):787–802.

The PIOPED Investigators. Value of the ventilation/perfusion scan in acute pulmonary embolism. Results of the prospective investigation of pulmonary embolism diagnosis (PIOPED). *JAMA.* 1990;263(20):2753–2759.

van Belle A, Büller HR, Huisman MV, et al. Effectiveness of managing suspected pulmonary embolism using an algorithm combining clinical probability, D-dimer testing, and computed tomography. *JAMA.* 2006;295(2):172–179.

Wells PS, Anderson DR, Rodger M, et al. Derivation of a simple clinical model to categorize patients probability of pulmonary embolism: increasing the models utility with the SimpliRED D-dimer. *Thromb Haemost.* 2000;83(3):416–420.

Wright RS, Anderson JL, Adams CD, et al. 2011 ACCF/AHA focused update of the guidelines for the management of patients with unstable angina/non-ST-elevation myocardial infarction (updating the 2007 guideline): a report of the American College of Cardiology Foundation/American Heart Association Task Force on Practice Guidelines. *Circulation.* 2011;123(18):2022–2060.

A 64-year-old Man With Increasing Dyspnea

Muhammad Farooq Asghar, MD

A 64-year-old man with a history of chronic obstructive pulmonary disease (COPD) is evaluated in the emergency department for increased dyspnea over the past 48 hours. There is no change in his baseline production of white sputum but he has increased nasal congestion and sore throat. His medications include inhaled tiotropium, combination fluticasone and salmeterol, and albuterol.

The patient is alert but in mild respiratory distress. The temperature is 38.6°C (101.5°F), blood pressure is 150/90 mm Hg, pulse rate is 108/min, and respiration rate is 30/min. Oxygen saturation with the patient breathing ambient air is 90%. Breath sounds are diffusely decreased with bilateral expiratory wheezes; he is using accessory muscles to breathe. He does not have any peripheral edema or elevated jugular venous distension (JVD). With the patient breathing oxygen, 2 L/min by nasal cannula, arterial blood gases (ABGs) are pH 7.27, P_{CO_2} 60 mm Hg, and P_{O_2} 62 mm Hg; oxygen saturation is 91%. His CBC shows leukocytosis of 11,000 and chest x-ray does not show any new infiltrates or pneumothorax.

1. What is your diagnosis?

2. How would you approach this patient?

Answers

1. This is a 64-year-old man with a known history of COPD who is on maintenance therapy. He has respiratory failure likely due to a COPD exacerbation precipitated by an upper respiratory tract infection.

   Diagnosis: COPD exacerbation.

2. Next step in therapy: The patient is already on supplemental oxygen and his oxyhemoglobin saturation (SaO_2) is >90%. Next, you should start the patient on a short-acting inhaled bronchodilator such as albuterol as well as an anticholinergic such as ipratropium bromide, IV corticosteroids, and empiric IV antibiotics. You should also consider placing the patient on noninvasive positive-pressure ventilation (NPPV).

CASE REVIEW

Acute exacerbations of COPD are common. When a patient with known COPD presents with respiratory failure, the first step is to differentiate it from other causes that may present similarly. Exacerbations of COPD must be distinguished from pneumonia, pneumothorax, pulmonary embolism (PE), and congestive heart failure (CHF). Pneumonia and pneumothorax usually can be diagnosed by the chest radiograph. PE can be difficult to diagnose in patients with COPD, and spiral CT angiography should be used if embolic disease is suspected. Your suspicion of PE should be high in those patients who have risk factors such as prolonged immobilization, a history of cancer, recent trauma, or a history of clotting disorders. PE should also be expected if the patient is in hypoxic respiratory failure rather than hypercarbic respiratory failure and in those patients who do not respond to appropriate treatment for COPD exacerbation. Patients with respiratory failure due to heart failure usually have a history of systolic or diastolic heart failure. On physical examination, they have bibasilar crackles, elevated JVD, and peripheral edema of their lower extremities. Their CXRs will show pulmonary vascular congestion and sometimes pulmonary edema. Elevated beta-natriuretic peptide (BNP) will further support this diagnosis.

Now if we look back at our patient, neither he has signs of heart failure nor does his CXR show any pulmonary vascular congestion or pulmonary edema. Pneumonia and pneumothorax can be excluded based on findings of chest auscultation and CXR. The patient does not have any risk factors for PE and his ABGs are consistent with a COPD exacerbation. Although PE cannot be fully excluded without a spiral CT scan of the chest, we should see the patient respond to initial treatment over the next couple of days.

COPD EXACERBATIONS

An acute exacerbation of COPD is defined as an acute increase in symptoms beyond normal day-to-day variation. This generally includes an acute increase in 1 or more of the following cardinal symptoms:

- Cough increases in frequency and severity.
- Sputum production increases.
- Dyspnea increases.

It is estimated that 70% to 80% of COPD exacerbations are due to respiratory infections. Viral and bacterial infections cause most exacerbations, whereas atypical bacteria are a relatively uncommon cause. The remaining 20% to 30% are due to environmental pollution or have an unknown etiology.

Diagnosis

Initial evaluation of a patient with a suspected exacerbation of COPD includes a medical history, physical examination, chest radiograph, and routine laboratory studies. ABG analysis should be performed in most patients to assess the severity of the exacerbation and to establish a baseline from which improvement or deterioration can be measured.

The first step is to triage the patient to inpatient or outpatient management following the initial evaluation. Patients having any of the following should be hospitalized:

- Inadequate response of symptoms to outpatient management
- Marked increase in dyspnea
- Inability to eat or sleep due to symptoms
- Worsening hypoxemia
- Worsening hypercapnia
- Changes in mental status
- Inability to care for oneself (ie, lack of home support)
- Uncertain diagnosis
- High-risk comorbidities including pneumonia, cardiac arrhythmia, heart failure, diabetes mellitus, renal failure, or liver failure

In addition, there is general consensus that acute respiratory acidosis justifies hospitalization.

Treatment

Successful management of acute exacerbations of COPD in either the inpatient or outpatient setting requires attention to a number of key issues:

1. Identifying and ameliorating the cause of the acute exacerbation
2. Assuring adequate oxygenation and secretion clearance
3. Optimizing lung function by administering bronchodilators and other pharmacologic agents
4. Averting the need for intubation, if possible
5. Preventing complications of immobility, such as thromboemboli and deconditioning
6. Addressing nutritional needs

Oxygen therapy

Supplemental oxygen is a critical component of acute therapy. A target of an arterial oxygen tension (Pao_2) of 60 to 70 mm Hg, with an SaO_2 of 90% to 94%, is optimal. There are numerous devices available to deliver supplemental oxygen during an acute exacerbation of COPD including nasal cannula, venturi masks, face masks, and non-rebreathing masks.

Adequate oxygenation must be assured, even if it leads to acute hypercapnia. Hypercapnia is generally well tolerated in patients whose arterial carbon dioxide tension ($Paco_2$) is chronically elevated. However, mechanical ventilation may be required if hypercapnia is associated with depressed mental status, profound acidemia, or cardiac dysrhythmias.

Pharmacologic treatment

The major components of managing an acute exacerbation of COPD include the use of inhaled short-acting bronchodilators (beta-adrenergic agonists and anticholinergic agents), glucocorticoids, and antibiotics.

Beta-adrenergic agonists

Inhaled short-acting beta-adrenergic agonists (eg, albuterol) are the mainstay of therapy for an acute exacerbation of COPD because of their rapid onset of action and efficacy in producing bronchodilation. These medications may be administered via a nebulizer or a metered dose inhaler (MDI) with a spacer device. Typical doses of albuterol for this indication are 2.5 mg (diluted to a total of 3 mL) by nebulizer every 4 hours and as needed, or 4 to 8 puffs (90 µg per puff) by MDI with a spacer every 1 to 4 hours and as needed.

Anticholinergic agents

Inhaled short-acting anticholinergic agents (eg, ipratropium) are used with inhaled short-acting beta-adrenergic agonists to treat exacerbations of COPD. Typical doses of ipratropium for this indication are 500 µg by nebulizer every 4 hours and as needed. Alternatively, 2 puffs (18 µg per puff) by MDI with a spacer every 4 hours and as needed may be used.

Glucocorticoids

Systemic glucocorticoids, when added to the bronchodilator therapies described above, improve symptoms and lung function, and decrease the length of hospital stay. Oral glucocorticoids are rapidly absorbed (peak serum levels achieved at 1 hour after ingestion) with virtually complete bioavailability and appear as equally efficacious as intravenous glucocorticoids for treating most exacerbations of COPD. However, intravenous glucocorticoids are typically administered to patients who present with a severe exacerbation, who respond poorly to oral glucocorticoids, who are unable to take oral medication, or who may have impaired absorption due to decreased splanchnic perfusion. Frequently used regimens range from prednisone 30 to 60 mg, once daily, to methylprednisolone 60 to 125 mg, 2 to 4 times daily. The optimal duration of systemic glucocorticoid therapy is not clearly established and often depends on the severity of the exacerbation and the observed response to therapy. As a rough guide, most exacerbations are treated with full-dose therapy (eg, prednisone 30–40 mg daily) for 7 to 10 days. After this time, glucocorticoid therapy may be discontinued if the patient has substantially recovered. Alternatively, the dose is tapered over another 7 days, as a trial to determine whether continued glucocorticoid therapy is required. Tapering solely because of concerns about adrenal suppression is not necessary if the duration of therapy is less than 3 weeks (a duration too brief to cause adrenal atrophy).

Antibiotics

A "risk stratification" approach should be used when selecting initial antibiotic therapy. Specifically, prescribe a broader antibiotic regimen for patients who have risk factors for a poor outcome. Risk factors include older age (>65 years), comorbid conditions (especially cardiac disease), severe underlying COPD (defined as FEV_1 <50%), frequent exacerbations (3 or more per year), and antimicrobial therapy within the past 3 months. Commonly used antibiotics include levofloxacin, azithromycin, and amoxicillin. In patients who are at high risk for *Pseudomonas* infection, antibiotic coverage should be broadened. These risk factors include recent hospitalization (≥2 days duration during the past 90 days), frequent administration of antibiotics (≥4 courses within the past year), severe COPD (FEV_1 <50% of predicted), isolation of *P. aeruginosa* during a previous exacerbation, colonization during a stable period, and systemic glucocorticoid use. The duration of antibiotic therapy for patients with a COPD exacerbation is usually 3 to 7 days, depending on the response to therapy.

Mechanical ventilation

Noninvasive positive-pressure ventilation Use of NPPV decreases the risk of endotracheal intubation and decreases intensive care unit (ICU) admission rates.

Indications for NPPV include severe dyspnea, acidosis (pH ≤7.35) and/or hypercapnia (Pco_2 >45 mm Hg), and respiratory rate >25 breaths/min. Contraindications to its use are an uncooperative patient, decreased level of consciousness, hemodynamic instability, inadequate mask fit, and severe respiratory acidosis. Increased airway pressure can be delivered by using inspiratory positive airway pressure, continuous positive airway pressure, or bilevel positive airway pressure (BiPAP), which combines the other modalities. When using NPPV, the nasal mask is usually tolerated the best, but patients must be instructed to keep their mouths closed while breathing with the nasal apparatus. A chin strap can be employed to help with this problem. Oxygen can be delivered at 10 to 15 L/min and started in spontaneous ventilation mode with an initial expiratory positive airway pressure setting of 3 to 5 cm H_2O and an inspiratory positive airway pressure setting of 8 to 10 cm H_2O. Adjustments in these settings should be made in 2 cm H_2O increments. It is important to monitor patients with frequent vital sign measurements, ABGs, or pulse oximetry.

Invasive ventilation Invasive mechanical ventilation should be administered when patients fail NPPV, do not tolerate NPPV, or have contraindications to NPPV. Other indications include severe dyspnea with evidence of increased work of breathing, acute respiratory acidosis with pH <7.25 and/or $Paco_2$ >60 mm Hg and Pao_2 <40 mm Hg, respiratory rate >35/min, *or* hemodynamic instability.

Follow-up After Resolution of Acute COPD Exacerbation

Once patients have recovered from an acute exacerbation of COPD and have completed a course of antibiotics and steroids, they should be managed according to the severity of their diseases as measured by the GOLD classification of COPD severity.

Stage I: Mild COPD, FEV_1/FVC <0.70, FEV_1 ≥80%.

Stage II: Moderate COPD, FEV_1/FVC <0.70, FEV_1 50% to 79%.

Stage III: Severe COPD, FEV_1/FVC <0.70, FEV_1 30% to 49%.

Stage IV: Very severe COPD, FEV_1/FVC <0.70, FEV_1 <30% or <50% with chronic respiratory failure present. Chronic respiratory failure is defined as Pao_2 <60 mm Hg or $Paco_2$ >50 mm Hg while breathing air at sea level.

The patient should be managed as follows:

Stage I: Smoking cessation:

Vaccinations (influenza and pneumococcal)

Short-acting beta-agonist prn

Stage II: All of the above plus:

Long-acting bronchodilators (salmeterol or tiotropium)

Pulmonary rehabilitation

Stage III: All of the above plus:

Inhaled corticosteroids

Oxygen if needed (Pao_2 <55 mm Hg or SaO_2 <88%)

Stage IV: All of the above plus:

Consider surgical treatment.

TIPS TO REMEMBER

- The cornerstones of treatment for a COPD exacerbation include supplemental oxygen, bronchodilators, IV steroids, and antibiotics.
- Indications for NPPV include severe dyspnea, acidosis (pH ≤7.35) and/or hypercapnia (Pco_2 >45 mm Hg), and respiratory rate >25 breaths/min.
- Cessation of smoking and supplemental oxygen (when indicated) are the only interventions that prolong survival in COPD patients.
- COPD exacerbation patients who require NPPV should be reassessed in a couple of hours by ABGs. If ABGs have not improved, intubation should not be delayed.
- After acute COPD exacerbation has resolved, patients should undergo PFTs (if not done recently) to stage their COPD, and they should be treated according to the stage of COPD that is found.

COMPREHENSION QUESTIONS

1. What are the cornerstones of treatment of COPD exacerbation?

2. When should NPPV be considered?

Answers

1. The cornerstones of treatment for a COPD exacerbation include supplemental oxygen, bronchodilators, IV steroids, and antibiotics.

2. Indications for NPPV include severe dyspnea, acidosis (pH ≤ 7.35) and/or hypercapnia (P_{CO_2} >45 mm Hg), and respiratory rate >25 breaths/min.

SUGGESTED READINGS

McPhee SJ, Papadakis M, Rabow MW. *Current Medical Diagnosis and Treatment*. New York: McGraw-Hill;2012:255–265.

Washington University School of Medicine Department of Medicine. *The Washington Manual of Medical Therapeutics*. 33rd ed. Philadelphia: Lippincott Williams & Wilkins; 2010:272–282.

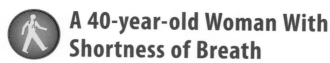

A 40-year-old Woman With Shortness of Breath

Siegfried W. B. Yu, MD, FACP

A 40-year-old female smoker is admitted to the inpatient service with shortness of breath. The shortness of breath is worse with exertion, chronic in nature, and has progressed in severity over the last year. She reports a history of asthma, but does not recall having any formal testing done for this in the past. At the time of admission, she is short of breath even with minimal activity. A chest x-ray is done that shows bilateral opacities that are interpreted as possible pneumonia. Treatment for this admission is started with intravenous (IV) corticosteroid therapy, antibiotics, and frequent nebulization with bronchodilators to treat asthma exacerbation with pneumonia.

By the fourth hospital day, despite aggressive treatment, she does not appear to have had any clinical improvement in her symptoms. In fact, she feels as if she has become worse, not better. On examination, she is anxious in appearance and in clear respiratory distress. She is able to communicate in only a few words at a time, between her labored breaths. She is afebrile, with a heart rate of 95 beats/min, and a blood pressure of 150/100 mm Hg. Her jugular venous pulse (JVP) is estimated at 16 cm. Lung examination is remarkable for very harsh breath sounds with coarse sounding expiratory wheezes bilaterally, and decreased breath sounds at the bases. Cardiac examination reveals a systolic murmur prominent at the apex. 2+ lower extremity pitting edema up to knees is found.

When questioned further, in addition to her history of shortness of breath with exertion, the patient notes frequent nighttime episodes of shortness of breath, requiring her to sit up in bed for extended periods before sleeping again to allow her to "catch her breath." A remote history of extended febrile illness is recalled from childhood, for which she does not recall getting specific treatment.

1. **In light of this patient's reported symptoms by history, what is the most likely primary diagnosis?**

2. **What may be the underlying factor in this case?**

3. **What management decision would you need to make at this time?**

Answers

1. The combination of the patient's historical features, physical examination findings, and lack of response to usual asthma therapy supports a diagnosis of congestive heart failure (CHF), not asthma.

2. The patient's murmur and remote history of untreated childhood febrile illness suggest the diagnosis of rheumatic heart disease.

3. If the patient has CHF, the IV corticosteroid therapy may be making her hypervolemia worse, and beta-agonist therapy may also be exacerbating her decreased cardiac function. Discontinuing these medications and initiating a trial of diuresis with a loop diuretic, while waiting on confirmatory testing for CHF, would be appropriate. The chest x-ray done at admission should be reviewed again for evidence of CHF. Additional testing may include an electrocardiogram (ECG), B-type natriuretic peptide (BNP), and an echocardiogram to definitively characterize cardiac function and the degree of structural heart disease that may be present.

CASE REVIEW

While asthma is typically episodic, this patient's history suggests she has had chronic progressive symptoms. Additionally, her nighttime attacks appear more consistent with paroxysmal nocturnal dyspnea (PND), not asthma. On examination, her elevated JVP of 16 cm, harsh breath sounds with "cardiac wheezing," decreased breath sounds at her bases, and lower extremity edema are all signs of a hypervolemic state. These features all suggest a diagnosis of CHF. Other physical examination findings that may be found include an S3 heart sound and a positive hepatojugular reflux. The patient's systolic heart murmur, possibly related to mitral regurgitation, and her remote history of an untreated childhood febrile illness, suggestive of rheumatic fever, make the diagnosis of rheumatic heart disease likely. Because she is demonstrating signs and symptoms of hypervolemia secondary to CHF, it would be reasonable to stop the asthma therapy and to start a trial of diuresis with a loop diuretic. Monitoring serum electrolytes is important in this situation. IV corticosteroid therapy has likely increased fluid retention and made her clinical status worse. Unnecessary beta-agonist therapy may also be putting more strain on her cardiac function if CHF is the primary etiology. These should be stopped. Because of the high prevalence of coronary artery disease (CAD) with any new diagnosis of CHF, it is also important to obtain an ECG. Depending on the clinical circumstances, an urgent cardiology consultation may also be appropriate. A CXR may be useful to assess for signs of CHF such as pulmonary edema, which may be confused with a pneumonic infiltrate outside of clinical context, and may help to estimate heart size. When the diagnosis of CHF is unclear, checking a BNP level can be supportive. An echocardiogram would provide more definitive information on structural heart disease, including wall thickness, left ventricular ejection fraction (EF), and degree of valvular involvement.

CONGESTIVE HEART FAILURE

CHF is a clinical syndrome of cardiac dysfunction that causes patients to develop clinical symptoms of dyspnea and fatigue, and physical signs of edema and rales, which ultimately lead to frequent hospitalizations, impaired quality of life, and a shortened life expectancy. CHF is the most common cause of hospitalization in US patients older than 65 years old, and leads to 300,000 deaths per year.

Pathophysiology

The American College of Cardiology (ACC) and American Heart Association (AHA) emphasize that symptoms due to CHF follow an initial asymptomatic stage of cardiac dysfunction (see Figure 9-1). CHF patients are also now broadly categorized into 2 groups: (1) systolic failure, CHF with a decreased EF (<40%), and (2) diastolic or non-systolic failure, CHF with a preserved EF (>40%). Notably, patients with preserved EF CHF are responsible for 50% of the hospitalization for CHF and have similar survival rates.

Any condition that can lead to an alteration in cardiac structure or function can predispose a patient to developing CHF (see Table 9-1). Depending on the cause of CHF, this will guide the course of treatment that is followed. In 20% to 30% of CHF patients with systolic failure, the exact etiology is unknown. These patients are referred to as having nonischemic, dilated, or idiopathic

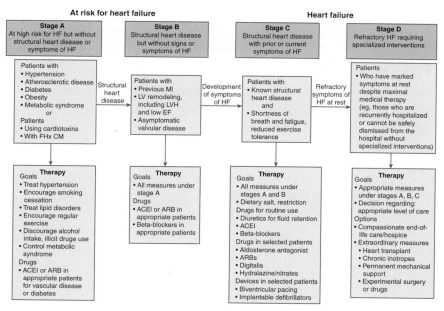

Figure 9-1. Stages in the development of heart failure/recommended therapy by stage. ACEI, angiotensin-converting enzyme inhibitors; ARB, angiotensin II receptor blocker; EF, ejection fraction; FHx CM, family history of cardiomyopathy; HF, heart failure; LVH, left ventricular hypertrophy; MI, myocardial infarction.

Table 9-1. Etiologies of Heart Failure

Depressed ejection fraction (<40%)	
Coronary artery disease	**Nonischemic dilated cardiomyopathy**
Myocardial infarction[a]	Familial/genetic disorders
Myocardial ischemia[a]	Infiltrative disorders[a]
Chronic pressure overload	Toxic/drug-induced damage
Hypertension[a]	Metabolic disorder[a]
Obstructive valvular disease[a]	Viral
Chronic volume overload	Chagas disease
Regurgitant valvular disease	**Disorders of rate and rhythm**
Intracardiac (left-to-right) shunting	Chronic bradyarrhythmias
Extracardiac shunting	Chronic tachyarrhythmias

Preserved ejection fraction (>40%–50%)	
Pathologic hypertrophy	**Restrictive cardiomyopathy**
Primary (hypertrophic cardiomyopathies)	Infiltrative disorders (amyloidosis, sarcoidosis)
Secondary (hypertension)	Storage diseases (hemochromatosis)
Aging	**Fibrosis**
Pulmonary heart disease	**Endomyocardial disorders**
Cor pulmonale	**Excessive blood-flow requirements**
Pulmonary vascular disorders	Systemic arteriovenous shunting
High-output states	Chronic anemia
Metabolic disorders	
Thyrotoxicosis	
Nutritional disorders (beriberi)	

[a]Conditions that can also lead to heart failure with a preserved ejection fraction.

cardiomyopathy. High-output states such as anemia and arteriovenous fistula, particularly in the presence of structural heart disease, may lead to overt CHF.

Depending on the classification of the cardiomyopathy causing the CHF, there are different associated anatomical and pathophysiologic processes that occur (see Table 9-2). It is important to note that hypertrophic cardiomyopathy has a bimodal age distribution, in the 20s and 50- to 60-year age groups, and is associated with LV outflow obstruction and sudden cardiac death due to

Table 9-2. Anatomical and Pathophysiologic Processes for Each Cardiomyopathy

Type	Left Ventricular Cavity Size	Left Ventricular Wall Thickness	Systolic Function	Diastolic Function	Other
Dilated cardiomyo-pathy	↑	N/↑	↓	↓	
Hypertrophic cardiomyo-pathy	↓/N	↑	↑	↓	Left ventricular outflow obstruction
Restrictive cardiomyo-pathy	N/↑	N/↑	N	↓	

N, normal; ↑, increased; ↓, decreased.

ventricular fibrillation. These patients benefit from implantable cardiac defibrillator (ICD) placement. The secondary form, hypertensive hypertrophic cardiomyopathy, does not carry the same risk, although it has similar pathophysiology.

CHF can be viewed as a progressive disorder that stems from an index event that either damages the myocardial muscle function or disrupts the ability of the myocardium to generate an adequate force for contraction. As patients progress to symptomatic CHF, there is a sustained activation of compensatory mechanisms that alter the myocardium, causing LV remodeling which is sufficient to lead to progression of CHF. The systems affected include activation of the sympathetic nervous system, the renin–angiotensin system, and the neurohormonal control of renal function.

Diagnosis

Heart failure can be made as a clinical diagnosis based on symptoms, physical findings, and radiography. Dyspnea, fatigue, and hypervolemia due to fluid retention are typical symptoms. Dyspnea may be exertional, worse with recumbency or at rest, depending on the severity of disease. The presence of dyspnea at varying levels of activity can be used to classify the patient by functional class (see Table 9-3).

In addition to the cardinal symptoms of shortness of breath, orthopnea and PND are important historical features present in CHF. Orthopnea is dyspnea occurring in the recumbent position. Nocturnal cough may be present. It is

Table 9-3. New York Heart Association Classification

Functional Capacity	Objective Assessment
Class I	Patients with cardiac disease but without resulting limitation of physical activity. Ordinary physical activity does not cause undue fatigue, palpitations, dyspnea, or anginal pain
Class II	Patients with cardiac disease resulting in slight limitation of physical activity. They are comfortable at rest. Ordinary physical activity results in fatigue, palpitation, dyspnea, or anginal pain
Class III	Patients with cardiac disease resulting in marked limitation of physical activity. They are comfortable at rest. Less-than-ordinary activity causes fatigue, palpitation, dyspnea, or anginal pain
Class IV	Patients with cardiac disease resulting in inability to carry on any physical activity without discomfort. Symptoms of heart failure or the anginal syndrome may be present even at rest. If any physical activity is undertaken, discomfort is increased

generally relieved by sitting upright or using additional pillows, and commonly quantified by how many pillows a patient needs. It can occur in other patient populations, including those with abdominal obesity or ascites, or with pulmonary diseases with mechanics that favor an upright position. PND refers to acute episodes of shortness of breath and coughing that awaken the patient from sleep, typically 1 to 3 hours after lying down. There may be coughing and wheezing, which often persists for some time even after assuming the upright position.

Physical examination findings may include evidence of a low cardiac output and volume overload: narrow pulse pressure, poor peripheral perfusion, jugular venous distention, hepatojugular reflux, peripheral edema, ascites, and decreased breath sounds at lung bases (suggestive of pleural effusion). An attempt should be made to evaluate the jugular venous pressure. Lung rales/crackles in chronic CHF may represent more atelectasis than fluid in the alveoli, which may be expected in acute CHF presentations. Although edema will usually affect the lower extremities, the abdomen may be involved too. Cardiac auscultation may be notable for S3 (in LV systolic failure) or S4 (in LV hypertrophy) gallop rhythms, with a sustained, enlarged, or displaced cardiac apex.

The symptoms and physical examination findings of CHF can be nonspecific; therefore, the Framingham criteria for the clinical diagnosis of CHF can

Table 9-4. Framingham Criteria for Clinical Diagnosis of Congestive Heart Failure

Major Criteria	Minor Criteria
Paroxysmal nocturnal dyspnea	Peripheral edema
Orthopenia	Night cough
Increased jugular venous pressure	Dyspnea on exertion
Rales	Hepatomegaly
Third heart sound	Pleural effusion
Chest radiography: cardiomegaly, pulmonary edema	Heart rate >120 beats/min
	Weight loss ≥4.5 kg in 5 days with diuretic

be very useful (see Table 9-4). An attempt should be made to search for precipitating factors in the new appearance or worsening of previous CHF symptoms (Table 9-5). Common findings that prompt hospitalization in CHF include hypotension, worsening renal function, altered mentation, dyspnea at rest, significant arrhythmias, electrolyte disturbances, and lack of adequate outpatient care.

When the diagnosis of CHF is suspected but not established, a BNP level is a useful test. The best use for this test in the setting of acute dyspnea is to determine the contribution of CHF versus pulmonary disease. It is a marker for ventricular

Table 9-5. Precipitating Factors in Heart failure

Diet (excessive sodium or fluid intake, alcohol)
Nonadherence with medication or inadequate dosing
Sodium-retaining medications (NSAIDs)
Infection (bacterial or viral)
Myocardial ischemia or infarction
Arrhythmia (atrial fibrillation, bradycardia)
Sleep-disordered breathing
Worsening renal function
Anemia
Metabolic (hyperthyroidism, hypothyroidism)
Pulmonary embolus

volume and pressure overload. The ACC and AHA recommend an ECG in any patient with new-onset or exacerbated CHF. It is important to compare this with baseline tracings, and this may reveal signs of hypertrophy, arrhythmia, conduction abnormalities, and prior or active myocardial infarction (MI). Tachycardia, which may be due to atrial fibrillation, atrial flutter, or persistent atrial tachycardia, may be a precipitating cause for CHF.

Two-dimensional echocardiography should be obtained in all patients with suspected CHF. The information obtained is very useful in establishing the presence of systolic failure, valvular abnormalities, hypertrophy, and wall motion abnormalities. Exercise treadmill stress testing may be considered to evaluate coronary ischemia, identify exercise-induced arrhythmias, and help determine functional capacity. In patients who cannot exercise, pharmacologic stress testing can be considered for ischemia and exercise-induced arrhythmia evaluation. A 6-minute walk test can also be considered for functional capacity. The peak oxygen consumption measured with exercise testing is cited as the most potent predictor of prognosis, but is not readily available in all centers. Cardiac catheterization may be necessary to complete evaluation of suspected ischemia, and also to clarify valvular abnormalities if echocardiography has been insufficient. In general, endomyocardial biopsy should not be done unless giant-cell myocarditis is being considered. In new-onset CHF, thyroid-stimulating hormone should be assessed to exclude hypothyroidism or hyperthyroidism, both of which can contribute to CHF. Anemia and infection can lead to high-output states and exacerbate existing CHF, so assessment of blood counts and appropriate cultures should be done. Because electrolyte abnormalities, renal insufficiency, and pulmonary disease can exacerbate heart failure, a metabolic assessment, as well as chest radiography to look for both overt pulmonary disease and pulmonary edema, should be done. If not already done, patients with CHF should be screened for hypertension, diabetes mellitus, anemia, and sleep-disordered breathing, because these conditions tend to exacerbate CHF.

Treatment

Based on the clinical presentation, with an assessment of perfusion status and congestion at rest, a classification can be made whether the problem is high-output (normal perfusion) or low-output (low perfusion) CHF, which can help further guide management decisions as to whether to pursue hospitalization and diuresis (see Table 9-6).

It is typical for CHF patients admitted to the hospital in an acute exacerbation to require IV doses of many of the same medications that are used in chronic CHF therapy, such as diuretics, ACE inhibitors, angiotensin II receptor blockers (ARBs), and beta-blockers. However, depending on their hemodynamic profile, they may also require the use of vasodilators, inotropes, or vasoconstrictors (see Table 9-7). Note that while inotropes, such as milrinone and dobutamine, can

Table 9-6. Management of High- and Low-Output Heart Failure

Warm and dry	Warm and wet
PCWP normal, CI normal (compensated)	PCWP increased, CI normal → *hospitalize* ± nesiritide or vasodilators, diuretics
Cold and dry	**Cold and wet**
PCWP low or normal, CI decreased → *hospitalize* Inotropic drugs	PCWP increased, CI decreased → *hospitalize* ± nesiritide or vasodilators, diuretics

Impaired perfusion/↓ CO/↑ SVR: yes, cold; no, warm. Congestion at rest/elevated LV filling pressure: no, dry; yes, wet. PCWP, pulmonary capillary wedge pressure (surrogate for LV filling pressure); CI, cardiac index; CO, cardiac output; SVR, systemic vascular resistance; vasodilators, nitroglycerin or nitroprusside; inotropic drugs, milrinone or dobutamine.

Table 9-7. Drug Treatment for Acute Heart Failure

	Initiating Dose	Maximal Dose
Vasodilators		
Nitroglycerin	20 µg/min	40–400 µg/min
Nitroprusside	10 µg/min	30–350 µg/min
Nesiritide	Bolus 2 µg/kg	0.01–0.03 µg/kg/min[a]
Inotropes		
Dobutamine	1–2 µg/kg/min	2–10 µg/kg/min[b]
Milrinone	Bolus 50 µg/kg	0.1–0.75 µg/kg/min[b]
Dopamine	1–2 µg/kg/min	2–4 µg/kg/min[b]
Vasoconstrictors		
Dopamine for hypotension	5 µg/kg/min	5–15 µg/kg/min
Epinephrine	0.5 µg/kg/min	50 µg/kg/min
Phenylephrine	0.3 µg/kg/min	3 µg/kg/min
Vasopression	0.05 U/min	0.1–0.4 U/min

[a]Usually <4 µg/kg/min.
[b]Inotropes also have vasodilatory properties.

improve cardiac output and decrease afterload in patients with severe CHF, they are associated with excess mortality and should be reserved for patients who have not responded to traditional CHF regimens. They may also be considered as palliative agents when a patient is not a candidate for cardiac transplantation or an LV assist device. They may also be used as a bridge to these therapies.

For unstable patients, it is very important to carefully monitor volume status with careful serial physical examinations, accurate input and output assessments, accurate weights, electrolyte status, and other parameters, such as ECG telemetry monitoring. The clinical manifestations of moderate to severe CHF are due in large part to excessive salt and water retention that leads to volume expansion and worsening congestive symptoms. Diuretics are the only pharmacologic agents that can restore and maintain normal volume status in patients with CHF. Loop diuretics (furosemide, torsemide, and bumetanide) reversibly inhibit the reabsorption of Na^+, K^+, and Cl^- in the loop of Henle. Thiazides and metolazone reduce Na^+ and Cl^- reabsorption. Potassium-sparing diuretics (spironolactone) act by inhibiting aldosterone receptors. Loop diuretics are generally necessary to attain normal volume status in patients with CHF. Thiazide diuretics lose their effectiveness in patients with moderate or severe renal insufficiency, however may be considered as an addition to loop diuretic monotherapy, when this alone has not achieved desired results. Acutely, dialysis may be helpful in the short term for patients who are not responding to therapy.

Ensuring adherence to appropriate fluid and salt restriction is important. Typically all CHF patients should be restricted to less than 3 g of sodium per day, and a restriction to less than 2 g may be necessary in moderate to severe CHF. Fluid restriction to less than 2 L per day should be considered if diuretic therapy and sodium restriction are not controlling symptoms well.

Once volume status is stabilized, it is important to consider the ongoing management of chronic CHF. In particular, when the volume status has been adequately controlled, consideration should be given to starting an ACE inhibitor (ARB therapy if ACE inhibitor intolerant) and beta-blocker therapy (see Figure 9-2 and Table 9-8). If symptoms continue, therapy with an aldosterone antagonist, hydralazine–nitrate combinations, and digoxin can also be used.

ACE inhibitors should be used in all patients with CHF with LV dysfunction, whether with current or prior symptoms of CHF, unless a contraindication, such as angioedema, or intolerance such as cough exists. Overall, the evidence shows that they reduce CHF mortality, readmissions, and worsening CHF. In general, therapy can be started at low doses using agents such as enalapril, captopril, lisinopril, or ramipril, and titrated upward to a target systolic BP as low as 90 mm Hg if tolerated. It is important to monitor for cough, worsening kidney function, and hyperkalemia.

ARBs are recommended for those patients with current or prior symptoms of CHF with LV dysfunction who are intolerant of ACE inhibitors. Studies show that they demonstrate comparable beneficial effects compared with ACE inhibitors.

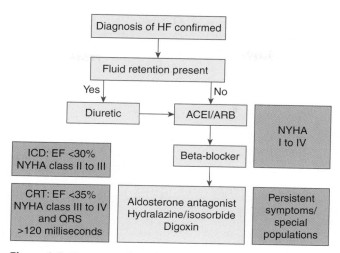

Figure 9-2. Treatment algorithm for CHF with a depressed EF.

In patients who cannot tolerate either ACE inhibitor or ARB therapy, combination therapy with hydralazine and isosorbide dinitrate can be effective, though not as effective as ACE inhibitors. Combination therapy with ACE inhibitors and ARBs has demonstrated decreased readmissions for CHF when compared with ACE inhibitor therapy alone. However, this combination does not reduce overall mortality, and is associated with more adverse advents, such as hypotension and worsening renal function.

Carvedilol, bisoprolol, and sustained-release metoprolol succinate are the 3 beta-blockers proven to reduce mortality in CHF, and should be used in patients with current or prior symptoms of CHF with LV dysfunction, if they are not volume overloaded and are stable on ACE inhibitor or other vasodilator therapy. In trials, they demonstrate significant reductions in mortality, CHF hospitalizations, and sudden death. Beta-blockers should be initiated at the lowest dose and adjusted every 2 to 4 weeks to the highest dose tolerated.

In CHF patients with LV dysfunction and NYHA class III to IV symptoms despite therapy with ACE inhibitors and beta-blockers, treatment with the aldosterone antagonist spironolactone may improve symptoms. Although digoxin provides no survival benefit in patients with CHF, it can be used in patients with NYHA class II to IV CHF to alleviate symptoms and decrease hospitalizations.

Device therapy with an ICD should be considered in patients with NYHA class I to III CHF, with an EF of less than 30% on optimal heart failure therapy, and a life expectancy greater than 6 months. Studies show a decrease in sudden death and overall mortality. Cardiac resynchronization therapy, also known as biventricular pacing, is another form of device that can improve quality of life and decrease hospitalizations in patients with CHF, an EF of less than 35%, and

Table 9-8. Drugs for the Treatment of Chronic Heart Failure (EF <40%)

	Initiating Dose	Maximal Dose
Diuretics		
Furosemide	20–40 mg qd or bid	400 mg/day[a]
Torsemide	10–20 mg qd bid	200 mg/day[a]
Bumetanide	0.5–1.0 mg qd or bid	10 mg/day[a]
Hydrochlorthiazide	25 mg qd	100 mg/day[a]
Metolazone	2.5–5.0 mg qd or bid	20 mg/day[a]
Angiotensin-converting enzyme inhibitors		
Captopril	6.25 mg tid	50 mg tid
Enalapril	2.5 mg bid	10 mg bid
Lisinopril	2.5–5.0 mg qd	20–35 mg qd
Ramipril	1.25–2.5 mg bid	2.5–5 mg bid
Trandolapril	0.5 mg qd	4 mg qd
Angiotensin receptor blockers		
Valsartan	40 mg bid	160 mg bid
Candesartan	4 mg qd	32 mg qd
Irbesartan	75 mg qd	300 mg qd[b]
Losartan	12.5 mg qd	50 mg qd
Beta-blockers		
Carvedilol	3.125 mg bid	25–50 mg bid
Bisoprolol	1.25 mg qd	10 mg qd
Metoprolol succinate CR	12.5–25 mg qd	Target dose 200 mg qd
Additional therapies		
Spironolactone	12.5–25 mg qd	25–50 mg qd
Eplerenone	25 mg qd	50 mg qd
Combination of hydralazine/isosorbide dinitrate	10–25 mg qd/10 mg tid	75/40 mg tid
Fixed dose of hydralazine/isosorbide dinitrate	37.5/20 mg (1 tablet) tid	75/40 mg (2 tablets) tid
Digoxin	0.125 mg qd	0.375 mg/day[b]

[a]Titrate dose to reduce congestive symptoms.
[b]Target dose not established.

a QRS interval greater than 120 milliseconds, with symptoms despite optimal medical therapy.

Advanced or end-stage CHF has become increasingly frequent due to the effective palliation for earlier stages of the disease, and prevention of sudden cardiac death with ICD therapy. Compassionate end-of-life care may be entirely appropriate for most patients. For relatively young patients without other serious comorbidities, extraordinary life-extending measures such as cardiac transplantation and mechanical assistance of the circulation (LV assist devices) may be considered.

TIPS TO REMEMBER

- The stages of CHF are like stages of cancer. When you reach one stage, you cannot go back to the stage before it.
- CHF with systolic dysfunction and preserved EF have similar survival rates.
- The major cause of CHF in the United States is ischemic heart disease.
- The BNP level is a very useful test to use when the diagnosis of CHF is unclear.
- In acute CHF, volume status should be corrected before ACE inhibitor and beta-blocker therapy are started.
- Digoxin can help improve symptoms, but does not improve survival.
- Although helpful in low cardiac output states, inotropes are associated with excessive mortality.
- ICD placement for CHF with systolic dysfunction should be considered only after optimal medical therapy has been achieved.
- Compassionate end-of-life palliative care is an appropriate treatment option for most patients with end-stage CHF; however, for relatively young patients with fewer comorbidities, extraordinary life-prolonging therapy using LV assist devices and cardiac transplantation may be considered.

COMPREHENSION QUESTIONS

1. A 22-year-old high school athlete presents to your clinic after passing out during a football game. He is in excellent health, however notes that his athletic older brother died suddenly when he was 23 years old. Sudden deaths are reported to have occurred in other close family members as well. An ECG is done in clinic and is normal. On examination, a crescendo-decrescendo murmur is heard along the left sternal border, which increases with a Valsalva maneuver, and does not radiate to the carotid arteries. What test will provide further evidence to make your diagnosis?
   A. Tilt-table test
   B. Echocardiography
   C. Exercise treadmill test
   D. BNP

2. A 55-year-old diabetic gentleman with a long-standing history of CAD and CHF presents to your clinic for follow-up. He has persistent dyspnea at rest despite apparently maximal medical therapy. More recently his echocardiogram demonstrates an EF of 20%, and an ECG shows a left bundle branch block with a QRS measured at 135 milliseconds. He feels terrible and tells you that he isn't "ready to go" yet. Of which of the following therapies would he benefit?

    A. ICD placement
    B. Cardiac catheterization with placement of multiple drug-eluting stents
    C. Cardiac transplant
    D. Cardiac resynchronization therapy

3. A 70-year-old woman is admitted to the hospital with severe exertional dyspnea and new-onset orthopnea. Her EF is found to be 20%, and attributed to a non-ischemic cardiomyopathy. She is treated with IV furosemide acutely, and over the next few days, she receives increasing doses of ACE inhibitor therapy, followed by beta-blocker therapy, and is discharged. She presents to your clinic with continued dyspnea with less-than-ordinary activity. She has a BP of 90/60 mm Hg, pulse of 75 beats/min, and on examination has a JVP of 13 cm, clear lungs, a displaced cardiac apex with an S3 heart sound, and 2+ lower extremity pitting edema to her knees. Discharge labs reveal a potassium level of 4.5 mEq/L and a creatinine of 1.2 mg/dL. Which of the following medication changes would be appropriate at this time?

    A. Add an ARB and a direct renin inhibitor to maximize inhibition of the renin–angiotensin system.
    B. Increase her diuretic dosing and counsel patient on fluid and salt restriction. Although her lungs are clear, you are not satisfied with her examination findings.
    C. Consider cardiac transplantation.
    D. Start vasodilator therapy with nitroglycerin.

4. Which of the following is true for CHF patients with preserved EF?

    A. They have much better survival when compared with patients with systolic dysfunction.
    B. They respond much better to renin–angiotensin system inhibition than those with systolic dysfunction.
    C. They constitute a minority of admissions of patients with CHF.
    D. They have similar survival rates compared with those with systolic dysfunction.

Answers

1. **B.** The patient has a history suggestive of hypertrophic cardiomyopathy, and an echocardiogram would help demonstrate structural heart disease, including

thickening of the intraventricular septum with resultant dynamic LV outflow obstruction, to support this diagnosis. It is typically inherited in an autosomal dominant fashion with variable penetrance, which is suggested by the family history. The murmur heard on the patient's examination is also consistent, and the decrease in systemic venous return caused by the Valsalva maneuver exacerbates the dynamic outflow obstruction, and its associated murmur.

2. **D.** The patient has NYHA class IV symptoms with a documented EF <35% and a QRS duration >120 milliseconds, making him a potential candidate for cardiac resynchronization therapy. ICD placement is indicated in patients with NYHA class I to III symptoms, and this patient has had persistent class IV symptoms despite optimal medical therapy. Placement of multiple drug-eluting stents would not be helpful based on his clinical presentation. Cardiac transplant may be something to consider, but would not be the first consideration in this case.

3. **B.** Although her lungs are clear, this patient's examination and symptoms reflect persistent volume overload, and she would benefit from further diuresis to correct this. Excessive use of multiple inhibitors of the renin–angiotensin system has not been found to be beneficial. Cardiac transplantation would not be appropriate based on her clinical presentation. Vasodilator therapy would not help correct her apparent volume overload.

4. **D.** The CHF population with a preserved EF makes up 50% of the admissions for heart failure, and has been shown to have very similar survival rates. Frustratingly, many of the proven medication regimens for CHF with systolic dysfunction have not shown similar benefit for those patients with CHF and preserved EF. They may still require these medications, however, for other indications.

SUGGESTED READINGS

Finn P. American Heart Association—scientific sessions 2005. 13–16 November 2005, Dallas, TX, USA. IDrugs. 2006;9:13–15.

Goldberg LR. Heart failure. *Ann Intern Med*. 2010;152:ITC61–ITC615 [quiz ITC616].

Hunt SA, Abraham WT, Chin MH, et al. 2009 focused update incorporated into the ACC/AHA 2005 guidelines for the diagnosis and management of heart failure in adults: a report of the American College of Cardiology Foundation/American Heart Association Task Force on Practice Guidelines: developed in collaboration with the International Society for Heart and Lung Transplantation. *Circulation*. 2009;119:e391–e479.

Jessup M, Abraham WT, Casey DE, et al. 2009 focused update: ACCF/AHA guidelines for the diagnosis and management of heart failure in adults: a report of the American College of Cardiology Foundation/American Heart Association Task Force on Practice Guidelines: developed in collaboration with the International Society for Heart and Lung Transplantation. *Circulation*. 2009;119:1977–2016.

Karon BL, Pereira NL. Cardiology. Part V: heart failure and cardiomyopathies. In: Ghosh AK, ed. *Mayo Clinic Internal Medicine Board Review*. 9th ed. New York: Oxford University Press; 2010: [chapter 3].

Klarich KW. Cardiology. Part I: cardiac examination, valvular heart disease, and congenital heart disease. In: Ghosh AK, ed. *Mayo Clinic Internal Medicine Board Review.* 9th ed. New York: Oxford University Press; 2010: [chapter 3].

Kuenzli A, Bucher HC, Anand I, et al. Meta-analysis of combined therapy with angiotensin receptor antagonists versus ACE inhibitors alone in patients with heart failure. *PLoS One.* 2010;5:e9946.

Mann DL, ed. Heart failure and cor pulmonale. In: Fauci AS, Braundwald E, Kasper DL, et al, eds. *Harrison's Principles of Internal Medicine.* 17th ed. New York: McGraw Hill; 2008:1443–1454: [chapter 227].

Mann DL, ed. Pathophysiology of heart failure. In: Libby P, Bonow RO, Mann DL, Zipes DP, eds. *Braunwald's Heart Disease: A Textbook of Cardiovascular Medicine.* 8th ed. Philadelphia: Saunders Elsevier; 2007:541–560: [chapter 22].

Phillips CO, Kashani A, Ko DK, Francis G, Krumholz HM. Adverse effects of combination angiotensin II receptor blockers plus angiotensin-converting enzyme inhibitors for left ventricular dysfunction: a quantitative review of data from randomized clinical trials. *Arch Intern Med.* 2007;167:1930–1936.

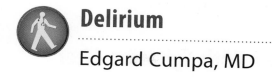

Delirium

Edgard Cumpa, MD

A 75-year-old Woman With Mental Status Changes

A 75-year-old woman with a history of chronic obstructive pulmonary disease is evaluated in the intensive care unit (ICU) for altered mental status. She had a repair of an aortic dissection and was extubated uneventfully. Three days later she developed changes in her mental status. In the ICU, she became agitated, pulling at her lines, attempting to climb out of bed, and asking to leave the hospital. Her arterial blood gas values are normal. The patient has no history of alcohol abuse. Calm reassurance and presence of family members have done little to reduce the patient's agitated behavior.

1. What is the diagnosis for the patient's altered mental status?

2. What is the most appropriate therapy for this patient's altered mental status?

Answers

1. This patient has a delirium.

2. The appropriate treatment is haloperidol. The recommended therapy for delirium is antipsychotic agents. There is no evidence that second-generation antipsychotics are superior to haloperidol for delirium. Haloperidol does not cause respiratory suppression. All antipsychotic agents increase the risk of torsades de pointes and extrapyramidal side effects as well as neuroleptic malignant syndrome.

A 79-year-old Woman With Agitation After Surgery

A 79-year-old woman was hospitalized 4 days ago after a right hip fracture from a fall. She had right hip replacement 3 days ago. She woke up from general anesthesia 12 hours after extubation. She has become increasingly agitated, yelling at the nurses; mechanical restraints were placed 1 day ago. The patient has a history of Alzheimer's dementia. She also has chronic atrial fibrillation treated with warfarin therapy. She has no other pertinent personal or family medical history. Current medications are donepezil, memantine, atenolol, warfarin, and low-molecular-weight heparin.

On physical examination today, temperature is 37.2°C (99.0°F), blood pressure is 100/68 mm Hg, pulse rate is 100/min and irregular, respiration rate is 18/min, and BMI is 21. The patient can move all 4 extremities. She is inattentive and disoriented to time and place and exhibits combativeness alternating with hypersomnolence. The remainder of the neurologic examination is unremarkable, without evidence of focal findings or meningismus.

1. What is the most likely diagnosis?

Answer

1. Acute worsening of confusion in elderly patients with chronic dementia usually results from an acute medical problem. Patients with chronic dementia are at greater risk for delirium after surgery with general anesthesia. This patient with a hip fracture and who had right hip surgery with general anesthesia most likely has a postoperative delirium.

DELIRIUM

Diagnosis

Delirium is defined as changes in the level of consciousness with difficulty focusing, sustaining, or shifting attention. The changes develop and occur over a short period of time, usually hours to days, and fluctuate during the course of the day. Delirium often involves other cognitive deficits, changes in level of arousal, altered sleep-wake cycle, and may include psychotic features such as hallucinations and/or delusions. It is a clinical syndrome precipitated by an underlying medical condition or medical issue.

Key features of delirium include:

- Altered level of consciousness
- Change in cognition
- Onset over hours to days
- Fluctuating course

- Behavioral changes
- Behavioral changes
- Sleep alterations

Common causes of delirium include certain commonly prescribed medications, including opioids, sedative–hypnotics, and polypharmacy. Medication withdrawal states and medication side effects such as quinolones in the elderly are also common precipitants. Other common causes include infections, metabolic abnormalities, and brain disorders. The infections that most commonly cause delirium include sepsis, pneumonia, and urinary tract infections. Electrolyte abnormalities, hypercarbia, hypoxemia, hyperglycemia, and hypoglycemia may also precipitate delirium. CNS infections, seizures, and hypertensive emergencies can cause delirium. Lack of sleep and poor sleep may also be contributing factors.

A mnemonic of some use to remember the possible etiologies of delirium is **I WATCH DEATH:**

Infectious: encephalitis, meningitis, syphilis, pneumonia, and urinary tract infection

Withdrawal: alcohol and sedative–hypnotics

Acute metabolic: acidosis, alkalosis, electrolyte disturbances, and hepatic or renal failure

Trauma: heat stroke, burns, and postoperative

CNS pathology: abscesses, hemorrhage, seizures, stroke, tumors, vasculitis, and normal pressure hydrocephalus

Hypoxia: due to anemia, carbon monoxide poisoning, hypotension, pulmonary embolus, and pulmonary or cardiac failure

Deficiencies: vitamin B_{12}, niacin, and thiamine

Endocrinopathies: hyperglycemia or hypoglycemia, hyperadrenocorticism or hypoadrenocorticism, hyperthyroidism or hypothyroidism, and hyperparathyroidism or hypoparathyroidism

Acute vascular: hypertensive encephalopathy, and shock

Toxins: medications, drugs, pesticides, and solvents

Heavy metals: lead, manganese, and mercury

The evaluation of a patient with delirium should always include a complete history. This is often quite challenging and sometimes must be obtained from alternative sources, including family members, friends, and/or nursing staff. A thorough review of the medical record may be quite helpful in helping to determine the underlying condition.

One key feature of the history is finding out whether or not the patient has a history of dementia or sundowning. This is essential, and requires clinicians to speak to someone close to the patient. This is a hard thing for busy residents to do on call nights, but its importance cannot be minimized. Often, dementia is not officially or formally diagnosed, so clinicians should ask family members and care-givers about general problems with memory, behavior, and mood as well as whether or not the patient had similar problems during other hospitalizations. Having a history of sundowning strongly predicts the presence of some underlying cognitive impairment. It is important to understand the relationship between dementia and delirium. Having a diagnosis of dementia predisposes a patient to developing delirium while hospitalized, and vice versa. If a patient develops delirium while in the hospital, he or she is at increased risk for a later diagnosis of dementia.

Other elements of the history should focus on any symptoms of infections, exposures, or metabolic abnormalities. One needs to take a detailed medication history, as well as a good diet and social history, including a detailed alcohol and drug use history.

The physical examination should be head-to-toe. Many causes of delirium may be missed without a thorough physical examination. Vitals are essential to take and review, including a pulse oximetry. The lung examination may uncover pneumonia or CHF as the etiology. Cardiac examination may lead you to consider cardiac ischemia, CHF, or an arrhythmia. Abdominal examination may cause you to consider bowel impaction, gastrointestinal bleeding, or ischemia. Urinary retention is a common contributor to delirium. A complete neurologic examination, as possible, may help diagnose encephalitis, meningitis, seizure, or stroke. Don't forget to do a good skin examination so a pressure ulcer or allergic reaction is not missed. Also don't forget to check the patient's hearing and vision as these, too, often contribute to altered mental status, and may be easily fixed with eyeglasses or hearing aids.

Delirium constitutes a medical emergency. Patients who present with acute delirium should be screened quickly for readily reversible causes such as hypoglycemia, hypoxia, and narcotic overdose. Further evaluation should be targeted based on your history and physical examination. Tests to consider include thyroid function tests, toxicology screen, drug levels, ammonia, cortisol, vitamin B$_{12}$, arterial blood gas, lumbar puncture, electroencephalography, neuroimaging, electrocardiography, and/or telemetry. Routine testing with a shotgun approach is not indicated or recommended. Additionally, there is no evidence to support routine use of head CT scanning. Head CT/MRI should only be done if there is history of head trauma, suspicion of encephalitis, or new focal neurologic finds, or if no other identifiable cause can be found.

Treatment

Assess and ensure patient safety first. Treatment should focus on the underlying acute illness as well as preventing possible complications. Management of the underlying condition and/or removal of suspected medications are important. Patients with an acute delirium are at risk for complications, including respiratory failure, malnutrition, pressure ulcers, and venous thromboembolism. Airway protection, nutritional support, skin care, and venous thromboembolism prophylaxis should be started. The patient's behavior should also be managed. Patients are at risk for falls, and removing feeding tubes and intravenous lines in the midst of the delirium. Physical restraints should be avoided. Sometimes putting the patient's eyeglasses on or hearing aids in will improve the confusion. Family involvement and use of sitters may be beneficial. Normal sleep-wake cycles should be encouraged; avoiding naps and having patients sleep in a quiet room with low lighting is suggested. Pharmacologic management is indicated in patients with severe agitation who are at a safety risk to themselves or staff. Start with the lowest dose possible and adjust to the patient's response. Low-dose haloperidol (0.5–1.0 mg orally or intramuscularly) or benzodiazepines (lorazepam 0.5–1.0 mg) may be used to control agitation or psychotic symptoms. Benzodiazepines are also indicated in cases of sedative drug and alcohol withdrawal. Thiamine supplementation should be considered in all patients with delirium (Figure 10-1).

Approach to Patient With Delirium

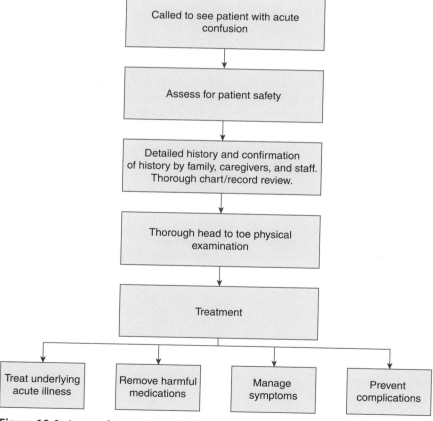

Figure 10-1. Approach to patient with delirium.

TIPS TO REMEMBER

- Delirium is an alteration of consciousness that develops over a short period of time.
- Recognizing that the disorder is present and uncovering the underlying etiology is essential.
- Delirium is a medical emergency.
- Pharmacologic management should only be used in patients with severe agitation who pose a safety risk to themselves or staff or for patients who are at risk for impeding essential medical care.
- Preventing complications of delirium is also a hallmark of treatment.

COMPREHENSION QUESTION

1. When called to see a patient with acute confusion, what are the 2 most important things to do?

Answer

1. Assess and ensure patient safety. Information gathering is essential. This information should include a comprehensive history and physical examination, including confirming the history with a thorough chart review and discussions with family members, caregivers, and staff. A good medication and substance use inquiry may provide the key.

SUGGESTED READINGS

Inouye SK. Delirium in older persons. *N Engl J Med.* 2006;354:1157–1165.
Marx JA, Hockberger RS, Walls RM, Rosen P. *Rosen's Emergency Medicine.* 7th ed. St. Louis, MO: Mosby; 2009.
Schneider LS, Tariot PN, Dagerman KS, et al. Effectiveness of atypical antipsychotic drugs in patients with Alzheimer's disease. *N Engl J Med.* 2006;355:1525–1538.
Sink KM, Holden KF, Yaffe K. Pharmacological treatment of neuropsychiatric symptoms of dementia. *JAMA.* 2005;293:596–608.

Diabetes Emergencies

Deepika Nallala, MD and
Michael Jakoby, MD, MA

A Case of Adult-onset Type 1 Diabetes Mellitus Presenting as Ketoacidosis

A 36-year-old woman presents to the emergency department for evaluation and management of refractory nausea, vomiting, and abdominal pain. Symptoms have persisted for 2 days, and the patient has felt somewhat short of breath and light-headed when standing for the past 12 hours. She was diagnosed with gestational diabetes mellitus 3 years ago and then type 2 diabetes when hyperglycemia persisted after delivery. The patient's only medication is metformin. Examination is notable for resting tachycardia, mild tachypnea, dry mucous membranes, and modest, diffuse pain on palpation of the abdomen. Capillary blood glucose (CBG) is >500 mg/dL.

Initial electrolyte panel revealed sodium 132 mEq/L, potassium 4.6 mEq/L, chloride 92 mEq/L, bicarbonate 12 mEq/L, blood urea nitrogen (BUN) 20 mg/dL, creatinine (Cr) 0.7 mg/dL, and glucose 520 mg/dL. Anion gap was computed to be 28. Arterial blood gas was notable for pH 7.21, pco_2 34 mm Hg, po_2 80 mm Hg, and calculated bicarbonate 14 mEq/L. Urinalysis was remarkable for large glucose and ketones, but nitrites and leukocyte esterase were undetectable. Complete blood count (CBC) showed modest leukocytosis and elevation of neutrophil count. Markers of liver function, amylase, lipase, EKG, and chest plain films were unremarkable.

1. How is diabetic ketoacidosis (DKA) diagnosed?

2. How should DKA patients be evaluated?

3. What are the appropriate steps in DKA management?

Answers

1. DKA is diagnosed by the simultaneous occurrence of hyperglycemia, ketonemia and ketonuria, and anion gap acidemia. The differential diagnosis of ketosis is

Table 11-1. Etiologies of Ketosis

Etiology	Glucose
Fasting (infancy, pregnancy)	N, D
Prolonged exercise	N, occ D
Ketogenic diet	N, occ D
DKA	I
Adrenal insufficiency	D
GH insufficiency (children)	D
Ketotic hypoglycemia	D
Alcoholic ketoacidosis	Varies
Isopropyl alcohol poisoning	N
Salicylate poisoning	Varies

N, normal; D, decreased; I, increased; occ, occasionally.

presented in Table 11-1, and American Diabetes Association (ADA) diagnostic criteria are presented in Table 11-2.

2. Metabolic confirmation of the diagnosis includes timely measurements of glucose, urine ketones, and electrolytes to allow computation of an anion gap ($Na-Cl-HCO_3$). Patients should also be evaluated for potential secondary causes of DKA. Pneumonia and urinary tract infections are the most common precipitating causes.

Table 11-2. American Diabetes Association (ADA) Diagnostic Criteria for DKA

	Mild	Moderate	Severe
Glucose (mg/dL)	>250	>250	>250
pH	7.25–7.30	7.00–7.24	<7.00
HCO_3^- (mM)	15–18	10–14	<10
Urine ketones	+	+	+
Serum ketones	+	+	+
Osmolality	Varies	Varies	Varies
Anion gap	>10	>12	>12
Sensorium	Alert	Drowsy	Stupor/coma

3. Successful management of DKA requires parenteral insulin, hydration, and potassium repletion. ADA recommendations are summarized in Table 11-4.

CASE REVIEW

DKA is a life-threatening complication of type 1 diabetes mellitus. The absence of endogenous insulin leads to unrestrained lipolysis in adipose tissue, ketogenesis and gluconeogenesis in liver, and severely reduced glucose uptake by skeletal muscle. These factors lead to hyperglycemia and ketoacidemia that are pathological hallmarks of DKA. Hyperglycemia and ketonemia also cause osmotic diuresis and hypovolemia. There are over 100,000 hospital admissions for DKA annually that account for more than $1 billion of health care costs, and mortality rates range from 2% to 5%. Potential etiologies of ketosis are presented in Table 11-1.

Diagnosis

Common symptoms of DKA include nausea, vomiting, abdominal pain, polyuria, polydipsia, blurry vision, lethargy, and shortness of breath. Tachycardia, hypotension, dry mucous membranes, poor skin turgor, and diffuse abdominal pain to palpation are usually found on physical examination. Patients are also often tachypneic and may exhibit Kussmaul breathing, characteristic rapid and deep respirations. The breath of DKA patients may smell of acetone.

The diagnosis of DKA is made by documenting anion gap acidemia in the setting of hyperglycemia. Potential causes of ketosis are presented in Table 11-1, and diagnostic criteria for DKA are summarized in Table 11-2. Although the patient's age may make type 1 diabetes seem unlikely, approximately 30% of type 1 diabetes cases are diagnosed in patients over age 18 years.

Workup of presumptive DKA should be directed at quickly confirming the diagnosis and identifying potential etiologies. Documenting hyperglycemia and an anion gap acidosis ($Na–Cl–HCO_3$ >10) confirms the diagnosis of DKA. The ADA recommends that all patients with DKA undergo an initial evaluation that includes arterial blood gas analysis, measurements of plasma glucose, electrolytes, Cr and BUN, CBC, and blood and urine cultures.

In 2 large series of patients (Table 11-3), medical noncompliance, newly diagnosed type 1 diabetes mellitus, or infections, particularly pneumonia or urinary tract infections, accounted for approximately 85% of all cases of DKA. In a recent series of adult patients, medical noncompliance was the cause of DKA in approximately 70% of hospital admissions. Other potential precipitating factors include myocardial infarction, stroke, pulmonary embolus, acute pancreatitis, alcohol or illicit substance abuse, and trauma. Patients managed with insulin pumps may develop DKA due to cannula site complications (inappropriate placement, fibrosis, or infection).

Table 11-3. Etiologies of DKA

Series	No. of Episodes	Infections (%)	Non-compliance (%)	New Onset (%)	Other Illness (%)	Unknown (%)
Kitabchi et al (1994)	202	38	28	22	10	4
Umpierrez et al (1997)	144	28	41	17	10	4

Treatment

Keys to successful management of DKA include prompt insulin therapy, hydration, and correction of total body potassium deficits. Parenteral insulin is preferred due to the ability to quickly achieve high insulin levels and suppress ketogenesis, although there are protocols for frequent administration of subcutaneous insulin aspart (NovoLog) or insulin lispro (Humalog) to manage mild DKA. Unless circulating potassium level is significantly low (<3.3 mEq/L), intravenous insulin should be started as a 0.1 U/kg bolus followed by 0.1 U/kg/h infusion or a 0.14 U/kg/h infusion without bolus. CBG is measured hourly, and dextrose is added to fluids when CBG is <200 to 250 mg/dL. Intravenous insulin should be continued until the anion gap has closed and serum bicarbonate is ≥17 mEq/L. Patients require basal insulin therapy with NPH, insulin glargine (Lantus), or insulin detemir (Levemir), and the insulin infusion must be overlapped 1 hour with the initial dose of NPH or 2 hours with the initial dose of glargine or detemir before termination to avoid recurrence of ketoacidosis.

Patients in DKA are significantly volume depleted (up to 0.1 L/kg) and require hydration with isotonic fluid (normal saline or Ringer's lactate) to correct volume status. After administration of at least 3 to 4 L of isotonic fluid and documented improvement in heart rate and blood pressure, patients can be hydrated with hypotonic fluid, usually half-normal saline, at a rate ranging from 4 to 14 mg/kg/h (typical rates are 250–500 mL/h). Although serum potassium level may be elevated on presentation due to acidemia, patients with DKA have large total body potassium deficits (3–5 mEq/kg) and require potassium repletion. Potassium may be withheld from fluids at levels >5.3 mEq/L, but 20 to 40 mEq of potassium chloride should be added to intravenous fluids at levels <5.3 mEq/L. An electrolyte panel should be checked every 2 hours to closely monitor changes in potassium levels, bicarbonate, and anion gap. A summary of recommendations for insulin dosing, hydration, and potassium repletion is presented in Table 11-4.

Table 11-4. Recommendations for Insulin, Fluids, and Potassium Management

Intervention	
Insulin	0.1 U/kg bolus, and then 0.1 U/kg/h infusion
	0.14 U/kg/h infusion w/o bolus
	0.14 U/kg bolus if CBG fails to fall by ≥10% from baseline first hour
	Hold insulin until potassium ≥3.3 mEq/L
Fluids	Severe hypovolemia—several liters normal saline (NS) at 1 L/h
	Mild hypovolemia and low sodium level— 250–500 mL/h NS
	Mild hypovolemia and normal or high sodium—250–500 mL/h half NS
	Add dextrose when CBG <200–250 mg/dL
	Switch to hypotonic fluid (half NS) when volume deficit corrected
Potassium	K^+ <3.3 mEq/L—hold insulin and administer KCl 40 mEq/h
	K^+ 3.3–5.2 mEq/L—administer KCl 20–40 mEq/h
	K^+ >5.2 mEq/L—monitor K^+ level every 2 h

Sodium bicarbonate may be administered when DKA is severe (pH <7.0). The recommended dose is 100 mEq of bicarbonate with 20 mEq potassium chloride in 400 mL sterile water over 2 hours, with the dose repeated every 2 hours as necessary until pH improves to >7.0. Bicarbonate is coadministered with potassium to help avoid hypokalemia. Treatment with sodium bicarbonate does not substitute for therapy with adequate insulin and hydration, and the utility of adding bicarbonate to insulin is unclear. In a study comparing administration of insulin and bicarbonate with insulin alone in patients with severe DKA (pH 6.90–7.14), time to resolution of acidemia was no faster in the group of patients who received bicarbonate in addition to parenteral insulin.

Hypophosphatemia is common in DKA, although administration of parenteral phosphate has not been shown to accelerate metabolic recovery. Serum phosphate levels fall significantly after stopping parenteral administration of supplemental phosphate, and the P_{50} curve for peripheral oxygen delivery is no different in treated or untreated patients. Hypophosphatemia usually resolves quickly once patients resume eating.

An Elderly Patient With Hyperglycemic Hyperosmolar Syndrome

A 74-year-old male is brought from his nursing home to the emergency department for evaluation of confusion and right hemiparalysis. The patient was recently transferred from the hospital to nursing home for inpatient rehabilitation after suffering a stroke complicated by residual right-sided weakness. Over the past 48 hours, the patient has grown progressively more confused and complained of thirst. Staff observed right-sided paralysis the morning of transfer. History is notable for type 2 diabetes, hypertension, and dyslipidemia. A thiazide diuretic was added to the patient's blood pressure regimen during hospital admission. Diabetes is managed with glyburide, but hemoglobin A1c (HbA1c) is unknown. CBG from the nursing home is reported as >400 mg/dL. Tachycardia and hypotension (BP 86/54 mm Hg) are noted. The patient is disoriented to place and time, has limited ability to follow commands, and does not spontaneously move his right extremities.

Admission electrolyte panel revealed serum sodium 124 mEq/L, chloride 92 mEq/L, bicarbonate 22 mEq/L, BUN 62 mg/dL, Cr 1.6 mg/dL, and glucose 820 mg/dL. Other serologies and CBC were unremarkable. Urinalysis was notable for large glucose and small ketones. No acute hemorrhages, ischemic changes, or masses were observed on computed tomography of the head. No infiltrates or effusions were visible on plain films of the chest. EKG showed sinus tachycardia and nonspecific ST segment changes.

1. **What are the diagnostic criteria for hyperglycemic hyperosmolar syndrome (HHS)?**
2. **What are important risk factors for HHS?**
3. **How should HHS patients be evaluated and managed?**

Answers

1. HHS is diagnosed when patients present with altered mental status of some degree in the setting of severe hyperglycemia (plasma glucose ≥600 mg/dL) and hyperosmolarity (≥320 mOsm/L). Unlike DKA, there is no metabolic acidemia.

2. Key risk factors are listed in Figure 11-1. Advanced age, residence in an institutional setting, infections, and cardiovascular events are all potential risk factors for HHS. Some patients may have undiagnosed type 2 diabetes at presentation. Occasionally, patients have been started on medications such as glucocorticoids that significantly exacerbate hyperglycemia.

3. Prompt fluid resuscitation, parenteral insulin, and potassium repletion are the most important factors in management. Specific dosing instructions are

- Age >70 years
- Nursing home resident
- Infection
- Myocardial infarction
- Stroke
- Undiagnosed/untreated Type 2 diabetes
- Drugs (glucocorticoids, diuretics, beta-blockers)

Figure 11-1. Risk factors for HHS.

summarized in Table 11-4. Since patients are not in ketoacidosis, insulin infusion rates are typically lowered as plasma glucose falls below 250 to 300 mg/dL to slow the rate of improvement and limit the possibility of cerebral edema.

CASE REVIEW

Hyperglycemic hyperosmolar state (HHS) occurs when severe elevation of plasma glucose leads to hyperosmolarity and altered mental status. Diagnostic criteria include plasma glucose $\geq$600 mg/dL, osmolarity $\geq$320 mOsm/L; and altered mental status, ranging from mild confusion to coma, in the absence of metabolic acidemia (pH $\geq$7.30, HCO_3 $\geq$18). Insulinopenia leads to impaired glucose uptake by skeletal muscle and inappropriate gluconeogenesis in liver, resulting in hyperglycemia that in turn induces osmotic diuresis and prerenal azotemia, further worsening hyperglycemia by limiting glucosuria. Attenuated thirst response, as a consequence of either aging or central nervous system injury, also plays a role. There is sufficient insulin to suppress lipolysis and ketogenesis, distinguishing HHS from DKA.

Risk factors for HHS are listed in Figure 11-1. HHS patients tend to be much older than DKA patients as HHS typically occurs in patients with type 2 diabetes mellitus. Patients may live in institutional settings and not have free access to water. In addition to altered mental status, they may exhibit neurological findings mimicking stroke that resolve with treatment of hyperosmolarity. Volume depletion is severe (0.1–0.2 L/kg), and signs such as tachycardia, hypotension, dry mucous membranes, and poor skin turgor are usually present on examination. Patients with poorly controlled hypertension may exhibit normotensive blood pressures that are an unusual change from baseline. Cardiopulmonary emergencies are well-known precipitants of HHS, and patients should be examined carefully for signs of coronary ischemia, heart failure, or chronic obstructive pulmonary disease (COPD) exacerbations. Infections also commonly trigger HHS, and patients require prompt evaluation for urinary tract infections and pneumonia. Glucocorticoids, thiazide diuretics, and beta-blockers may worsen preexisting diabetes or hyperglycemia, and medications should be carefully reviewed.

Diagnosis and Treatment

Initial evaluation of patients with presumptive HHS is similar to workup of patients with DKA. Key laboratories include electrolytes, markers of renal and hepatic function, CBC, and amylase or lipase. Urinalysis and cultures of blood and urine should be obtained. Given the high risk of cardiopulmonary disease, EKG, chest films, and cardiac enzymes should also be screened.

The mortality rate for patients with HHS is as high as 10% to 15%. In a large study of nearly 500 patients presenting with HHS, age, severity of altered mental status on presentation, degree of hyperosmolarity, and renal function were independent predictors of mortality risk. Goals of therapy are to correct volume deficits and hyperglycemia with parenteral fluids and insulin, respectively, and in turn correct hyperosmolarity. Patients are also total body potassium depleted and require careful monitoring of potassium levels and therapy with supplemental potassium in intravenous fluids. Inciting events (eg, infection, coronary ischemia) also need to be identified and treated promptly.

Fluids, insulin, and supplemental potassium are initiated and managed mostly as discussed in management of DKA and summarized in Table 11-4. However, when plasma glucose falls below 300 mg/dL, dextrose is added to intravenous fluids and insulin rate is reduced (0.02–0.05 U/kg/h) to maintain plasma glucose in the range of 200 to 300 mg/dL until patients recover to baseline mental status as a protection against possible cerebral edema. Capillary glucose is monitored hourly and electrolytes every 2 hours while patients are managed with intravenous insulin. Patients require subcutaneous insulin to prevent recurrence of severe hyperglycemia, and intravenous insulin is overlapped 1 to 2 hours with the first dose of subcutaneous insulin.

TIPS TO REMEMBER

- DKA and HHS are life-threatening emergencies of type 1 and type 2 diabetes, respectively. DKA occurs due to an absence of insulin activity that results in both hyperglycemia and ketogenesis. Insulinopenia and prerenal azotemia lead to severe hyperglycemia in HHS, but there is sufficient insulin activity to prevent ketogenesis.

- DKA is distinguished by the biochemical triad of hyperglycemia, ketonemia, and anion gap acidemia. Medical noncompliance, infection, and newly recognized type 1 diabetes mellitus are the 3 most common etiologies of DKA.

- Severe hyperglycemia, hyperosmolarity, and altered mental status are the defining manifestations of HHS. There are several risk factors for HHS including advanced age, residence in an institutional setting, cardiovascular disease, infection, and medications that exacerbate hyperglycemia such as glucocorticoids or thiazide diuretics.

- Intravenous insulin, hydration, and supplemental potassium are the key interventions for successful management of both DKA and HHS. Patients require frequent monitoring of CBG and serum electrolytes during treatment.

- Subcutaneous insulin is required to prevent recurrence of ketoacidosis in DKA and control hyperglycemia in both DKA and HHS after acute metabolic derangements have been successfully managed. Insulin infusion should overlap the first dose of subcutaneous insulin by 1 to 2 hours depending on the basal subcutaneous insulin chosen.

SUGGESTED READINGS

American Diabetes Association. American Diabetes Association clinical practice recommendations. Standards of medical care in diabetes—2012. *Diabetes Care*. 2012;35:S11–S63.

Fisher JN, Kitabchi AE. A randomized study of phosphate therapy in the treatment of diabetic ketoacidosis. *J Clin Endocrinol Metab*. 1983;57:177–180.

Fisher JN, Shahshahani MN, Kitabchi AE. Diabetic ketoacidosis: low-dose insulin therapy by various routes. *N Engl J Med*. 1977;297:238–247.

Graves EJ, Gillum BS. National Hospital Discharge Survey: annual summary, 1994. *Vital Health Stat 13*. 1997;(128):i–v, 1–50.

Kitabchi AE, Fisher JN, Murphy MB, Rumbak MJ. Diabetic ketoacidosis and the hyperglycemic hyperosmolar nonketotic state. In: Kahn CR, Weir GC, eds. *Joslin's Diabetes Mellitus*. 13th ed. Philadelphia: Lea & Febiger; 1994:738–770.

Kitabchi AE, Umpierrez GE, Miles JM, Fisher JN. Hyperglycemic crises in adult patients with diabetes. *Diabetes Care*. 2007;32:1335–1343.

Morris LR, Murphy MB, Kitabchi AE. Bicarbonate therapy in diabetic ketoacidosis. *Ann Intern Med*. 1986;105:836–840.

Musey VC, Lee JK, Crawford R, Klatka MA, McAdams D, Phillips LS. Diabetes in urban African Americans: cessation of insulin therapy is the major precipitating cause of diabetic ketoacidosis. *Diabetes Care*. 1995;18:483–489.

Umpierrez GE, Cuervo R, Karabell A, Latif K, Freire AX, Kitabchi AE. Treatment of diabetic ketoacidosis with subcutaneous insulin aspart. *Diabetes Care*. 2004;27:1873–1878.

Umpierrez GE, Kelly JP, Navarrete JE, Casals MM, Kitabchi AE. Hyperglycemic crises in urban blacks. *Arch Intern Med*. 1997;157:669–675.

Umpierrez GE, Latif K, Stoever J, et al. Efficacy of subcutaneous insulin lispro versus continuous intravenous regular insulin for the treatment of patients with diabetic ketoacidosis. *Am J Med*. 2004;117:291–296.

Wachtel TJ, Tetu-Mouradjian LM, Goldman DL, Ellis SE, O'Sullivan PS. Hyperosmolarity and acidosis in diabetes mellitus: a three-year experience in Rhode Island. *J Gen Intern Med*. 1991;6:495–502.

A 64-year-old Male Requiring Diabetes Management in the Hospital

Michael Jakoby, MD, MA and
Owaise M. Y. Mansuri, MD

A 64-year-old male is admitted to the hospital to manage a heart failure exacerbation. History is notable for type 2 diabetes mellitus diagnosed 7 years ago and managed with glipizide and metformin. He insists on full compliance with all prescribed medications. The patient is unaware of any microvascular complications. Hemoglobin A1c (HbA1c) checked shortly before admission was 8.5%.

Initial evaluation reveals the patient to be in mild-to-moderate respiratory distress but capable of eating. Weight and height are recorded as 90 kg and 173 cm, respectively. Admission plasma glucose (glc) is 234 mg/dL, and serum creatinine is 1.1 mg/dL. The admitting service writes orders for lispro (LP; Humalog) with meals and glargine (Glarg) at bedtime as presented in Figure 12-1. The night nurse calls the on-call intern to report bedtime capillary blood glucose (CBG) is 254 mg/dL and outside call parameters.

The patient responds well to therapy with diuretics and vasodilators. His CBG pattern (mg/dL) by the morning of hospital day 2 is shown in Table 12-1.

Glycemic control improves after advancing LP doses. However, on hospital day 4, the patient feels sweaty and tremulous in the morning, and CBG before breakfast is measured at 64 mg/dL. At bedtime on hospital day 3, CBG was 95 mg/dL.

1. What is the best approach to manage the patient's type 2 diabetes?

2. How can the patient's unanticipated exacerbation of hyperglycemia on the night of admission be corrected?

3. How should insulin be adjusted on hospital day 2 to improve glycemic control?

4. How should hypoglycemia occurring the morning of hospital day 4 be addressed?

Answers

1. A basal/bolus insulin regimen is the preferred approach to diabetes management on non–critical care hospital services. Typically, a basal insulin analog such as Glarg (Lantus®) is combined with a prandial insulin analog such as LP (Humalog®).

2. Correction factor (CF) insulin should be dosed as summarized in Figure 12-2. Rapid-acting insulin analogs are preferred as CF insulin. CBG correction target is usually 140 or 150 mg/dL.

3. Persistently elevated CBG measurements during the day but stable CBG from night to morning indicate a need to increase prandial insulin doses. See

---

Since BMI is greater than 25, estimate daily calories with Mifflin–St. Jeor equation:

$(9.99 \times 90 \text{ kg}) + (6.25 \times 173 \text{ cm}) - (4.92 \times 64) + 5 = 1670 \text{ kcal/day}$

Carbohydrates (g/meal) = 1670/24 = 70

TDI = 0.6 U/kg x 90 kg = 54 U

Prandial insulin (U/meal) = TDI $\times$ 1/6 = 54/6 = 9 U/meal

Basal insulin (U/day) = TDI/2 = 54/2 = 27 U/day

Figure 12-1. Initial diet and insulin orders.

Figure 12-3 or Appendix 1 for instructions regarding prandial insulin adjustments. In this case, insulin LP should be increased by 20% at each meal to 11 U.

4. Fall in CBG from night to morning indicates that the patient's basal insulin requirement is reduced. Lantus dose should be reduced by approximately 20% as indicated in Appendix 1. Reducing the Glarg dose by 20% to 24 U at bedtime is likely to avoid additional morning hypoglycemia.

CASE REVIEW

Diabetes mellitus is a common comorbidity of patients admitted to the hospital and has a significant impact on clinical outcomes. In the 15-year period from 1993 to 2007, the number of hospital discharges listing diabetes mellitus with or without complications as one of the diagnoses increased more than 2-fold to over 7 million in 2007. A study of 2030 consecutive admissions to Georgia Baptist Medical Center in Atlanta, Georgia, in 1998 found a 26% prevalence of preexisting diabetes and 12% prevalence of newly recognized hyperglycemia. Diabetes mellitus and hyperglycemia have been linked to poor clinical outcomes in both the critical care and non–critical care settings and for several specific clinical presentations including myocardial infarction, stroke, pneumonia, and heart failure.

A growing body of evidence indicates that basal/bolus insulin is the superior approach to managing diabetes on non–critical care hospital services. In the

Table 12-1. Capillary Blood Glucose Measurements

Day	0300	Breakfast	Lunch	Dinner	Bedtime
Admission					254
Day 1	185	173	158	174	162
Day 2	—	155			

ISF = 1500/TDI = 1500/54 = 28

CF insulin = (measured CBG – 140)/ISF = (254 – 140)/28 = 4 U of lispro

Figure 12-2. Correction factor insulin dosing.

RABBIT-2 trial, patients with type 2 diabetes mellitus admitted to general medicine services were randomized to a basal/bolus insulin protocol with glulisine
(Apidra) dosed at meals and Glarg (Lantus) administered daily for basal insulin or a sliding scale insulin protocol (regular insulin dosed depending on CBG
measurements). Glycemic control was significantly better for basal/bolus insulin–
managed patients than for sliding scale insulin–managed patients. A basal/bolus
insulin protocol study at Carle Foundation Hospital in Urbana, Illinois, documented significant improvements in both glycemic control and hospital length
of stay for patients on general medicine. Basal/bolus insulin was compared with
sliding scale regular insulin for general surgery patients in the RABBIT-2 Surgery trial, and basal/bolus insulin–managed patients had better blood glc control,
fewer surgical morbidities, and shorter stay in the surgical intensive care unit than
patients managed with sliding scale insulin.

Treatment

Most basal/bolus insulin protocols stop outpatient diabetes medications and
make estimates of the patient's total daily insulin (TDI) requirements based on
weight in kilograms. TDI is divided equally between prandial and basal insulin,
although patients receiving glucocorticoids have a disproportionate need for
prandial insulin and may have better glycemic control if TDI is divided as two
thirds prandial and one third basal insulin. Protocols often include orders for supplemental insulin to correct elevated blood glc levels. If no protocol is available,
CF insulin can be estimated using the "rule of 1500" as discussed later in the chapter. American Diabetes Association glycemic targets are <140 mg/dL before meals
and <180 mg/dL between meals. Renal failure may lower TDI requirements, and
TDI should be reduced by 25% when glomerular filtration rate (GFR) is below
50 mL/min/1.73 m^2 and by 50% when GFR is below 10 mL/min/1.73 m^2.

CBG stable from bedtime to morning, no basal insulin adjustment

CBG 141 to 179 mg/dL throughout the day, increase prandial insulin by 20%

New lispro dose = 9 × 1.2 = 11 U

Figure 12-3. Insulin dosing adjustments.

Diet orders are also important to effective hospital diabetes management. Caloric requirements for height/weight proportionate patients can be estimated as 20 to 25 kcal/kg per day, with 50% of calories provided as carbohydrate. Caloric requirements for overweight or obese patients (BMI >25) can be estimated using the Mifflin-St. Jeor equations. Orders should be written so that equal amounts of carbohydrate are provided at each meal (consistent carbohydrate diet). An example of diet and initial insulin orders for the patient under consideration is presented in Figure 12-1.

When unanticipated high blood glc occurs, potential causal factors should be investigated and corrected if possible. CBG may be increased above target due to delayed or omitted insulin dose, delayed meal with measurement of postprandial glc, inadequate standing insulin doses, unplanned carbohydrate consumption between meals or before bedtime, dextrose-containing fluids or parenteral medications, and initiation of glucocorticoid therapy.

Most formulas for estimating insulin sensitivity factor (ISF) and determining CF insulin dose have been developed for patients with type 1 diabetes. The SIU Hospital Diabetes Team typically uses the "rule of 1500" to estimate ISF and supplemental insulin doses when CBG is elevated and CF insulin is required. A target-corrected CBG of 140 to 150 mg/dL is typically chosen, and the difference between measured and target CBG is then divided by ISF to determine the dose of CF insulin as illustrated in Figure 12-2. When administered at meals, it is important to clarify with nursing staff that CF insulin is administered in addition to standing prandial insulin. If CF insulin is administered at bedtime, CBG should be rechecked 3 to 4 hours later to determine CF insulin dose efficacy and screen for possible hypoglycemia due to overcorrection.

Stable CBG from bedtime to morning indicates that basal insulin (Glarg) is dosed appropriately and does not need to be adjusted. When CBG increases from bedtime to morning, basal insulin should be increased. If CBG falls significantly from night to morning, basal insulin dose is excessive and should be reduced.

Persistent elevation of CBG values during the day implies that prandial insulin doses (LP) should be increased. The CBG after a dose of mealtime insulin is a measure of how well the dose covered carbohydrate at that meal; for example, lunch CBG is a measure of the efficacy of breakfast prandial insulin. The SIU Pocket Insulin Dosing Card presented in Appendix 1 gives guidance for adjusting prandial and basal insulin doses. Insulin dosing adjustments for this clinical vignette are presented in Figure 12-3.

CBG <70 mg/dL is considered mild hypoglycemia, and CBG <40 mg/dL or an episode of low blood glc requiring third-party intervention for resolution is considered severe hypoglycemia. Hypoglycemia should be treated immediately to avoid potential complications such as confusion, loss of consciousness, or seizures.

Mild hypoglycemia should be managed according to the "rule of 15's": 15 g of oral glc followed by repeat CBG monitoring in 15 minutes. Appropriate sources of supplemental glc include 4 oz of fruit juice, 6 oz of regular soda, 1 to 2 teaspoons of honey, 3 to 4 glc tablets, or a tube of glc gel. Goal of treatment is to raise CBG above 80 mg/dL without causing rebound hyperglycemia. A small snack may be required after initial treatment to avoid recurrent hypoglycemia.

When patients are too impaired to consume an oral source of glc safely, either parenteral glc or glucagon should be administered. A half (12.5 g dextrose) or full (25.0 g dextrose) ampule of 50% dextrose can be administered as an intravenous bolus, or glucagon 0.5 to 1.0 mg can be administered by the subcutaneous, intramuscular, or intravenous routes.

TIPS TO REMEMBER

- Prevalence of diabetes mellitus and hyperglycemia in the hospital is high, and management of hyperglycemia has a significant impact on outcomes such as hospital length of stay.

- Ambulatory medications should be stopped and basal/bolus insulin substituted for patients admitted to general medicine who are able to eat. Many hospitals have basal/bolus insulin protocols, and there are protocols published in the peer-reviewed literature.

- CF insulin should be administered to treat unanticipated high blood glc. If a supplemental insulin dosing protocol is unavailable, the "rule of 1500" can be used to estimate insulin sensitivity and determine CF insulin dose.

- Insulin should be adjusted to achieve premeal blood glc <140 mg/dL and random glc <180 mg/dL.

- Mild hypoglycemia should be treated according to the "rule of 15's": 15 g of glc and repeat capillary glc measurement in 15 minutes. Severe hypoglycemia should be managed with parenteral glc or glucagon.

Appendix 1. SIU Pocket Insulin Dosing Guide

Stop all outpatient diabetes medications.

Diabetic diet with 20 to 25 kcal/kg total calories.

Oral medications/new hyperglycemia:

Admit glc <200 mg/dL: 0.5 U/kg per day TDI; admit glc ≥200 mg/dL: 0.6 U/kg per day TDI

Basal insulin + oral medications as outpatient:

Admit glc <200 mg/dL: 0.6 U/kg per day TDI; admit glc ≥200 mg/dL: 0.7 U/kg per day TDI

Basal and prandial insulin as outpatient:

Admit glc <200 mg/dL: greater of TDI = 0.7 U/kg per day or outpatient TDI × 1.2

Admit glc ≥200 mg/dL: greater of TDI = 0.8 U/kg per day or outpatient TDI × 1.3

(continued)

Appendix 1. SIU Pocket Insulin Dosing Guide (*Continued*)

Standard dosing:

Lantus (Glarg) dose = TDI/2; Humalog (LP) dose (each meal) = TDI/6

Steroid treated:

Lantus (Glarg) dose = TDI/3; Humalog (LP) dose (each meal) = (TDI × 2)/9

Adjustments if glc high:

AM glc >QHS glc	Increase Glarg
AM glc ~QHS glc	Increase supper LP
Lunch glc high	Increase breakfast LP
Supper glc high	Increase lunch LP
QHS glc high	Increase supper LP

If glc 141 to 179 mg/dL, increase by 20%.

If glc 180 to 219 mg/dL, increase by 25%.

If glc ≥220 mg/dL, increase by 35%.

Daily adjustments if glc <70 mg/dL:

Use guide for glc high to determine insulin dose to adjust.

If glc <70 mg/dL, decrease by 20%.

If glc <50 mg/dL, decrease by 35%.

Appendix 2. Insulin Preparations and Pharmacokinetics

Insulin	Onset	Peak	Duration
Prandial			
Lispro (Humalog)	5–15 min	30–90 min	5 h
Aspart (NovoLog)	5–15 min	30–90 min	5 h
Glulisine (aspart)	5–15 min	30–90 min	5 h
Regular	30–60 min	2–3 h	5–8 h
Basal			
NPH	2–4 h	4–10 h	10–16 h
Glargine (Lantus)	2–4 h	None	20–24 h
Detemir (Levemir)	2–4 h	None	16–22 h[a]

[a]Dose dependent.

Appendix 3. Mifflin-St. Jeor Equations

Men = [9.99 × actual weight (kg)] + [6.25 × height (cm)] − [4.92 × age] + 5

Women = [9.99 × actual weight (kg)] + [6.25 × height (cm)] − [4.92 × age] − 161

Add 10% to estimated calories if recent surgery, fever/infection, or wound debridement.

SUGGESTED READINGS

Agency for Healthcare Research and Quality. HCUPnet Provides Trend Information for the 15 Year Period: 1993-2007. <http://hcupnet.ahrq.gov/HCUPnet.jsp>; Retrieved April 8, 2010.

American Diabetes Association. American Diabetes Association clinical practice recommendations. Standards of medical care in diabetes—2012. *Diabetes Care.* 2012;35(suppl 1):S11–S63.

Capes SE, Hunt D, Malmberg K, Pathak P, Gerstein HC. Stress hyperglycemia and prognosis of stroke in nondiabetic and diabetic patients: a systematic overview. *Stroke.* 2001;32:2426–2432.

Davidson PC, Hebblewhite HR, Steed RD, Bode BW. Analysis of guidelines for basal–bolus insulin dosing: basal insulin, correction factor, and carbohydrate to insulin ratio. *Endocr Pract.* 2008;14:1095–1101.

Gebreegziabher Y, McCullough PA, Bubb C, et al. Admission hyperglycemia and length of hospital stay in patients with diabetes and heart failure: a prospective cohort study. *Congest Heart Fail.* 2008;14:117–120.

Goyal A, Mehta SR, Diaz R, et al. Differential clinical outcomes associated with hypoglycemia and hyperglycemia in acute myocardial infarction. *Circulation.* 2009;120:2429–2437.

Jakoby M, Alnijoumi M, Soriano S, et al. Impact of a pocket insulin dosing guide on utilization of basal/bolus insulin by internal medicine resident physicians. *Diabetes.* 2012;61(suppl 1):A21–A22.

Jakoby M, Kumar J, Six B, Hall M. Basal/bolus insulin is superior to prevalent methods of diabetes management on the general medicine service at a regional medical center. *Carle Selected Papers.* 2007;50:1–7.

King AB, Armstrong DU. A prospective evaluation of insulin dosing recommendations in patients with type 1 diabetes at near normal glucose control: bolus dosing. *J Diabetes Sci Technol.* 2007;1:42–46.

Krinsley JS. Association between hyperglycemia and increased hospital mortality in a heterogeneous population of critically ill patients. *Mayo Clin Proc.* 2003;78:1471–1478.

McAlister FA, Majumdar SR, Blitz S, Rowe BH, Romney J, Marrie TJ. The relation between hyperglycemia and outcomes in 2,471 patients admitted to the hospital with community acquired pneumonia. *Diabetes Care.* 2005;28:810–815.

Mifflin MD, St. Jeor ST, Hill LA, Scott BJ, Daugherty SA, Koh YO. A new predictive equation for resting energy expenditure in health individuals. *Am J Clin Nutr.* 1990;51:241–247.

Moghissi ES, Korytkowski MT, Dinardo M, et al; American Association of Clinical Endocrinologists; American Diabetes Association. American Association of Clinical Endocrinologists and American Diabetes Association consensus statement on inpatient glycemic control. *Diabetes Care.* 2009;32:1119–1131.

Snyder RW, Berns JS. Use of insulin and oral hypoglycemic medications in patients with diabetes mellitus and advanced kidney disease. *Semin Dial.* 2004;17:365–370.

Umpierrez GE, Isaacs SD, Bazargan N, You X, Thaler LM, Kitabchi AE. Hyperglycemia: an independent marker of in-hospital mortality in patients with undiagnosed diabetes. *J Clin Endocrinol Metab.* 2002;87:978–982.

Umpierrez GE, Smiley D, Jacobs S, et al. Randomized study of basal–bolus insulin therapy in the inpatient management of patients with type 2 diabetes undergoing general surgery (RABBIT 2 Surgery). *Diabetes Care.* 2011;34:256–261.

Umpierrez G, Smiley D, Zisman A, et al. Randomized study of basal–bolus insulin therapy in the inpatient management of patients with type 2 diabetes (RABBIT 2 Trial). *Diabetes Care.* 2007;30:2181–2186.

Diarrhea in Hospitalized Patients

Sayeeda Azra Jabeen, MD, FACP

A 72-year-old Man With Diarrhea

A 72-year-old man is admitted to the hospital 7 days ago with a fall resulting in a left hip fracture. He underwent successful surgery to repair the hip fracture with an open reduction internal fixation procedure. He has been progressing well with physical therapy. His pain is well controlled with hydrocodone. Other medications include metoprolol, hydrochlorothiazide, simvastatin, docusate, ranitidine, and enoxaparin. He received antibiotics intraoperatively (ceftriaxone). He has no known drug allergies. He is a nonsmoker and does not drink alcohol. You were called by the nurse today because the patient has developed diarrhea that is described as loose, nonbloody stools. He had 2 episodes yesterday and 1 episode today. His vital signs are normal. His abdominal examination is unremarkable. Rectal examination reveals brown liquid stool in the vault that is Hemoccult negative.

1. **What is the most likely etiology of his diarrhea? How would you treat his diarrhea?**

Answer

1. His diarrhea is likely medication induced. It is unlikely antibiotic-related given that he only received the ceftriaxone intraoperatively and the surgery was 7 days ago. The most likely offending medications include docusate as well as metoprolol and ranitidine. Non-antibiotic-associated diarrhea (non-AAD) generally improves with removal of the offending medication(s). No additional treatment is usually needed.

A 78-year-old Woman With Profuse Diarrhea

A 78-year-old woman was admitted to the hospital 2 weeks ago with a community-acquired pneumonia. She was initially started on levofloxacin IV. Despite antibiotics, her condition deteriorated, and she required intubation and mechanical ventilation. In the ICU, her antibiotics were changed to piperacillin, tazobactam, and cefuroxime. Tube feeds were initiated while she was on the ventilator. She improved clinically and was extubated 3 days ago. Since transfer to the general medical floor, she developed profuse, watery, nonbloody diarrhea that is foul smelling. Episodes occur 6 to 8 times per day. She has no fever or chills. Her white blood cell count is elevated to 14,000.

1. **What is the most likely etiology of her diarrhea? How would you treat her diarrhea?**

Answer

1. *Clostridum difficile*–induced diarrhea is the most likely etiology given her antibiotic usage. The description of the diarrhea is also consistent with *C. difficile*–induced diarrhea. Although she was on tube feeds, the clinical course and the elevated white blood cell count make tube feed–induced diarrhea unlikely. She should be started on oral metronidazole while awaiting the results of stool testing for *C. difficile* toxin.

HOSPITAL-ACQUIRED DIARRHEA

Hospital-acquired diarrhea is defined as 3 or more loose bowel movements per day, for at least 2 days and occurring after 72 hours of admission.

Diarrhea acquired in the hospital can be broadly classified into 2 major categories:

    A. Non-AAD

    B. AAD

Non-antibiotic-associated Diarrhea

This diarrhea is caused by agents, other than antibiotics, started during hospitalization. The classic presentation is diarrhea that is benign and self-limited. It is recognized by a lack of constitutional symptoms such as fever, large-volume diarrhea, dehydration, abdominal pain, or leukocytosis. Diarrhea resolves once the offending agent is discontinued.

The pathogenesis of non-AAD is due to nonosmotic means or as a result of recognized side effects of medications. Many drugs contain inert carriers for the active compound. These inert carriers, however, are osmotically active. Inert carriers, such as sorbitol, magnesium, and docusate sodium, may cause diarrhea. Table 13-1 shows the most commonly used medications and agents that cause diarrhea.

Diagnosis

Most episodes of non-AAD do not require any investigation or imaging. A good history, a thorough physical examination, including rectal examination (to assess

Table 13-1. Medications That Cause Diarrhea

Common Medications Causing Diarrhea Through Nonosmotic Effect	Magnesium-containing Medications	Medications Containing Osmotic Agents	Others Agents Causing Diarrhea
• Colchicine • Chemotherapeutic agents • Cholinergic agents • Digoxin • H$_2$ blockers • Metformin • Metoclopramide • Misoprostol • NSAIDs • Olsalazine • Proponolol • Quinidine • Serotonin receptor uptake inhibitors	• Nutritional supplements • Antacids • Laxatives	• Ingestion of elixir containing sorbitol or mannitol (such as acetaminophen or theophylline)	• Tube feeds (occur in 30% of patients on general medical and surgical floors) • Bowel preparation • Contrast agents • Fecal impaction/overflow incontinence

for fecal impaction), and a thorough chart review to look for any offending agents should be performed. Non-AAD is noninfectious and self-limited, and investigations should be performed only if the results will influence management and outcome. Routine stool examination for enteric pathogens, ova, and parasites is usually unrewarding and not cost-effective. One does not need to and should not order stool studies for ova and parasites in patients with hospital-acquired diarrhea, especially in immunocompetent patients.

Treatment

Identify and remove the offending agent. Most patients do not require specific therapy, as the diarrhea is self-limiting. Therapy should mainly be directed at preventing dehydration.

Antibiotic-associated Diarrhea

AAD is the most common cause of diarrhea in hospitalized patients, representing an important source of morbidity, mortality, and cost. It is estimated that 10% to 15% of all hospitalized patients treated with antibiotics will develop AAD.

The pathogenesis is due to prolonged use of multiple antibiotics, especially broad-spectrum agents with poor intestinal absorption or high biliary excretion. These antibiotics induce a change in the composition and function of the intestinal flora and therefore result in a higher incidence of AAD. A decrease in the colonic anaerobic flora interferes with carbohydrate and bile acid metabolism. Osmotic or secretary diarrhea may occur. Overgrowth of opportunistic pathogens takes place as a result of microbiologic and metabolic alterations.

AAD can be classified into 2 distinct categories:

  i. Diarrhea related to the direct effects of antibiotics

  ii. Diarrhea related to an enteric pathogen (primarily C. difficile)

Diarrhea related to the direct effects of antibiotics

Diagnosis This diarrhea often presents as an annoyance, presenting with frequent loose and watery stools without fever, leukocytosis, or severe abdominal cramps. Diarrhea occurs due to a change in the composition and function of intestinal flora. Additionally, nonantimicrobial effects of antibiotics can occur. Erythromycin can act as a motilin receptor agonist and accelerate the rate of gastric emptying, thus causing diarrhea. The clavulanate in amoxicillin–clavulanate appears to stimulate small bowel motility, thus causing diarrhea. In rare instances, penicillins may cause segmental colitis, resulting in diarrhea. Some antibiotics, such as clindamycin, cephalosporins, ampicillin, amoxicillin, and amoxicillin–clavulanate, can cause both types of diarrhea.

Typically, no pathogens are identified. There is no diagnostic test specific for benign, self-limiting AAD. One should not order routine stool culture for ova and parasites in patients with hospital-acquired diarrhea, especially in immunocompetent patients with a benign presentation.

Treatment Effective treatment is generally limited to discontinuation of the implicated agent, with or without therapy with antiperistaltic agents. Probiotics such as live culture yogurt may be helpful.

Diarrhea related to enteric pathogens (primarily due to C. *difficile* infection)

Enteric pathogen-related diarrhea accounts for 15% to 20% of all AAD cases (Table 13-2).

The cardinal symptom of the disease is diarrhea, which can range from a mild illness to life-threatening pseudomembranous colitis. C. difficile infection (CDI) manifests with a profuse, mucous, foul-smelling diarrhea associated with cramps and tenesmus. Frank bleeding is rare, although fecal occult blood and leukocytes are frequently detected. Constitutional symptoms are common, and include nausea, vomiting, dehydration, and low-grade fever. Mild leukocytosis is frequently present and may occur even in the absence of diarrhea. An occasional leukemoid reaction can be seen. Diarrhea commonly develops during treatment but may appear as late as 8 weeks after discontinuation of antibiotics. CDI should be highly suspected in patients with leukocytosis of unknown etiology even in the absence of diarrhea, especially in the severely ill elderly, hospitalized patient on

Table 13-2. Antimicrobial Agents That May Induce *Clostridium difficile* Diarrhea or Colitis

Frequently Associated	Occasionally Associated	Rarely Associated
Fluoroquinolones, clindamycin, penicillins (broad spectrum), cephalosporins (broad spectrum)	Macrolides Trimethoprim Sulfonamides	Aminoglycosides, tetracyclines, chloramphenicol, metronidazole, vancomycin (drugs used to treat *C. difficile* can rarely cause *C. difficile* diarrhea)

antimicrobials or those who have recently completed a course of antimicrobials, including antifungal agents.

   C. difficile causes diarrhea via toxin-mediated effects on the large bowel. Both *C. difficile* toxins A and B exhibit potent enterotoxic and cytotoxic effects that are responsible for the clinical manifestations. Toxic megacolon and subsequent perforation are possible complications if the CDI goes untreated. A dramatic clinical picture of marked colonic distention, peritoneal irritation, fever, and elevated white blood count may occur. Hypoalbuminemia, hypovolemia, and ascites are common features.

Diagnosis Cytotoxin assay or tissue culture assays are considered to be the gold standard with 94% to 100% sensitivity and 99% specificity, but cell culture tests are expensive, time-consuming, and rarely used in clinical practice. The most preferred diagnostic method in *C. difficile* colitis is the enzyme-linked immunosorbent assay (ELISA). ELISA is fast, relatively inexpensive, and has an excellent specificity (99%). Its sensitivity, however, is 60% to 95%. Serial stool determinations on different days are suggested for suspected cases with initial negative results. Polymerase chain reaction (PCR) appears to be a rapid, more sensitive and specific test compared with ELISA, which is important for prompt implementation of treatment and infection control. Major clinical laboratories are adopting PCR as the primary tool to detect *C. difficile*. Repeat PCR within 7 days is of no utility, unless patients develop new symptoms. Imaging is usually not required in mild cases. Abdominal CT scan in patients with pseudomembranous colitis demonstrates pronounced colonic wall thickening. If suspecting toxic megacolon, a plain abdominal x-ray may show marked colonic distention (>7 cm) or thumbprinting, with or without pneumatosis intestinalis. CT often reveals colonic wall thickening, lumen obliteration, pericolonic fat stranding, and ascites with toxic megacolon.

Treatment Indication for treatment:

1. Patients with typical CDI manifestations and a positive diagnostic assay.
2. Empirical therapy is indicated in patients with a high suspicion of CDI pending diagnostic test results.

Treatment is *not* indicated in patients who have a positive diagnostic assay, but are asymptomatic.

The initial step in the treatment of CDI is tapering the antibiotic regimen and cessation of the inciting antibiotic as soon as possible given other comorbid illness. Infection control practices must be implemented, including contact precautions and hand hygiene. Hand hygiene should include washing using soap and water, as this is more effective than alcohol-based agents in removing *C. difficile* spores.

Treatment of initial episode of nonsevere *C. difficile* infection

Metronidazole can be used for initial treatment of nonsevere CDI. The recommended regimen is 500 mg 3 times daily or 250 mg 4 times daily for 10 to 14 days. An alternative agent is oral vancomycin 125 mg orally 4 times daily for 10 to 14 days.

Oral vancomycin should be reserved for the following conditions:

• The patient has failed therapy with metronidazole.

• The patient's organism is resistant to metronidazole.

• The patient is allergic to, or cannot tolerate, metronidazole.

• The patient is pregnant.

Metronidazole is preferred due to low cost and comparable efficacy, and to limit the spread of vancomycin-resistant enterococci (VRE). Patients with underlying infections, along with *C. difficile* diarrhea, with prolonged use of antibiotics should continue CDI treatment throughout the course of antibiotic plus 1 additional week after its completion. Routine stool assay is not recommended during the course or following treatment of CDI, in patients who are recovering or symptom-free. Up to 50% of these patients have a positive test.

Treatment of severe *C. difficile* infection

Patients with acute CDI may develop signs of systemic toxicity with or without profuse diarrhea warranting admission to an intensive care unit or emergency surgery. There is no general consensus on the definition of severe CDI.

The following definition has been described in the literature:

1. White blood cell count of >15,000 cells/μL or a serum creatinine level $\geq$1.5 times the premorbid condition.

2. White blood cell count >20,000 cells/μL and an elevated serum creatinine as potential indicators of complicated disease.

3. One point each was given for age >60 years, temperature >38.3°C, serum albumin <2.5 mg/dL (25 g/L), or peripheral white blood cell count >15,000 cells/μL within 48 hours of enrollment. Two points were given for endoscopic evidence of pseudomembranous colitis or treatment in the intensive care unit. Patients with 2 or more points were considered to have severe disease.

4. Severe disease is defined as having >10 bowel movements per day, WBC >20,000 cells/µL, or severe abdominal pain.

Decisions regarding treatment are left up to the clinician to decide based on the severity of the disease. Any or all of the above criteria can be used to rate the severity of the disease.

Oral vancomycin 125 or 500 mg (many physicians tend to use a higher dose, although there is no evidence 500 mg is better than 125 mg) orally 4 times daily, *plus* intravenous metronidazole 500 mg every 8 hours for 10 to 14 days, is suggested. Fecal concentrations in the therapeutic range are achieved with this regimen because of biliary and intestinal excretion of metronidazole. Fidaxomicin (bactericidal) 200 mg twice daily for 10 days is recommended in patients who cannot tolerate vancomycin. In patients with significant ileus, intracolonic vancomycin is recommended. One needs to be aware though that this method involves the risk of perforation. Enemas should be given with caution.

Relapse is defined as complete resolution of symptoms while a patient is on CDI treatment and reappearance of diarrhea and other symptoms after completion of CDI treatment.

1. First relapses can occur in 25% of patients. Repeat treatment similar to the first episode with oral metronidazole or vancomycin is indicated as suggested above.

2. For a second relapse, intermittent and tapering vancomycin therapy is suggested. Alternatively, fidaxomicin 200 mg orally twice daily for 10 days can be used.

3. Subsequent relapses can occur in 65% of cases. Use vancomycin 125 mg orally 4 times daily for 14 days, followed by rifaximin 400 mg twice daily for 14 days. Alternatively, fidaxomicin 200 mg orally twice daily for 10 days can be used.

Other potential agents such as new antibiotics, binding resins, probiotics, intravenous immunoglobulins (IVIG), and fecal bacteriotherapy require further investigation prior to routine use. Urgent surgical evaluation for elderly patients (≥65 years) with a white blood cell count ≥20,000 cells/mL and/or a plasma lactate between 2.2 and 4.9 mEq/L is recommended. In addition, surgical intervention is advisable in the setting of peritoneal signs, severe ileus, or toxic megacolon.

TIPS TO REMEMBER

- Diarrhea acquired in the hospital can be broadly classified into 2 major categories: non-AAD and AAD.

- Laboratory evaluation should only include assessment for *C. difficile* and only in patients at risk. Additional stool studies are not needed.

● Metronidazole should be the initial treatment of nonsevere CDI.
    Treatment is not indicated in patients who have a positive *C. difficile* diagnostic assay, but are asymptomatic.

● Oral vancomycin should be used only if the patient is *pregnant or allergic to metronidazole*, has failed metronidazole therapy, or the organism is resistant to metronidazole.

SUGGESTED READINGS

Aranda-Michel J, Giannella RA. Acute diarrhea: a practical review. *Am J Med.* 1999;106(6):670–676 [Epub 1999/06/23].

Bartlett JG. Clinical practice. Antibiotic-associated diarrhea. *N Engl J Med.* 2002;346(5):334–339 [Epub 2002/02/01]. doi:10.1056/NEJMcp011603.

Gilligan PH. Diarrheal disease in the hospitalized patient. *Infect Control.* 1986;7(12):607–609 [Epub 1986/12/01].

Kelly C, Lamont T. Treatment of *Clostridium difficile* infection in adults. In: Calderwood S, Baron E, eds. *UpToDate.* 2012.

Kyne L, Moran A, Keane C, O'Neill D. Hospital-acquired diarrhea in elderly patients: epidemiology and staff awareness. *Age Ageing.* 1998;27(3):339–343. doi:10.1093/ageing/27.3.339.

Lamont T. Clinical manifestations and diagnosis of *Clostridium difficile* infection in adults. In: Calderwood S, Baron E, eds. *UpToDate.* 2012.

Lamont T. Epidemiology, microbiology, and pathophysiology of *Clostridium difficile* infection in adults. In: Calderwood S, Baron E, eds. *UpToDate.* 2012.

Pimental R. *Antibiotic-associated Diarrhea and Clostridium difficile.* 2010. <http://www.clevelandclinicmeded.com/medicalpubs/diseasemanagement/gastroenterology/antibiotic-associated-diarrhea/>.

Stern S, Cifu A, Altkorn D. Diarrhea, acute. In: Benoit J, Stein S, eds. *Symptom to Diagnosis: An Evidence Based Guide.* 2nd ed. New York: McGraw-Hill (Lange Clinical Medicine); 2010.

Thielman NM, Guerrant RL. Clinical practice. Acute infectious diarrhea. *N Engl J Med.* 2004;350(1):38–47 [Epub 2004/01/02]. doi:10.1056/NEJMcp031534.

Yamada T. Approach to the patient with diarrhea. In: Yamada T, ed. *Handbook of Gastroenterology.* Philadelphia: Lippincott Williams & Wilkins; 1998:84–96: [chapter 12].

An 86-year-old Woman With Fever and Chills

Muhammad Farooq Asghar, MD

An 86-year-old African American female with a history of hypertension, COPD, CHF with an ejection fraction (EF) of 40%, and coronary artery disease was admitted to the hospital 4 days ago with respiratory failure due to decompensation of her systolic heart failure. She was intubated in the ER and was transferred to the ICU for further management. In the ICU she required a central line due to poor IV access. A Foley catheter was placed for urine output monitoring. She was diuresed with Lasix successfully, and after 48 hours in the hospital she was extubated. She was maintaining her oxygen saturation of more than 90% on 4 L of O_2. She was then transferred to a regular floor. Her current medications include Lasix 80 mg IV bid, lisinopril 40 mg daily, amlodipine 10 mg daily, metoprolol 50 mg bid, aspirin 325 mg bid, Spiriva inhaler qday, and enoxaparin 40 mg SQ daily. Now, 4 days after the admission, the patient is complaining of fever and chills since last night. She denies any cough, sputum production, postnasal drip, diarrhea, abdominal pain, suprapubic tenderness, or flank pain.

Her vitals are temperature 39.2°C, BP 135/85 mm Hg, pulse 110/min, and respiratory rate 18/min. She is awake, alert, and oriented; central line in the internal jugular vein is without evidence of any discharge or surrounding erythema. There is 1+ pedal edema bilaterally. Cardiac examination shows a normal S1 and S2 without any gallops or murmur; respiratory examination shows vesicular breathing with bibasilar crackles (which have improved since admission 4 days ago). Abdomen is soft and nontender and bowel sounds are normal. Neurologic examination is nonfocal. Skin examination does not reveal any abnormalities. The patient still has a Foley catheter in place.

1. What is your diagnosis?

2. What is your next step in evaluation?

Answers

1. The patient has a nosocomial fever at present, which by definition is a fever of at least 38.3°C occurring in a hospitalized patient at least 48 hours after admission in whom neither fever nor infection was present on admission.

2. Once we have confirmed the fever, the next step is figuring out its source. The patient has had a thorough history and physical examination, which failed to reveal any etiology of fever, so we will start our evaluation with CBC, CMP, blood cultures × 2, urinalysis, and a chest x-ray.

Fever is a sign of inflammation, not infection. It is not a specific response to infection, but rather is a response to any form of tissue injury that is sufficient

153

enough to trigger an inflammatory response. This might explain why some hospitalized patients with fever have no apparent infection. The distinction between inflammation and infection is an important one, not only for the evaluation of fever but also for curtailing the use of antibiotics to treat a fever. The severity of the fever is not an indication of the presence or severity of infection. High fevers can be associated with noninfectious processes (eg, drug fever), while fever can be mild or absent in patients with life-threatening infections.

FEVER IN HOSPITALIZED PATIENTS

For several reasons, fever that develops in the hospitalized patients warrants a thoughtful evaluation. First, hospitalized patients are usually severely ill and often have complex underlying illnesses. Second, organisms commonly found in nosocomial infections in seriously ill patients include *Staphylococcus aureus*, *Enterococcus*, gram-negative bacilli, and fungi. Infections due to these organisms are characterized by necrotizing destruction of tissue, high rates of associated blood invasion, and relative resistance to antibiotic treatment. Third, hospital-acquired organisms are likely to exhibit broad resistance to antimicrobials, making empiric and even definitive selection of treatment difficult. Finally, fever may herald exacerbation or progression of the disease that prompted hospitalization.

Diagnosis

If the patient is able to communicate, he or she should be interviewed to identify localizing complaints. The patient and hospital chart should be reviewed thoroughly for a history of relevant antecedent problems (eg, prior postoperative staphylococcal infections, renal disease, allergic reactions to drugs). If the patient is unable to communicate, the chart and medical personnel can provide helpful information concerning duration of intravascular accesses, amount and purulence of sputum or wound drainage, changes in skin condition, apparent abdominal or musculoskeletal pain or tenderness, difficulty in handling respiratory secretions and feeding, and changes in supplemental oxygen.

A thorough physical examination is mandatory.

- Skin examination may demonstrate findings suggestive of drug reaction, vasculitis, endocarditis, or soft tissue necrosis.

- All intravenous and intra-arterial line sites should be inspected; a tender intravenous access site, with or without purulence, can indicate septic thrombophlebitis. Spreading erythema, warmth, and tenderness that appear to indicate cellulitis of an extremity also can be the hallmarks of deep venous thrombophlebitis, pyarthrosis, or gout.

- After the first 24 hours postoperatively, wounds should be examined; this may require fenestrating or changing a cast to allow examination of a fractured extremity if no other source of fever is found.

- Head and neck examination can provide important signs of systemic and localized infection.
- Purulent sinusitis can occur in the nasally or orally intubated patient and may have a paucity of associated symptoms.
- Cardiac examination may demonstrate a pericardial friction rub due to Dressler syndrome in a patient with an acute myocardial infarction or a new or changing murmur possibly due to endocarditis.
- Abdominal findings can be misleadingly unremarkable in the elderly, in the patient with obtunded sensorium, and in the patient receiving sedatives. They may be confounding in the patient with recent abdominal or thoracic surgery. Abdominal pain and tenderness may be localized (cholecystitis, intra-abdominal abscess, diverticulitis) or generalized (diffuse peritonitis, ischemic bowel, antibiotic-associated colitis). Examination of the genitalia and rectum may demonstrate unsuspected epididymitis, prostatitis, prostatic abscess, or perirectal abscess.

Blood cultures are the only mandatory diagnostic tests in patients with a new fever; the rationale is that clinical findings cannot reliably exclude bacteremia and mortality is high without appropriate treatment. Further investigation may be indicated depending on the clinical assessment.

- Sputum: Sputum Gram stain and culture are indicated for febrile patients with any of the following findings—new sputum production; a change in the color, amount, or thickness of their sputum; a new or progressive pulmonary infiltrate; an increased respiratory rate; or requiring more inspired oxygen.
- Urine: Urinalysis and urine culture are indicated for febrile patients with a urethral catheter, urinary obstruction, renal calculi, recent genitourinary surgery or trauma, or neutropenia.
- Chest imaging: A chest radiograph is easily obtainable in the hospital and worthwhile in many patients with respiratory symptoms or signs. It may detect a new or progressive pulmonary infiltrate and identify a respiratory source of fever other than pneumonia or tracheobronchitis that would otherwise be missed because it may not be associated with sputum production.
- Laboratory studies: Transaminase, bilirubin, alkaline phosphatase, amylase, lipase, and lactate measurements are indicated for patients with abdominal pain or whose abdominal examination cannot be reliably assessed. Serum sodium, potassium, glucose, and cortisol levels should be drawn if adrenal insufficiency is in the differential. Thyroid-stimulating hormone (TSH), T3, and T4 levels should be drawn if thyroid storm is possible. Blood should be drawn for measurement of direct antiglobulin, plasma free hemoglobin, and haptoglobin, as well as a repeat blood type and crossmatch if an acute hemolytic transfusion reaction is suspected.

- Abdominal imaging: Abdominal imaging is indicated for patients with symptoms or signs of an intra-abdominal process, but for whom laboratory testing has not identified the cause of the symptoms or signs. It is also indicated for patients who have a reason to have an intra-abdominal infection and no alternative source of the fever has been identified, even if there are no symptoms or signs of an abdominal process. Finally, abdominal imaging may be indicated if laboratory testing suggests a possible intra-abdominal process, but the results are insufficient to identify the exact abnormality.

- Sinus evaluation: Evaluation for sinusitis is appropriate for patients who were recently mechanically ventilated and who have purulent nasal drainage or whose evaluation has otherwise been completely negative. The evaluation begins with a radiographic evaluation looking for sinus opacification. CT is the preferred modality, but sinus radiographs and sinus ultrasound are reasonable alternatives. Culture of sinus fluid obtained by endoscopic-guided middle meatus aspiration is indicated for patients with sinus opacification and no other cause for fever.

- It is important for the clinician to keep several things in mind when investigating a fever. First, clinicians should remain mindful that hospitalized patients often have more than 1 infection. Second, evidence of infection and inflammation (eg, leukocytosis, pus) may be altered if the patient is immunosuppressed.

Treatment

Treatment of fever should be directed at its underlying causes, which are discussed in separate chapters in this book.

Perhaps the 2 most common clinical decisions that need to be made when a patient develops a new fever in the hospital are whether or not empiric antibiotic therapy is warranted and whether or not the patient's offending intravascular catheter needs to be removed:

- Hospitalized patients who develop a new fever should be treated with empiric antibiotics if they are deteriorating, in shock, neutropenic, or have a ventricular assist device. Empiric therapy should also be started for patients who have a temperature ≥38.9°C because most fevers in this range will be infectious. For most other patients, further diagnostic workup with ongoing clinical assessment prior to the initiation of antibiotic therapy is reasonable.

- Whether or not to routinely remove an intravascular catheter (or other device) in a febrile patient is a controversial and evolving issue. Generally speaking, considerations in the decision include the severity of illness, age of the catheter, and probability that the catheter is the source of fever.

- Fever itself does not generally require treatment with antipyretics (eg, acetaminophen) or external cooling (eg, cooling blanket, ice packs). Exceptions to this are when the fever may be detrimental to the outcome (eg, increased intracranial pressure) or is ≥41.0°C. If body temperature exceeds the "critical thermal maximum," which is thought to be 41.6°C, life-threatening complications can ensue (eg, rhabdomyolysis).

Fever in hospitalized patients can be categorized into infectious and noninfectious causes.

Common causes of fever in hospitalized patients include:

A. *Infections*:

  1. Pneumonia

  2. UTI

  3. Catheter-related bloodstream infections (CRBSIs)

  4. Surgical site infection

  5. *C. difficle* colitis

  6. Sinusitis

  7. Abdominal abscess

  8. Other infections

B. *Noninfectious causes*:

  1. Drug-induced fever

  2. Reaction to blood products

  3. Deep venous thrombophlebitis

  4. Pulmonary embolism (PE)

  5. Infarctions

  6. Acute pancreatitis

  7. Acalculous cholecystitis

  8. Adrenal insufficiency

  9. Malignant hyperthermia

  10. Neuroleptic malignant syndrome (NMS)

  11. Serotonin syndrome (SS)

  12. Postoperative fever

  13. Fever related to procedures

Infections in hospitalized patients

Hospital-acquired pneumonia Hospital-acquired (or nosocomial) pneumonia (HAP) is pneumonia that occurs 48 hours or more after admission and did not appear to be incubating at the time of admission.

The most common organisms responsible for HAP are *P. aeruginosa*, *S. aureus including MRSA, Enterobacter, K. pneumoniae, Escherichia coli, Proteus, Serratia marcescens, H. influenzae,* and streptococci. Additional information can be found in Chapter 22. The symptoms and signs associated with HAP include fever, cough, increasing oxygen requirements, purulent sputum, and abnormal breath sounds.

UTI in hospitalized patients Nosocomial urinary tract infections are a common complication in hospitalized patients. The use of urinary catheters is the major risk factor for the development of these infections. Urinary tract infection should be suspected as a cause of nosocomial fever in any patient who has had an indwelling bladder catheter for more than a few days. The diagnosis of urinary tract infection is difficult in chronically catheterized patients because the urine in these patients often contains large numbers of bacteria. Therefore, a positive urine culture is not always evidence of infection in a chronically instrumented patient. Additional information can be found in Chapter 42.

Catheter-related bloodstream infection Infections caused by indwelling vascular catheters should be suspected in any case of unexplained fever when a catheter has been in place for more than 48 hours, or when purulence is found at the catheter insertion site. Other clinical manifestations include hemodynamic instability, altered mental status, catheter dysfunction (as occurs with intraluminal clot), and clinical signs of sepsis that start abruptly after catheter infusion. Complications related to a bloodstream infection (such as suppurative thrombophlebitis, endocarditis, osteomyelitis, metastatic infection) may also be observed. Paired blood samples drawn from the catheter and a peripheral vein should be obtained for culture prior to initiation of antibiotic therapy.

Microbiologic confirmation of CRBSI may be made based on blood cultures obtained prior to initiation of antibiotic therapy based on fulfilling at least 1 of the following criteria:

A. The same organism from both the culture of the catheter tip and at least 1 percutaneous blood culture

B. Culture of the same organism from at least 2 blood samples (1 from a catheter hub and the other from a peripheral vein or second lumen) meeting criteria for quantitative blood cultures or differential time to positivity

Most laboratories do not perform quantitative blood cultures, but many laboratories are able to determine differential time to positivity. Quantitative blood cultures demonstrating a colony count from the catheter hub sample ≥3-fold higher than the colony count from the peripheral vein sample (or a second lumen) support a diagnosis of CRBSI. Semiquantitative cultures demonstrating >15 cfu/mL of the same microbe from the insertion site, hub site, and peripheral blood culture also support a diagnosis of CRBSI. Differential time to positivity refers to growth detected from the catheter hub sample at least 2 hours before growth detected from the peripheral vein sample. Sensitivity and specificity for this technique are very good (85% and 91%, respectively).

In general, the first step for treatment of systemic intravenous catheter-related infection requires a determination regarding catheter management.

Catheter removal is warranted in the following circumstances:

- Severe sepsis
- Hemodynamic instability
- Endocarditis or evidence of metastatic infection
- Erythema or exudate due to suppurative thrombophlebitis
- Persistent bacteremia after 72 hours of antimicrobial therapy to which the organism is susceptible

Catheters that have been left in place should be removed if cultures confirm the presence of catheter-related septicemia. There are 2 situations in which catheters can be left in place if the patient shows a favorable response to antimicrobial therapy:

A. When catheter removal is not easily accomplished (eg, tunneled catheters)

B. When the responsible organism is *Staphylococcus epidermidis*

However, relapse after systemic antimicrobial therapy is higher when catheters have been left in place, and this relapse is less likely when antibiotic lock therapy is used.

Empiric antibiotic therapy for CRBSI in health care settings should include activity against methicillin-resistant *S. aureus*; vancomycin is a reasonable agent. Patients with neutropenia or sepsis should also receive empiric antibiotic therapy for gram-negative organisms (including *Pseudomonas*). Patients known to be colonized with drug-resistant organisms should receive empiric antibiotic therapy selected accordingly; therapy should be tailored based on subsequent culture data. Following initiation of empiric treatment, antibiotic therapy should be tailored to culture and susceptibility results once data are available.

In general, transesophageal echocardiogram (TEE) should be pursued in the setting of *S. aureus* bacteremia to rule out infective endocarditis (IE). Possible exceptions include patients whose fever and bacteremia resolve within 72 hours following catheter removal and who have no underlying cardiac predisposing conditions or clinical signs of endocarditis.

In general, for uncomplicated CRBSI with negative blood cultures following catheter removal and institution of appropriate antibiotic therapy, the duration of therapy is 10 to 14 days (day 1 is the first day on which negative blood cultures are obtained). Patients with persistent bacteremia >72 hours following catheter removal should receive treatment for at least 4 to 6 weeks. For patients with complications related to bacteremia (such as suppurative thrombophlebitis, endocarditis, osteomyelitis, or metastatic infection), the duration of therapy should be tailored accordingly depending on the nature of infection. Patients with CRBSI must be monitored closely during and following therapy to detect relapses or signs of metastatic infection. Blood cultures should be drawn after treatment has been initiated to demonstrate clearance of bacteremia. Repeatedly positive blood cultures and/or persistent symptoms 72 hours after catheter removal with appropriate antibiotic therapy should prompt evaluation for sequelae of CRBSI such as those listed above.

Surgical site infection In hospitalized patients who have undergone surgical procedures, fever may develop due to surgical site infection. Wound infections typically appear at 5 to 7 days after surgery. Most infections do not extend beyond the skin and subcutaneous tissues, and can be managed with debridement and antimicrobial therapy to cover *Streptococcus*, *Staphylococcus*, and anaerobes.

Necrotizing wound infections are produced by Clostridia or β-hemolytic streptococci. Unlike other wound infections, which appear 5 to 7 days after surgery, necrotizing infections are evident in the first few postoperative days. There is often marked edema around the incision, and the skin may have crepitus and fluid-filled bullae. Spread to deeper structures is rapid and produces progressive rhabdomyolysis and myoglobinuric renal failure. Treatment involves extensive debridement and intravenous penicillin. The mortality is high (above 60%) when treatment is delayed.

Clostridium difficile colitis Enterocolitis from *C. difficile* should be suspected for cases of nosocomial fever accompanied by diarrhea in patients who have received antibiotics or chemotherapy within 2 weeks prior to the onset of the fever. The diagnosis requires documentation of *C. difficile* toxin in stool samples or evidence of pseudomembranes on proctosigmoidoscopy. A stool sample should be submitted for *C. difficile* toxin assay, and if it is negative, a second stool sample should be submitted.

Empiric antibiotics should not be necessary unless the diarrhea is severe or the patient appears toxic. Therapy can include oral or intravenous metronidazole or oral vancomycin for 10 to 14 days. Although rarely necessary, surgical intervention is required when *C. difficile* colitis is associated with progressive sepsis and multiorgan failure, or signs of peritonitis, despite antibiotic therapy. The procedure of choice is subtotal colectomy. Additional information can be found in Chapter 13.

Sinusitis Fever due to sinusitis should be considered in patients who were recently intubated or have indwelling nasogastric or nasotracheal tubes. Evaluation for sinusitis is appropriate for patients who have purulent nasal drainage or whose evaluation has otherwise been completely negative. The evaluation begins with a radiograph looking for sinus opacification. CT is the preferred modality, but sinus radiographs and sinus ultrasound are reasonable alternatives. Culture of sinus fluid obtained by endoscopic-guided middle meatus aspiration is indicated for patients with sinus opacification and no other cause for fever. Additional information can be found in Chapter 41.

Abdominal abscess An abdominal abscess may present with fever. Patients who undergo abdominal surgeries are at risk. Abdominal abscesses typically become symptomatic 1 to 2 weeks after laparotomy. Septicemia occurs in approximately 50% of cases. CT of the abdomen will reveal the localized collection in more than 95% of cases. Initial antimicrobial therapy should be directed at gram-negative enteric pathogens, including anaerobes (eg, *Bacteroides fragilis*), but definitive treatment requires surgical or percutaneous drainage.

Other infections Other infections that should be considered in selected patient populations are endocarditis (in patients with prosthetic valves), meningitis (in neurosurgical patients and those with human immunodeficiency virus infection), and spontaneous bacterial peritonitis (in patients with cirrhosis and ascites).

Noninfectious causes

Drug-induced fever Drug-induced fever can be the result of a hypersensitivity reaction, an idiosyncratic reaction, or an infusion-related phlebitis. The therapeutic agents most often implicated in drug fever are amphotericin, cephalosporins, penicillins, phenytoin, procainamide, quinidine, vancomycin, cimetidine, carbamazepine, hydralazine, and rifampin. The onset of the fever varies from a few hours to a few weeks after the onset of drug therapy. The fever can appear as an isolated finding or can be accompanied by other manifestations such as rigors, myalgias, leukocytosis, eosinophilia, rash, and hypotension. Approximately half of patients have rigors, and about 20% develop hypotension, indicating that patients with a drug fever can appear to be seriously ill. Evidence of a hypersensitivity reaction (ie, eosinophilia and rash) is absent in most cases of drug fever.

Drug fever is a diagnosis of exclusion. Suspicion of drug fever usually occurs when there are no other probable sources of fever. In the majority of patients, the only way to know if a patient has a drug fever is by stopping the drug(s). The usual approach is to discontinue the most probable offending drug first, followed sequentially by cessation of other drugs if fever persists. Discontinuing all medications at once may eliminate the fever but may also put the patient at risk from the underlying disease and prevent identification of the causative drug. In most, but not all, cases, resolution of drug fever will occur within 72 to 96 hours of discontinuing the offending drug.

Reaction to blood products Hospitalized patients who receive blood products can develop fever either due to acute hemolytic or nonhemolytic febrile reactions or sometimes due to transmission of infections. Additional information can be found in Chapter 28.

Deep venous thrombosis Sometimes DVT can present with fever, although more common manifestations of DVT include asymmetric extremity edema, pain, or erythema. In a febrile patient, if no other etiology for fever is identified and the patient is at high risk for DVT, the patient should be evaluated with venous Dopplers of both lower extremities. Additional information can be found in Chapter 29.

Pulmonary embolism Fever in hospitalized patients can be associated with PE. The most common symptoms of acute PE are dyspnea (at rest or with exertion), pleuritic pain, cough, >2-pillow orthopnea, calf or thigh pain or swelling, and wheezing. The most common signs are tachypnea, tachycardia, rales, decreased breath sounds, an accentuated pulmonic component of the second heart sound, and jugular venous distension. Additional information can be found in Chapter 29.

Infarctions Ischemic injury in any organ will trigger a local inflammatory response and this can produce a fever. Myocardial and cerebrovascular infarctions are usually heralded by other symptoms, but bowel infarction can be clinically silent in the elderly, debilitated patients or patients with depressed consciousness. The only sign of a bowel infarction may be an unexplained fever or metabolic (lactic) acidosis. Additional information can be found in Chapters 1, 3, and 26.

Acute pancreatitis Fever can be a prominent symptom in acute pancreatitis. Additional information can be found in Chapter 1.

Acalculous cholecystitis Acalculous cholecystitis is an uncommon but serious disorder reported in up to 1.5% of critically ill patients. The clinical manifestations of acalculous cholecystitis include fever, nausea and vomiting, abdominal pain, and right upper quadrant tenderness. Abdominal findings can be minimal or absent, and fever may be the only presenting manifestation. Elevations in serum bilirubin, alkaline phosphatase, and amylase can occur but are variable. Additional information can be found in Chapter 1.

Adrenal insufficiency An adrenal crisis usually occurs in patients with previously undiagnosed adrenal insufficiency when subjected to a serious infection or other major stress, patients with known adrenal insufficiency who do not take more glucocorticoid during a serious infection or other major stress, patients with acute bilateral adrenal infarction or hemorrhage, or patients whose chronic glucocorticoid therapy is abruptly withdrawn. Distributive shock is the predominant manifestation of an adrenal crisis, but fever, nausea, vomiting, abdominal pain, weakness, fatigue, lethargy, hypoglycemia, confusion, or coma may also be present. Acute adrenal crisis is more commonly seen in primary adrenal insufficiency (Addison disease) than in disorders of the pituitary gland causing secondary adrenocortical hypofunction.

An early morning low serum cortisol concentration (less than 3 μg/dL [80 nmol/L]) is strongly suggestive of adrenal insufficiency especially if accompanied by simultaneous elevation of plasma ACTH level (usually >200 pg/mL). The diagnosis is made by a simplified cosyntropin stimulation test, which is performed as follows: (1) synthetic $ACTH_{1-24}$ (cosyntropin), 0.25 mg, is given parenterally and (2) serum is obtained for cortisol between 30 and 60 minutes after cosyntropin is administered. Normally, serum cortisol should rise to at least 20 μg/dL. Failure of an appropriate rise in cortisol levels in response to ACTH indicates primary adrenal insufficiency.

If the diagnosis is suspected acutely, draw a blood sample for cortisol determination and treat with hydrocortisone, 100 to 300 mg intravenously, and saline *immediately*, without waiting for the results. Thereafter, give hydrocortisone phosphate or hydrocortisone sodium succinate, 100 mg intravenously immediately, and continue intravenous infusions of 50 to 100 mg every 6 hours for the first day. Give the same amount every 8 hours on the second day, and then adjust the dosage in view of the clinical picture.

When the patient is able to take food by mouth, give oral hydrocortisone, 10 to 20 mg every 6 hours, and reduce the dosage to maintenance levels as needed. Most patients ultimately require hydrocortisone twice daily (AM, 10–20 mg; PM, 5–10 mg). Mineralocorticoid therapy is not needed when large amounts of hydrocortisone are being given, but as the dose is reduced it is usually necessary to add fludrocortisone acetate, 0.05 to 0.2 mg daily. Some patients never require fludrocortisone or become edematous at doses of more than 0.05 mg once or twice weekly. Once the crisis has passed, the patient must be evaluated to assess the degree of permanent adrenal insufficiency and to establish the cause if possible.

Malignant hyperthermia A rare but important cause of elevated body temperatures in the immediate postoperative period is malignant hyperthermia. It is an inherited disorder with an autosomal dominant pattern, and it is characterized by excessive release of calcium from the sarcoplasmic reticulum in skeletal muscle in response to halogenated inhaled anesthetic agents (eg, halothane, isoflurane, sevoflurane, and desflurane) and depolarizing neuromuscular blockers (eg, succinylcholine). The calcium influx into the cell cytoplasm somehow leads to an uncoupling of oxidative phosphorylation and a marked rise in metabolic rate.

The clinical manifestations of malignant hyperthermia include hypercapnia, muscle rigidity, increased body temperature, depressed consciousness, and autonomic instability. The generalized muscle rigidity can progress rapidly to widespread myonecrosis (rhabdomyolysis) and subsequent myoglobinuric renal failure. The heat generated by the muscle rigidity is responsible for the marked rise in body temperature (often above 40°C) in malignant hyperthermia. The altered mental status in malignant hyperthermia can range from confusion and agitation to obtundation and coma. Autonomic instability can lead to cardiac arrhythmias, fluctuating blood pressure, or persistent hypotension.

The first suspicion of malignant hyperthermia should prompt immediate discontinuation of the offending anesthetic agent. Specific treatment for the muscle rigidity is available with dantrolene sodium, a muscle relaxant that blocks the release of calcium from the sarcoplasmic reticulum. When given early in the course of malignant hyperthermia, dantrolene can reduce the mortality rate from 70% or higher (in untreated cases) to 10% or less. Treatment is extended to 3 days to prevent recurrences. Patients should be aggressively hydrated to keep adequate urine output, and cooling blankets should be used to keep body temperature below 38.5°C. Patients' electrolytes and renal functions as well as CBCs should be monitored closely because these patients can have deranged electrolytes and renal failure due to rhabdomyolysis. They are also prone to develop DIC.

Neuroleptic malignant syndrome NMS is strikingly similar to malignant hyperthermia in that it is a drug-induced disorder characterized by 4 clinical features: increased body temperature, muscle rigidity, altered mental status, and autonomic instability. As the name implies, NMS is caused by neuroleptic agents. Note that drugs other than neuroleptic agents can trigger NMS, so the name of this syndrome is misleading.

Most cases of NMS begin to appear 24 to 72 hours after the onset of drug therapy, and almost all cases are apparent in the first 2 weeks of drug therapy. The onset is usually gradual, and can take days to fully develop. In 80% of cases, the initial manifestation is muscle rigidity or altered mental status. The change in mental status can range from confusion and agitation to obtundation and coma. Hyperthermia (body temperature can exceed 41°C) is required for the diagnosis of NMS, but the increase in body temperature can be delayed for 8 to 10 hours after the appearance of muscle rigidity or change in mental status. Autonomic instability can produce cardiac arrhythmias, labile blood pressure, or persistent hypotension.

The serum CK level should be higher than 1000 U/L in NMS. The leukocyte count in blood can increase to 40,000/μL with a leftward shift in NMS, so the clinical presentation of NMS (fever, leukocytosis, altered mental status, hypotension) can be confused with sepsis. The serum CK level will distinguish NMS from sepsis.

The single most important measure in the management of NMS is immediate removal of the offending drug. If NMS is caused by discontinuation of dopaminergic therapy, it should be restarted immediately with plans for a gradual reduction in dosage at a later time. General measures, including volume resuscitation and evaluation for multiorgan involvement (eg, rhabdomyolysis), are the same as described for malignant hyperthermia.

Dantrolene sodium (the same muscle relaxant used in the treatment of malignant hyperthermia) can be given intravenously for severe cases of muscle rigidity. The risk of liver injury should be considered when using dantrolene in NMS because there are alternative treatments.

Bromocriptine is a dopamine agonist that has been successful in treating NMS when given orally in a dose of 2.5 to 10 mg 3 times daily. Some improvement in muscle rigidity can be seen within hours after the start of therapy, but the full response often takes days to develop. Hypotension is a troublesome side effect. There is no advantage of bromocriptine over dantrolene, except in patients with advanced liver disease (where dantrolene is not advised). Treatment of NMS should continue for about 10 days after clinical resolution because of delayed clearance of many neuroleptics (when depot preparations are implicated, therapy should continue for 2–3 weeks after clinical resolution).

Serotonin syndrome Another important cause of fever in hospitalized patients is SS. Overstimulation of serotonin receptors in the central nervous system produces a combination of mental status changes, autonomic hyperactivity, and neuromuscular abnormalities that are known as the SS. The severity of illness can vary widely in cases of SS, and the most severe cases can be confused with any of the other hyperthermia syndromes.

There are several serotonergic drugs that are capable of producing SS. These include:

- Drugs that decrease serotonin breakdown such as MAOIs (including linezolide)
- Drugs that increase serotonin release such as amphetamines, MDMA ("ecstasy"), cocaine, and fenfluramine
- Drugs that decrease serotonin reuptake such as SSRIs, TCAs, dextromethorphan, meperidine, fentanyl, and tramadol
- Serotonin receptor agonists such as lithium, sumatriptan, buspirone, and LSD

The onset of SS is usually abrupt (in contrast to NMS, where the full syndrome can take days to develop), and over half of the cases are evident within 6 hours after ingestion of the responsible drug(s). The clinical findings include mental status changes (eg, confusion, delirium, coma), autonomic hyperactivity (eg, mydriasis, tachycardia, hypertension, hyperthermia, diaphoresis), and neuromuscular abnormalities (eg, hyperkinesis, hyperactive deep tendon reflexes, clonus, and muscle rigidity). The clinical presentation can vary markedly. Mild cases may include only hyperkinesis, hyperreflexia, tachycardia, diaphoresis, and mydriasis. Moderate cases often have additional findings of hyperthermia (temperature >38°C), clonus, and agitation. The clonus is most obvious in the patellar deep tendon reflexes, and horizontal ocular clonus may also be present. Severe cases of SS often present with delirium, hyperpyrexia (temperature >40°C), widespread muscle rigidity, and spontaneous clonus. Life-threatening cases are marked by rhabdomyolysis, renal failure, metabolic acidosis, and hypotension.

The first step in the diagnostic evaluation is to establish recent ingestion of 1 or more serotonergic drugs. Hyperthermia and muscle rigidity can be absent in mild cases of the illness. The features that most distinguish SS from other hyperthermia syndromes are hyperkinesis, hyperreflexia, and clonus. However, in severe cases of SS, muscle rigidity can mask these clinical findings. Severe cases of SS can be difficult to distinguish from malignant hyperthermia and neuromuscular malignant syndrome, and the history of drug ingestion is important in these cases (although the same drugs can be implicated in NMS and SS).

As is the case with all drug-induced hyperthermia syndromes, removal of the precipitating drug(s) is the single most important element in the management of SS. The remainder of the management includes measures to control agitation and hyperthermia, and the use of serotonin antagonists. Many cases of SS will resolve within 24 hours after initiation of therapy, but serotonergic drugs with long elimination half-lives can produce more prolonged symptomatology.

Benzodiazepines are considered essential for the control of agitation and hyperkinesis in SS. Physical restraints should be avoided because they encourage isometric muscle contractions and this can aggravate skeletal muscle injury and promote lactic acidosis.

Cyproheptadine is a serotonin antagonist that can be given in severe cases of SS.

Neuromuscular paralysis may be required in severe cases of SS to control muscle rigidity and extreme elevations of body temperature (41°C). Nondepolarizing agents (eg, vecuronium) should be used for muscle paralysis because succinylcholine can aggravate the hyperkalemia that accompanies rhabdomyolysis.

Dantrolene is not effective in reducing the muscle rigidity and hyperthermia in SS.

Postoperative fever Surgery always involves some degree of tissue injury, and major surgery can involve considerable tissue injury. Because inflammation and fever are the normal response to tissue injury, fever is a likely consequence of major surgery. Fever in the first day following major surgery is reported in 15% to 40% of patients, and in most of these cases, there is no associated infection. These fevers are short-lived, and usually resolve within 24 to 48 hours. If the fever is very high, the patient has other systemic symptoms, or fever lasts beyond 48 hours, a thorough evaluation looking for an infectious process should be done.

Fever related to procedures The following procedures or interventions can be accompanied by noninfectious fever:

A. Hemodialysis: Febrile reactions during hemodialysis are attributed to endotoxin contamination of the dialysis equipment, but bacteremia occurs on occasion. Blood cultures are recommended for all patients who develop fever during hemodialysis, but the dialysis does not have to be terminated unless the patient shows signs of sepsis (eg, mental status changes or hypotension). Empiric antibiotics are recommended only for patients who appear septic. Vancomycin plus ceftazidime should suffice pending culture results. (One gram of each antibiotic given after dialysis will provide adequate serum levels pending culture results.)

B. Bronchoscopy: Fiber-optic bronchoscopy is followed by fever in 5% of cases. The fever usually appears 8 to 10 hours after the procedure, and it subsides spontaneously in 24 hours. The probable cause is release of endogenous pyrogens from the lung during the procedure. The fever is often associated with leukocytosis, but pneumonia and bacteremia are rare. There is no need for blood cultures or empiric antimicrobial therapy unless the fever does not subside or the patient shows signs of sepsis (eg, mental status changes or hypotension).

TIPS TO REMEMBER

- History and physical examination are the most important parts of your evaluation of a hospitalized patient with fever.
- Etiologies include infectious and noninfectious causes.
- Blood cultures are the only mandatory test in hospitalized patients with new-onset fever.
- Additional workup should be targeted based on the clinical scenario and clues obtained from your history and physical examination.

COMPREHENSION QUESTIONS

Refer back to the 86-year-old patient with fever described at the beginning of the chapter.

The patient has several risk factors for the development of nosocomial infections. These include: Foley catheter, central venous catheter, recent intubation, and mechanical ventilation. The patient's laboratory studies show a WBC count of 16,000 with a neutrophilia of 85%. Renal function, AST, ALT, and alkaline phosphatase are all within normal range. Her urine is positive for high leukocyte esterase, and has WBCs of 42 per high power and many bacteria. Her CXR shows improving pulmonary edema and infiltrates and was negative for any consolidation. Blood cultures did not grow anything.

1. What is your next step?
2. When should a catheter-related bacteriuria be treated?
3. If a patient has a vascular catheter and develops fever, under which circumstances should the catheter be removed?

Answers

1. Once established that the patient has a UTI, urine cultures should be sent, the Foley catheter removed, and antibiotics started empirically. The antibiotics can be changed once culture results are available. This patient was started on ciprofloxacin and her urine cultures later grew >100,000 colonies of enterococci that were sensitive to ciprofloxacin. Her blood cultures remained negative. The patient completed a 10-day course of ciprofloxacin. Her fever subsided after 48 hours of starting the antibiotics.

2. All symptomatic catheter-related bacteriuria should be treated. Symptomatic catheter-related bacteriuria (usually referred to as UTI since a clinically significant infection is inferred) is defined as the presence of fever >38°C, suprapubic tenderness, costovertebral angle tenderness, or otherwise unexplained systemic symptoms such as altered mental status, hypotension, or evidence of a systemic inflammatory response syndrome, together with 1 of the following laboratory profiles:

- Urine culture with >100,000 cfu/mL irrespective of urinalysis results
- Urine culture with >1000 cfu/mL with evidence of pyuria (dipstick positive for leukocyte esterase and/or nitrite, microscopic pyuria or presence of microbes seen on Gram stain of unspun urine)

Patients who are no longer catheterized but had indwelling urinary catheters within the past 48 hours are also considered to have catheter-associated UTI if they meet these definitions.

3. Catheter removal is warranted in the following circumstances:
- Severe sepsis
- Hemodynamic instability
- Endocarditis or evidence of metastatic infection
- Erythema or exudate due to suppurative thrombophlebitis
- Persistent bacteremia after 72 hours of antimicrobial therapy to which the organism is susceptible

Catheters that have been left in place should be removed if cultures confirm the presence of catheter-related septicemia. There are 2 situations where catheters can be left in place if the patient shows a favorable response to antimicrobial therapy:

A. When catheter removal is not easily accomplished (eg, tunneled catheters)
B. When the responsible organism is S. epidermidis

However, relapse after systemic antimicrobial therapy is higher when catheters have been left in place, and this relapse is less likely when antibiotic lock therapy is used.

SUGGESTED READINGS

Irwin RS, Rippe JM, eds. *Irwin and Rippe's Intensive Care Medicine*. 6th ed. Philadelphia: Lippincott Williams and Wilkins; 2007:1015–1022.
Marino PL, Sutin KM. *The ICU Book*. 3rd ed. Philadelphia: Lippincott Williams and Wilkins; 2006:713–733.

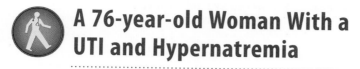

A 76-year-old Woman With a UTI and Hypernatremia

Mohamad Alhosaini, MD

A 76-year-old female nursing home resident was admitted to the hospital for complicated urinary tract infection and hypernatremia. The patient is confused and has a blood pressure of 80/40, heart rate of 110 bpm, temperature of 38.5°C, respiratory rate of 16/min, and saturation of 95% on room air. Her initial labs are significant for white blood cell count of 15,000 with 10% bands, sodium of 169, bicarbonate of 18, blood urea nitrogen of 32, and creatinine of 2.0 (baseline creatinine is normal).

1. What is the best intravenous fluid solution to administer and at what rate in this case?

Answer

1. This patient is hypotensive secondary to severe sepsis or possible septic shock. She also has hypernatremia most likely related to dehydration. Half-normal saline and dextrose 5% are the best fluids for patients with hypernatremia. However, this patient is in shock and she needs aggressive volume resuscitation. Half-normal saline or 5% dextrose does not support the blood pressure as isotonic fluids do. The best fluid in this case is normal saline. The initial rate should be given as boluses until the central venous pressure is >8 and the mean arterial blood pressure is >65. Of note, the sodium concentration in NS is 154 mEq/L, which is lower than this patient's serum sodium concentration, so NS will not worsen her hypernatremia. Once the patient is stable, fluids can be changed to 1/2 NS or D5W to correct the hypernatremia.

FLUID MANAGEMENT

Intravenous fluids are "medications" that have side effects. Using them in inappropriate settings can cause serious complications and prolong hospitalization stays. For example, patients with acute respiratory distress syndrome (ARDS) do better when they are on conservative fluid management. Loading patients with a high volume of fluids can cause pulmonary edema even in patients with no history of heart failure.

The most important indications for intravenous fluids will be summarized (Table 15-1) and the suggested type of fluids to use for each of them will be suggested. Table 15-2 summarizes the compositions of different intravenous fluids.

Table 15-1. Indications for Intravenous Fluids

1. Maintenance fluid
2. Volume resuscitation
3. Hyponatremia
4. Hypernatremia
5. Hypercalcemia/tumor lysis syndrome/rhabdomyolysis
6. Contrast-induced nephropathy prophylaxis
7. Persistent hypoglycemia
8. Spontaneous bacterial peritonitis management
9. After large-volume paracentesis in cirrhosis patients

Maintenance Fluids

Hospitalized patients are frequently placed on nothing by mouth for various reasons (surgeries, imaging, etc). During that time they must be provided with ongoing requirements of water, sodium, and potassium.

Water requirements can be calculated by the 4/2/1 rule. Four milliliters of water is needed per hour for each kilogram of the first 10 kg, 2 mL/kg for the second 10 kg, and 1 mL/kg for the rest of the weight. Daily sodium and potassium

Table 15-2. Intravenous Fluids Composition

Parameter	Human Serum	D5W	0.45 NS	0.9 NS	Lactated Ringers	Albumin	Hypertonic Saline
Na (mmol/L)	135–150	0	75	154	131	140	513
Cl (mmol/L)	95–105	0	75	154	111	128	513
K (mmol/L)	3.5–5.0	0	0	0	5	0	0
Ca (mmol/L)	2.2–2.6	0	0	0	2	0	0
HCO_3 (mmol/L)	24–28	0	0	0	29	0	0
Glucose (mg/dL)	70–100	5000	0	0	0	0	0
Albumin (g/L)	30–50	0	0	0	0	50	0
pH	7.3–7.4		5.4	6.0			
Osmolality	270–290	0	150	308	276	265	900

requirements are 1 to 2 and 0.5 to 1 mmol/kg, respectively. All the above are rough estimates, and one must use judgment when dealing with different patients. For example, patients with heart failure should get minimum fluids or perhaps none at all and patients with chronic kidney disease (CKD) should not be placed on potassium.

The best maintenance fluid is half-normal saline. If the patient does not have diabetes, D5 half-normal saline is the best choice as it provides some calories to prevent starvation-induced ketoacidosis. Don't forget to add potassium to the fluid order.

Basic maintenance fluids with potassium are not enough for patients on fasting states for prolonged periods of time (more than 48–72 hours). Other minerals, vitamins, amino acids, and fatty acids should be given to these patients by tube feedings or by total parenteral nutrition.

Volume Resuscitation

Patients who have lost volume or have become dehydrated are in need of fluids that expand the extracellular space to support blood pressure. Isotonic fluids do not cross cell membranes and thus stay in the extracellular space. They will support blood pressure and increase organ perfusion in shock patients.

Isotonic fluids include normal saline, lactated Ringers, and albumin. Albumin provides high oncotic pressure and brings fluids to the intravascular space. Theoretically, albumin should therefore support blood pressure more than the other 2 fluids; however, there is no evidence that shows albumin does better than normal saline, and it is much more expensive. Both lactated Ringers and normal saline are cheap and effective fluids. Be aware, however, that using large volumes of lactated Ringers may cause hyperkalemia, and so normal saline may often be the best choice of the 2.

When giving volume to resuscitate patients, start with boluses of 500 mL to 1 L over 30 minutes. If patients have end-stage renal disease or advanced heart failure, boluses of 250 mL may be used to avoid precipitating acute pulmonary edema. Boluses should be repeated until the central venous pressure (if internal jugular vein central line monitoring is available) and the mean arterial blood pressure improve. After blood pressure is stabilized, isotonic fluid rates can be lowered to a fixed rate per hour. Follow up the heart rate and the urine output to adjust the rate. Patients should make at least 0.5 mL/kg/h of urine.

Treatment of hypercalcemia/prevention of AKI in tumor lysis syndrome/prevention of AKI in rhabdomyolysis

High serum calcium, uric acid, and myoglobin have significant toxicities. Hypercalcemia causes mental status changes, kidney salt wasting with dehydration, vomiting, and serious arrhythmia. High uric acid can precipitate in the tubules and causes anuric acute kidney injury. Myoglobin has significant kidney toxicity as well. Intravenous hydration is a major part of the prevention and treatment of these 3 disorders. Aggressive hydration increases the glomerular filtration rate and thus increases the urinary excretion of these substances. Isotonic saline is the fluid that is most commonly used for this purpose.

Patients with hypercalcemia should be placed on 200 to 300 mL/h of NS. The urine output should be at least 100 to 150 mL/h. Hydration alone will not decrease the calcium level, and therefore bisphosphonate with or without calcitonin should be used as well.

Tumor lysis syndrome is seen in patients with high cell burden tumors who are on chemotherapy. Tumor cell death will lead to the release of potassium, phosphate, and nucleic acids. The metabolism of such a high load of purines will cause hyperuricemia. Patients at risk for tumor lysis syndrome are usually those with aggressive lymphomas and leukemia. Before starting chemotherapy these patients should be started on isotonic saline at 2 to 3 $L/m^2/24$ h. Urine output should be at least 100 mm/h. Lasix may be added to increase the urine output. Allopurinol or rasburicase is used to decrease uric acid production. Uric acid, kidney function, and electrolytes should be monitored closely.

Trauma, immobility, and drugs are the most common etiologies of rhabdomyolysis. The myoglobin released from myocytes can precipitate acute kidney injury. Patients with serum creatinine kinases (CK) of more than 5000 and those with rapidly increasing CKs from baselines lower than 5000 are at high risk for AKI. Aggressive hydration with NS to keep urine output to at least 200 to 300 mL/h is recommended. Hydration may be stopped when CKs stop rising.

Alkalinization of the urine is thought to increase uric acid solubility and thus decrease its precipitation in the tubules. Alkalinization may also decrease free ion release from myoglobin (this in turn decreases its toxicity to the kidney). However, there is no clear clinical evidence to support the use of alkalinization. Some clinicians still recommend using sodium bicarbonate in the fluids to achieve a urine pH of at lease 6.5 in these patients. If this is done, closely monitor the serum bicarbonate and the arterial pH (serum bicarbonate of 30 or arterial pH of 7.5 indicates the need to stop this process).

Hydration in these disorders is aggressive, and the risk of pulmonary edema should always be kept in mind. Serial lung and lower extremity examinations are recommended to watch for signs of fluid overload. The hydration rate should be adjusted downward for patients with baseline cardiac dysfunction.

Contrast-induced nephropathy prevention

Contrast material used for CT imaging and in arterial angiography procedures has the potential to cause acute kidney injury. Contrast-induced nephropathy has a significant effect on morbidity and mortality; therefore, prevention of contrast-induced AKI should be a goal. There are conflicting data regarding who should get prophylaxis and what are the best prophylaxis procedures. However, patients with estimated glomerular filtration rates of less than 60 mL/1.73 m^2 are at high risk, and intravenous fluids (especially normal saline or sodium bicarbonate) definitely decrease the risk of contrast nephropathy. It is probably wise to give prophylactic fluids to patients with CKD stage III or more. Isotonic sodium bicarbonate fluid can be made by adding 3 ampules of $NaHCO_3$ (a total of 150 mL) to 850 mL of D5W. Give 3 mL/kg/h of sodium bicarbonate fluid 1 hour before contrast administration and continue for 6 hours after. An alternate protocol is to give 1 mL/kg of NS 6 hours prior to the contrast and to continue that for 6 to 12 hours after.

Persistent Hypoglycemia

Sometimes patients get too much insulin. Most of the time orange juice or a half ampule of dextrose 50% will take care of the hypoglycemia. If the patient has renal dysfunction, sometimes the hypoglycemia will persist for hours. This is also true if an elderly patient or a patient with CKD takes too much sulfonylurea and does not eat enough. Hypoglycemia in these cases can last for a few days. In cases like these, it becomes impractical to give dextrose ampules alone. A better approach is to start the patient on continuous intravenous dextrose 5% or 10% and follow the Accu-Checks.

Spontaneous Bacterial Peritonitis

Cirrhosis patients with spontaneous bacterial peritonitis (SBP) are at high risk for acute kidney injury. This is because of the decreased effective arterial circulation that results in decreased kidney perfusion. Albumin infusion has been shown to decrease this risk and in turn decrease the mortality in these patients.

Once SBP is diagnosed, start the patient on a 1-time dose of 1.5 g/kg intravenous albumin. Give another 1 g/kg on day 3.

Post-large-volume Paracentesis

Patients with diuretic-resistant cirrhotic ascites need frequent paracenteses. Sometimes, a large volume of ascites fluid needs to be removed. Following removal of a large volume of fluid, patients will be at risk for circulatory collapse and renal failure. Infusion of albumin may decrease this risk. When paracentesis of more than 5 L is performed, it is reasonable to give 6 to 8 g of intravenous albumin for each liter removed.

TIPS TO REMEMBER

- Intravenous fluids should be used only when indicated. The "liberal" use of IV fluids can have adverse reactions.
- Half-normal saline with dextrose and potassium supplements is probably the best maintenance fluid to use for patients fasting for short periods of time.
- Normal saline and lactated Ringers are the fluids of choice for shock patients.

- Isotonic fluids are used in patients with hypercalcemia to keep the urine output to at least 100 cm^3/h.
- Patients at risk for tumor lysis syndrome should be on isotonic fluids to prevent uric acid–induced AKI. Urine output should be at least 100 cm^3/h.
- Patients at risk for myoglobin-induced AKI should be on isotonic fluids to keep the urine output to at least 200 cm^3/h.
- Sodium bicarbonate or normal saline should be used in patients with CKD stage III or more to prevent contrast nephropathy.
- Intravenous albumin use is currently indicated only in patients with SBP or after paracentesis of at least 5 L of ascites fluid.

COMPREHENSION QUESTIONS

1. A 55-year-old female had a right total knee replacement done 1 day ago. She was started on lactated Ringers at 120 mL/h. The patient has a history of hypertension, diastolic heart failure, and CKD stage III. Her current medications are morphine, atenolol, and ondansetron. The patient has been doing fine except for the pain at her surgery site. Her appetite is still poor due to her morphine-induced nausea. Her vitals are within normal limits and the physical examination is not significant. Her labs show the following:

> Sodium: 138
> Potassium: 5.8
> Chloride: 100
> Bicarbonate: 24
> Blood urea nitrogen: 20
> Creatinine: 2.2 (baseline is 2.3)
> Glucose: 98
> Calcium: 8.9

Which of the following is the most appropriate regarding this patient's fluid management?

> A. Continue the same management.
> B. Stop lactated Ringers.
> C. Stop lactated Ringers and start normal saline.
> D. Stop lactated Ringers and start dextrose 5% half-normal saline.

2. A 63-year-old male patient was admitted by vascular surgery for evaluation of worsening peripheral vascular disease in his right leg. The patient is prepared to have arterial angiography the next day. He has a history of DM, hypertension, CKD stage IV, congestive heart failure, and left below-the-knee amputation 3 years ago for advanced peripheral vascular disease. The patient complains of right foot pain on walking for 2 blocks that has worsened over the last 2 months.

He noted that his torsemide dose was increased 2 weeks ago because of worsening dyspnea on exertion. Since that time his dyspnea has been controlled. The patient is not in acute distress and his vital signs are within normal limits. Physical examination is significant for 3+ edema in the right leg, and a cold hairless shin. His right dorsalis pedis and posterior tibial pulses are weak.

Which of the following is the most appropriate for this patient?
    A. Stop diuretics prior to angiography.
    B. Give bicarbonate sodium fluid prior to angiography.
    C. Continue diuretics.
    D. Give half-normal saline fluid prior to angiography.

Answers

1. **D.** Lactated Ringers is the most likely cause of the hyperkalemia in this patient with a history of CKD. Thus, it should be stopped. The patient is nauseated and her oral intake is still poor, so she needs maintenance fluid. The best maintenance fluid in this patient would be D5 1/2 NS. There is no evidence of hypovolemia on examination, so NS is better to be avoided, especially given this history of heart failure in this patient.

2. **C.** This patient is at high risk for contrast nephropathy because of his advanced CKD. Sodium bicarbonate decreases the risk of contrast nephropathy. However, this patient has evidence of hypervolemia (edema in his right leg) and his diuretic dose was recently increased. Starting fluids, whether hypotonic or isotonic, or discontinuing the diuretics will put him at risk for acute exacerbation of his congestive heart failure. This risk most likely outweighs the benefit of giving isotonic fluid. Diuretics will help make this patient euvolemic and improve the stroke volume; this in turn will increase the kidney perfusion and help decrease the risk of contrast nephropathy in this patient.

SUGGESTED READINGS

Dale D, Federman D. *ACP Medicine*. Vol. 2. 3rd ed. New York: WebMD Inc; 2007:1976–1979.
McPhee S, Papadakis M. *Current Medial Diagnosis and Treatment*. 50th ed. New York: McGraw-Hill; 2011:867–868.

Gastrointestinal Bleeding

Zak Gurnsey, MD, FACP

A 47-year-old Man Vomiting Bright Red Blood

Mr Donaldson is a 47-year-old male who presents to the emergency department with a 12-hour history of vomiting bright red blood. He has had 4 episodes of emesis during this time span. He also complains of nausea, fatigue, and light-headedness. He had 1 episode of melena shortly before arrival. He denies abdominal pain, diarrhea, or fevers. He has a history of hypertension and chronic back pain secondary to a car accident. His medications include hydrochlorothiazide, amlodipine, and ibuprofen. He smokes 1 pack per day. He also drinks 6 to 8 beers per day, with more being consumed on the weekends and holidays. He has drunk this amount of alcohol for 22 years. On examination, he appears drowsy, with a blood pressure of 94/46 mm Hg, heart rate of 122 bpm, respiratory rate of 24 breaths/min, and oxygen saturation of 96% on room air. He is afebrile. His eyes are slightly icteric. His oral mucosa is slightly dry. Chest auscultation reveals clear lungs and a regular heart rhythm. Abdominal examination reveals mild distention and evidence of hepatomegaly. His rectal examination reveals heme-positive stool.

Laboratory data show hemoglobin 9.8, hematocrit 29, and platelets 98,000. BUN is 28 and creatinine is 1.2. INR is 1.6. AST is 102 and ALT is 68.

1. What is the most likely diagnosis?
2. What is the initial goal of evaluation and patient care?
3. What else is on the differential diagnosis?

Answers

This is a 47-year-old male with risk factors for GI bleeding (alcohol abuse and NSAID usage) who presents with several episodes of hematemesis. His vitals, physical examination, and laboratory data suggest volume loss and hemodynamic instability. He requires rapid evaluation and treatment, including volume resuscitation and workup for the cause of his bleeding.

1. The most likely diagnosis is bleeding from esophageal varices.

2. The initial goals of his care revolve around volume resuscitation and hemodynamic stability with an urgent GI consult.

3. The differential diagnosis includes peptic ulcer disease, esophagitis, gastric varices, and Mallory-Weis tear.

Analysis: This case represents the approach to a patient with an upper GI bleed with a focus on initial assessment and resuscitation, as well as a discussion of the differential diagnoses.

UPPER GI BLEED

Diagnosis

Historical clues
A focused history should revolve around such questions as history of length of time and progression of bleeding, associated symptoms (nausea, retching, abdominal pain), prior history of GI bleeding, and medication usage.

Physical clues
Vital signs revealing hypotension, tachycardia, tachypnea, and hypoxia can help determine the degree of blood loss. Other physical examination findings to look for include dry mucus membranes, poor skin turgor, and evidence of chronic liver disease (jaundice, ascites, hepatomegaly, spider angiomas, and caput medusae).

Laboratory clues
The laboratory evaluation should focus on blood and volume status as well. The hemoglobin and hematocrit should be assessed for degree of anemia. Keep in mind, though, that an acute bleeding episode will not have an immediate impact on the hemoglobin level due to lack of equilibrizing. Low platelet levels may indicate underlying liver disease. BUN and creatinine should be assessed for renal complications due to volume loss. An exceedingly high BUN:creatinine ratio (>20) may indicate GI bleeding. This is because the blood is digested in the GI tract, with by-products being reabsorbed and causing the BUN to rise. PT/INR and PTT should be assessed to look for any underlying coagulopathies, which may impact the ability to reverse the bleeding. Liver enzymes should be assessed to determine underlying acute and/or chronic liver disease.

Initial assessment
As in all urgent/emergent situations, the first approach revolves around the ABCs (airway, breathing, circulation). Patients with upper GI bleeding may develop the inability to protect their airways. This may be due to persistent vomiting and/or associated lethargy due to blood loss with inadequate perfusion of vital organs. If this occurs, the patient needs to be intubated for airway protection.

Treatment

Volume resuscitation

As in all cases of sudden volume loss, patients with GI bleeding need adequate vascular access. This is ideally accomplished with 2 large-bore (18 gauge or larger) peripheral IV sites. This will allow rapid infusion of volume (such as normal saline or Ringer lactate) and blood products (such as packed red blood cells, fresh frozen plasma, and platelets).

Patients should be kept NPO (nothing to eat or drink by mouth).

Blood products

Packed red blood cells should be considered for transfusion based on degree of reported or witnessed blood loss, degree of anemia, and degree of hemodynamic instability. Transfusion of other blood products, such as fresh frozen plasma and platelets, should be considered based on the laboratory evaluation and/or underlying coagulopathies.

Other medications

Besides IV fluids and blood products, other medications should be considered. Home medications should be discontinued (in line with the patient's NPO status). Proton-pump inhibitors should be ordered for all patients with GI bleeding, in either continuous or bolus intravenous routes. Octreotide infusion should be used for upper GI bleeding cases with a suspected cause of esophageal varices. Octreotide is a somatostatin analog that reduces the pressure in the portal venous system.

Bed status

Patients with upper GI bleeding should be monitored in an ICU or IMC setting with frequent evaluations of hemodynamic status.

Consults

A gastroenterology consult should be obtained in all cases of upper GI bleeding. For those patients with hemodynamic instability, this consult needs to be obtained urgently/emergently.

Diagnostic approach

Upper endoscopy is the mainstay of definitive diagnosis in cases of upper GI bleeding. Angiography may also help localize an area of bleeding.

Treatments for Upper GI Bleeding (Depending on Diagnosis)

Esophageal varices

Esophageal varices are dilated veins in the submucosa of the esophagus caused by portal hypertension. They are asymptomatic until they present as an upper GI bleed. Diagnosis is made via endoscopy. Treatment options include banding, sclerotherapy, balloon tamponade with a Sengstaken–Blakemore tube, transjugular intrahepatic portosystemic shunt (TIPS), and liver transplantation. Nonselective beta-blockers are used to prevent bleeding or rebleeding in patients with esophageal varices. They are not, however, used to prevent the initial formation of esophageal varices.

Gastric varices

Gastric varices are dilated veins in the submucosa of the stomach caused by portal hypertension. They are asymptomatic until they present as an upper GI bleed. Diagnosis is made via endoscopy. Gastric varices are extremely difficult to treat or eradicate. They often rebleed and have a high mortality rate. Treatment options include gastric variceal obliteration with cyanoacrylate, intragastric balloon tamponade, TIPS, and liver transplantation.

Peptic ulcer disease

Peptic ulcer disease most commonly occurs in the duodenum, but may also occur in the esophagus or stomach. Abdominal pain is usually an associated symptom. Causes generally include *Helicobacter pylori* infection, NSAID usage, and antiplatelet medication usage (eg, aspirin or clopidogrel). Malignancy is also a potential cause. Diagnosis may be considered on clinical suspicion, but is confirmed with endoscopy. Treatment focuses on the underlying cause. Any offending medications are discontinued. *H. pylori* infections are treated with a combination of 2 antibiotics and a proton-pump inhibitor. Multiple biopsies should be taken to help rule out malignancy.

Esophagitis

Esophagitis is inflammation of the lining of the esophagus. Common causes include GERD (acid reflux), chemical ingestions, alcohol, infections (*Candida*, HSV, CMV), and eosinophilic esophagitis. Diagnosis may be considered on clinical suspicion, but is confirmed with endoscopy. Treatment focuses on the underlying cause. Any offending medications are discontinued. Proton-pump inhibitors are generally prescribed regardless of the cause. Antimicrobials directed toward any confirmed infectious cause should be used. Inhaled corticosteroids swallowed down the esophagus are used to treat eosinophilic esophagitis.

Gastritis

Gastritis is inflammation of the lining of the stomach. Common causes include alcohol, NSAID usage, severe illness (stress, burns, trauma, sepsis), and *H. pylori* infection. Diagnosis may be considered on clinical suspicion, but is confirmed with endoscopy. Treatment focuses on the underlying cause. Any offending medications are discontinued. Proton-pump inhibitors are generally prescribed regardless of the cause. Other potential medications to use include sucralfate, bismuth, and misoprostol.

Mallory-Weis tear

Mallory-Weis tears occur in the mucosa at the gastroesophageal junction after episodes of severe retching and vomiting. The bleeding usually stops on its own in 1 to 2 days, but endoscopic treatment via cauterization or epinephrine injection can be used.

Portal gastropathy

Portal gastropathy occurs as a result of portal hypertension and subsequent engorgement of the gastric mucosa vasculature. The mucosa becomes quite friable, lending itself to bleeding from underlying vessels. Treatment is geared toward reducing portal venous pressure with the use of nonselective beta-blockers. Endoscopic treatment of individual bleeding vessels can also be used.

Angiodysplasias

Angiodysplasias are small vascular malformations seen in the lining of the GI tract during endoscopy. They are a common cause of unexplained or recurrent GI bleeding. They are usually multiple and may occur throughout the upper and lower GI tracts. Treatment is usually via argon plasma coagulation during endoscopy.

Aortoenteric fistula

Aortoenteric fistulas usually occur as a result of erosion of an abdominal aortic aneurysm into the duodenum. Prior aortic vascular surgery also increases the risk. This situation requires emergent surgical intervention. These patients have a high mortality rate.

Dieulafoy lesions

Dieulafoy lesions are caused by large arterioles in the submucosa. The larger size and pulsatile nature of the arteriole cause the small layer of overlying submucosa to erode, leading to bleeding into the stomach or GI lumen. Even with endoscopy, they are difficult to diagnose because of an intermittent bleeding pattern. Endoscopic treatment options include epinephrine injection, electrocoagulation, sclerotherapy, photocoagulation, hemoclipping, and banding.

Cameron lesions

Cameron lesions are small, linear erosions or ulcers seen at the gastroesophageal junction. They are associated with hiatal hernias. They are usually asymptomatic. They may lead to iron deficiency anemia due to chronic bleeding of small amounts.

A 62-year-old Woman With Bright Red Blood Per Rectum

Mrs Lincoln is a 62-year-old female who presents to the emergency department after developing bright red blood per rectum (BRBPR) that started last night. She has had a total of 8 episodes of BRBPR. She denies any abdominal pain, rectal pain, weight loss, or fevers. She does complain of fecal incontinence with these episodes. She has never had any previous episodes of GI bleeding. She has a history of diabetes mellitus type 2 and hyperlipidemia. Her home medications include metformin and simvastatin. She denies any tobacco or alcohol use. She had a colonoscopy 3 years ago that revealed diverticulosis without any other significant findings. On examination, she is awake and pleasant with a blood pressure of 136/74 mm Hg, heart rate of 84 bpm, respiratory rate of 16 breaths/min, and oxygen saturation of 98% on room air. She is afebrile. Her HEENT, cardiovascular, and respiratory examinations are all normal. Her abdomen is soft without any tenderness or distention. Bowel sounds are normal. Rectal examination reveals some red blood on the examination finger.

Laboratory data show hemoglobin 12.5, hematocrit 37, and platelets 215,000. BUN is 15 and creatinine is 1.1. INR is 0.9. AST is 34 and ALT is 30.

1. What is the most likely diagnosis?

2. What is the initial goal of evaluation and patient care?

3. What else is on the differential diagnosis?

Answers

This is a 62-year-old female with sudden onset of BRBPR that began last night. She has no other symptoms. A previous colonoscopy was negative for polyps or malignancy. Her vitals and physical examination show that she is hemodynamically stable. She has mild anemia. She requires further workup for these episodes of lower GI bleeding.

1. The most likely diagnosis is diverticular bleeding.

2. The initial goals of her care revolve around monitoring volume status and anemia levels. She will require a nonurgent GI consult.

3. The differential diagnosis includes malignancy, inflammatory bowel disease (IBD), hemorrhoids, and angiodysplasias.

LOWER GI BLEED

Diagnosis

Unlike upper GI bleeding, most patients with lower GI bleeding will show (at least temporarily) spontaneous resolution of the bleeding.

Historical clues

A focused history should revolve around such questions as history of length of time and progression of bleeding, associated symptoms (such as abdominal pain, rectal pain, and weight loss), prior history of GI bleeding, and medication usage.

Physical clues

Vital signs revealing hypotension, tachycardia, tachypnea, and hypoxia can help determine the degree of blood loss. Other physical examination findings to look for include dry mucus membranes, poor skin turgor, and evidence of hemorrhoids or rectal masses.

Laboratory clues

The laboratory evaluation should focus on blood and volume status as well. The hemoglobin and hematocrit should be assessed for degree of anemia. Keep in mind, though, that an acute bleeding episode will not have an immediate impact on the hemoglobin level due to lack of equilibrizing. BUN and creatinine should be assessed for renal complications due to volume loss. PT/INR and PTT should be assessed to look for any underlying coagulopathies, which may impact the ability to reverse the bleeding.

Volume resuscitation

As in all cases of sudden volume loss, patients with GI bleeding need adequate vascular access. This is ideally accomplished with 2 large-bore (18 gauge or larger) peripheral IV sites. This will allow rapid infusion of volume (such as normal saline or Ringer lactate) and blood products (such as packed red blood cells, fresh frozen plasma, and platelets).

Patients should be kept NPO (nothing to eat or drink by mouth).

Blood products

Packed red blood cells should be considered for transfusion based on degree of reported or witnessed blood loss, degree of anemia, and degree of hemodynamic instability. Transfusion of other blood products, such as fresh frozen plasma and platelets, should be considered based on the laboratory evaluation and/or underlying coagulopathies.

Medications

Besides IV fluids and blood products, other medications should be considered. Home medications should be discontinued (in line with the patient's NPO status). This is especially true for such medication classes as NSAIDs, anticoagulants, and antiplatelet drugs.

Consults

A gastroenterology consult should be obtained.

Diagnostic approach

Colonoscopy will help visualize and localize an area of bleeding. It also allows for direct intervention. Radionuclide scanning may help localize bleeding to a particular quadrant of the abdomen. It is performed by tagging red blood cells with a radionuclide tracer. It has drawbacks in that it requires a bleeding rate of approximately 0.5 mL/min and does not allow for therapeutic intervention. Angiography is another option. It does not require bowel preparation and does allow for intervention via embolization. Drawbacks include a bleeding rate requirement of approximately 1.0 mL/min and the use of IV contrast.

Treatments for Lower GI Bleeding (Depending on Diagnosis)

Diverticulosis

Diverticula may develop along the colonic wall. These small outpouches occur through weaknesses in the colonic wall musculature. They are most common in the sigmoid colon. They are usually asymptomatic. If stretched too far, the blood vessels within the outpouches may bleed. Treatment is generally supportive, with fluid resuscitation and, at times, blood transfusions. If diverticular bleeding is a recurrent problem, the ultimate treatment may be surgical removal of the section of colon with predominant diverticular disease.

Angiodysplasias

Angiodysplasias are small vascular malformations seen in the lining of the GI tract during endoscopy. They are a common cause of unexplained or recurrent GI bleeding. They are usually multiple and may occur throughout the upper and lower GI tracts. Treatment is usually via argon plasma coagulation during endoscopy.

Colorectal malignancy

Colon cancer may present as rectal bleeding or anemia. Associated symptoms of weight loss and change in bowel habits should be investigated. Colon cancer usually occurs later in life. General screening recommendations suggest age 50 as the starting point for surveillance colonoscopy. Diagnosis requires histopathologic samples from endoscopic biopsies. Treatment depends on the stage, and may include surgery, chemotherapy, and/or radiation therapy.

Inflammatory bowel disease

IBD has 2 main forms: Crohn disease and ulcerative colitis. It should be suspected in younger patients with lower GI bleeding with associated symptoms of fever, malaise, and abdominal pain. Diagnosis is made via autoimmune and genetic serum markers and via endoscopic biopsies. Treatment typically involves systemic steroids and other immunosuppressive agents.

Ischemic colitis

Ischemic colitis occurs due to lack of blood flow to an area of the colon. This is usually due to decreased blood pressure (ie, volume loss or septic shock) or a stoppage in blood flow (ie, atherosclerotic disease or thromboembolic disease). Treatment starts with supportive care, including fluid resuscitation and pain management. Surgical excision of the ischemic area may be needed if the area develops gangrene or perforation.

Hemorrhoids

Hemorrhoids can occur internally or externally, in relation to the dentate line. Bleeding typically occurs with a bowel movement. External hemorrhoids will be painful as well. Diagnosis is via digital rectal examination or endoscopy. Treatment begins with supportive care, but may ultimately include rubber band ligation or surgical excision.

Upper GI bleeding

Cases of upper GI bleeding that exhibit very rapid transit of the blood through the GI tract may present as BRBPR. These patients are likely to have significant hemodynamic instability. If upper GI bleeding is suspected as the cause of BRBPR, the approaches outlined in the first half of this chapter should be employed. The much more common appearance of stool in relation to upper GI bleeding is that of melena, or black tarry stools.

TIPS TO REMEMBER

- Adequate vascular access and sufficient volume resuscitation are necessary in all cases of GI bleeding.
- Proton pump inhibitors should be empirically started in all cases of upper GI bleeding.
- Endoscopy is the standard for diagnosis in cases of upper GI bleeding.
- Most cases of lower GI bleeding will resolve spontaneously.

COMPREHENSION QUESTIONS

1. A 54-year-old male with a history of alcoholism presents to the emergency department after experiencing hematemesis of 200 mL bright red blood at home. He complains of fatigue and is pale in appearance. His blood pressure is 98/46 and heart rate is 112. What is the next step in this patient's management?
   - A. Nasogastric tube placement
   - B. Gastroenterology consult
   - C. Transfusion of 2 U of packed red blood cells
   - D. Placement of 2 large-bore peripheral IV sites and initiation of IV fluid boluses

2. An 80-year-old female with a history of atrial fibrillation, hypertension, and coronary artery disease presents with a 1-day history of abdominal pain and rectal bleeding with bright red blood. The pain is dull and vague, located in the left lower quadrant, and has been getting worse over time. Her warfarin therapy was stopped several months ago due to concerns regarding frequent falls. Her blood pressure is 136/78 and heart rate is 64. On examination, she has severe tenderness on palpation of the left lower quadrant with some associated guarding. What is the most likely diagnosis?
   - A. Hemorrhoids
   - B. Peptic ulcer disease
   - C. Diverticulosis
   - D. Ischemic colitis

3. A 26-year-old male with no prior medical history complains of a 3-day history of nausea with vomiting and diarrhea. He has several episodes of each per day. His fiancé had similar symptoms that resolved spontaneously 2 days ago. Earlier today, he developed hematemesis of bright red blood during his episodes of nausea with vomiting. His vital signs and physical examination are essentially normal. What is the most likely diagnosis?

> A. Esophageal varices
> B. Peptic ulcer disease
> C. Esophagitis
> D. Mallory-Weis tear

Answers

1. **D.** This patient has several indicators of volume loss, including the amount of hematemesis, pale appearance, and hypotension with compensatory tachycardia. The other options are all likely to occur in the urgent management of this patient, but appropriate vascular access and aggressive volume resuscitation are the initial concerns in an attempt to stabilize this patient so that further interventions (ie, blood transfusions, endoscopy) may occur.

2. **D.** This elderly female most likely has ischemic colitis. Her history of atrial fibrillation without current anticoagulation treatment places her at an increased risk of developing thromboembolic disease. Her abdominal pain is also characteristic of ischemic colitis, as it is worse on physical examination than reported during the history and it is located in a typical area for ischemic colitis. Abdominal pain would not be expected with hemorrhoids or diverticulosis. Peptic ulcer disease should present with upper GI bleeding or melena, but not typically with bright red lower GI bleeding.

3. **D.** This patient has likely developed a Mallory-Weis tear due to recurrent vomiting and retching. He has no noted history of alcohol abuse or liver disease, acid reflux, or abdominal pain that would make the other choices more likely.

SUGGESTED READINGS

Cappell MS, Friedel D. Initial management of acute upper gastrointestinal bleeding: from initial evaluation up to gastrointestinal endoscopy. *Med Clin North Am.* 2008;92:491–509.

Gralnek IM, Barkun AN, Bardou M. Current concepts: management of acute bleeding from a peptic ulcer. *N Engl J Med.* 2008;359:928–937.

Longo DL, Fauci AS, Kasper DL, Hauser SL, Jameson JL, Loscalzo J, eds. *Harrison's Principles of Internal Medicine.* 18th ed. New York: McGraw-Hill; 2012.

Manning-Dimmitt LL, Dimmitt SG, Wilson GR. Diagnosis of gastrointestinal bleeding in adults. *Am Fam Physician.* 2005;71(7):1339–1346.

McQuaid KR. Gastrointestinal disorders. In: McPhee SJ, Papadakis MA, eds. *Current Medical* Diagnosis *& Treatment.* New York: McGraw-Hill; 2012:chap 15.

Sepe PS, Yachimski PS, Friedman LS. Gastroenterology. In: Sabatine M, ed. *Pocket Medicine: The Massachusetts General Hospital Handbook of Internal Medicine*. 2nd ed. Philadelphia: Lippincott Williams & Wilkins; 2004:1–26:chap 3.

Washington University School of Medicine, Cooper DH, Krainik AJ, Lubner SJ, Reno HEL. *The Washington Manual of Medical Therapeutics*. 32nd ed. Philadelphia: Lippincott Williams & Wilkins; 2007.

Zuckerman GR, Prakash C. Acute lower intestinal bleeding. Part I: clinical presentation and diagnosis. *Gastrointest Endosc*. 1998;48:606.

Zuckerman GR, Prakash C. Acute lower intestinal bleeding. Part II: etiology, therapy and outcomes. *Gastrointest Endosc*. 1998;49:228.

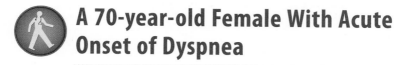

A 70-year-old Female With Acute Onset of Dyspnea

Thamilvani Thiruvasahar, MD

A 70-year-old female was evaluated in the emergency department for acute onset of dyspnea with severe frontal headaches and diaphoresis. She was diagnosed with a left adrenal pheochromocytoma a week ago, and surgery is scheduled next week. Her PMH is otherwise not significant. Current medications include phenoxybenzamine and propranolol. On physical examination, the patient appears anxious, dyspneic, and diaphoretic. Blood pressure (BP) is 220/120 mm Hg; heart rate is 130/min; respiratory rate is 30/min; oxygen saturation is 92% on room air. On auscultation, lungs reveal bibasilar crackles and heart examination reveals tachycardia. She has 2+ pedal edema. CBC and BMP are normal. Chest x-ray (CXR) shows cardiomegaly and pulmonary congestion. EKG shows no evidence of ischemia.

1. What is the most likely diagnosis?
2. What is the next appropriate initial treatment for this patient's hypertension?

Answers

1. This is a hypertensive crisis, specifically a hypertensive emergency.
2. When BP exceeds 180/110 mm Hg, think about 3 categories of patients:

   A. Severe hypertension—BP >180/110 in the absence of symptoms beyond mild or moderate headache without evidence of acute target organ damage.

   B. Hypertensive urgency—BP exceeds 180/110 mm Hg with significant symptoms, such as severe headache or dyspnea, but absent or only minimal acute target organ damage.

   C. Hypertensive emergency—BP >220/140 mm Hg accompanied by evidence of life-threatening end-organ dysfunction.

Hypertensive crises include hypertensive emergencies and urgencies. Among the 65 million Americans with hypertension, hypertensive crises occur in less than 1% of individuals. Even though crises are infrequent, significantly elevated BP is a common clinical scenario.

Hypertensive emergencies include accelerated hypertension, defined as progressive hypertension with the funduscopic vascular changes of malignant hypertension but without papilledema, and malignant hypertension, defined as a severe hypertensive state with papilledema of the ocular fundi and vascular hemorrhagic

Table 17-1. Target Organ Manifestations

Organ System	Manifestations
Vascular	Aneurysmal dilation
	Accelerated atherosclerosis
	Aortic dissection
Cardiac	
Acute	Pulmonary edema, myocardial infarction
Chronic	Clinical or EKG evidence of coronary artery disease (CAD); left
	Ventricular hypertrophy (LVH) by EKG or echocardiogram
Cerebrovascular	
Acute	Intracerebral bleeding, coma, seizures, mental status changes, transient ischemic attack (TIA), stroke
Chronic	TIA, stroke
Renal	
Acute	Hematuria, azotemia
Chronic	Serum creatinine >1.5 mg/dL, proteinuria >1+ on dipstick
Retinopathy	
Acute	Papilledema, hemorrhages
Chronic	Hemorrhages, exudates, arterial nicking

lesions, thickening of the small arteries and arterioles, left ventricular hypertrophy, and a poor prognosis (Table 17-1).

DIAGNOSIS

As is the case with most patients, a targeted history, targeted physical examination, and selected testing are the important elements of the initial assessment in patients with extremely elevated BPs. When taking the history, the physician should assess the duration and the severity of the HTN as well as symptoms suggesting end-organ damage including headache, chest pain, dyspnea, edema, acute fatigue, focal weakness, epistaxis, seizures, and change in level of consciousness. Adherence to antihypertensive medications should also be assessed. It is important to ask about any recent use of medications including oral contraceptives,

NSAIDs, prednisone, monoamine oxidase inhibitors, cyclosporine, and stimulant or appetite suppressant agents. The focused past medical history should specifically include asking about chronic kidney disease, prior stroke, and prior heart disease, especially myocardial infarction. It is very important that the social history include questioning about recreational drugs, especially cocaine, amphetamines, and phencyclidine (PCP). The review of systems may offer important clues about possible secondary causes of hypertension. Tachycardia, diaphoresis, and tremors should cause you to consider a pheochromocytoma. Unintentional weight gain, a buffalo hump, thinning skin, and easy bruising should lead you to consider Cushing syndrome.

Physical examination should include repeating the BP measurement, while ensuring the appropriate technique and cuff size is used. BPs should be measured in both arms, as coarctation of the aorta may be present. If the pedal pulses are diminished, BPs should also be measured in the lower extremities. The remainder of the physical examination should focus on target organs. A funduscopic examination is essential to assess for papilledema, hemorrhages, and exudates. Cardiovascular examination should be thorough. It should include assessing for jugular venous distention, abdominal bruits, and lower extremity pulses. These are parts of the examination commonly not assessed. Lung examination should be done to assess for pulmonary edema. A thorough neurologic examination should be done to assess for any evidence of stroke. This should include an assessment of mental status.

Laboratory studies should focus on assessing for target organ damage as well as possible secondary causes of the hypertension. It is reasonable to check a complete blood count, a metabolic panel, a urinalysis, an electrocardiogram, and a CXR. A computed tomography (CT) scan of the head is only indicated if there are focal neurologic symptoms, complaints of acute speech or swallowing problems, mental status changes, or findings on neurologic examination suggestive of stroke.

TREATMENT

There is no proven benefit to the rapid reduction of BP in patients with severe asymptomatic HTN. The initial goal of therapy in these patients should be to achieve a diastolic BP of 100 to 110 mm Hg. A rapid decrease in BP may cause cerebral hypoperfusion or coronary insufficiency. The target BP can be achieved over several days.

Hypertensive emergencies warrant admission to an ICU and treatment with parenteral agents. In an emergency situation, control of acute or ongoing end-organ damage is more important than the absolute level of BP. BP control with rapidly acting IV agent should be administered within 1 hour to reduce permanent organ damage or death. A reasonable target is a 20% to 25% reduction of mean arterial pressure (MAP) or reduction of diastolic BP to 100 to 110 mm Hg over a period of minutes to hours. Precautions should be taken in patients who

Table 17-2. Triage of Patients With Very Elevated Blood Pressure

	Severe Hypertension	Hypertensive Urgency	Hypertensive Emergency
Blood pressure	>180/110 mm Hg	>180/110 mm Hg	Often >220/140 mm Hg
Clinical features and symptoms	May be asymptomatic; headache	Severe headache, dyspnea, edema	Chest pain, severe dyspnea, altered mental status, focal neurologic deficit
Clinical features: findings	No acute target organ damage	Acute target organ damage usually absent, but may include elevated serum creatinine	Life-threatening target organ damage (eg, acute myocardial infarction, stroke, encephalopathy, acute renal failure, heart failure)
Immediate goal	Lower blood pressure within days	Lower blood pressure within 24–72 h	Immediate blood pressure reduction; decrease by 15%–25% within 2 h
Treatment setting	Outpatient	Usually outpatient	Inpatient, intensive care unit
Medications	Long-acting, oral	Oral medications with rapid onset of action; occasionally intravenously	Intravenous medication
Follow-up	Within 3–7 days	Within 24–72 h	As appropriate after hospital management

are elderly, volume depleted, or receiving other antihypertensive agents to avoid cerebral hypoperfusion (Tables 17-2 to 17-4).

COMPLICATIONS

Acute aortic dissection is a life-threatening condition, and timely diagnosis and aggressive treatment are essential. Severe HTN and tachycardia are typically present. The goal is to reduce the BP and heart rate to reduce the shear stress, which in turn will decrease the propagation of the dissection. The drugs of choice are labetalol, esmolol, and nitroprusside.

Table 17-3. Preferred Medications for Hypertensive Urgencies

Agent	Dose	Onset of Action	Precautions
Labetalol	200–400 mg po	20–120 min	Bronchoconstriction, heart block, aggravates heart failure
Clonidine	0.1–0.2 mg po	30–60 min	Rebound hypertension with abrupt withdrawal
Captopril	12.5–25 mg po	15–60 min	Can precipitate acute renal failure in setting of bilateral renal artery stenosis
Nifedipine, extended release	30 mg po	20 min	Avoid short-acting oral or sublingual nifedipine due to risk of stroke, acute myocardial infarction, severe hypotension
Amlodipine	5–10 mg po	30–50 min	Headache, tachycardia, flushing, peripheral edema
Prazosin	1–2 mg po	2–4 h	Syncope (first dose), tachycardia, postural hypotension

Acute coronary syndromes include unstable angina and acute MI. The drugs of choice are IV nitroglycerin and beta-blockers.

Acute pulmonary edema may occur and drugs that decrease preload and left ventricular volume are the treatment of choice for acute heart failure with pulmonary edema secondary to uncontrolled hypertension. These include sodium nitroprusside, fenoldopam, and loop diuretics.

Neurologic complications of hypertensive emergencies include encephalopathy, stroke, subarachnoid hemorrhage, or Cushing reflex. With hypertensive encephalopathy, papilledema will be found on funduscopic examination. Nitroprusside is the drug of choice. Acute and aggressive lowering of BP may confer a risk of stroke in patients with hypertensive emergency. BP reduction should be done cautiously with close neurologic surveillance.

With new or acutely worsening renal dysfunction, fenoldopam is the drug of choice because of its efficacy and the fact that it increases renal blood flow and urine output.

Adrenergic crises may occur in pheochromocytomas, with cocaine use, amphetamine use, and clonidine withdrawal. Treatment should be with pure alpha-blockers, such as phentolamine. Beta-blockers may be added if inadequate BP control is obtained. Clonidine withdrawal should be handled with a combination of alpha- and beta-blockers, such as labetalol and clonidine.

Table 17-4. Preferred Medications for Hypertensive Emergencies

Agent	Dose	Onset/Duration of Action (After Discontinuation)	Precautions
Parenteral vasodilators			
Sodium nitroprusside	0.25–10.00 µg/kg/min as intravenous infusion; maximal dose for 10 min only	Immediate/2–3 min after infusion	Nausea, vomiting, muscle twitching; with prolonged use, may cause thiocyanate intoxication, methemoglobinemia acidosis, cyanide poisoning; bags, bottles, and delivery sets must be light-resistant
Glyceral trinitrate	5–100 µg as intravenous infusion	2–5/5–10 min	Headache, tachycardia, vomiting, flushing, methemoglobinemia; requires special delivery systems due to the drug's binding to polyvinyl chloride tubing
Nicardipine	5–15 mg/h intravenous infusion	1–5/15–30 min, but may exceed 12 h after prolonged infusion	Tachycardia, nausea, vomiting, headache, increased intracranial pressure, possible protracted hypotension after prolonged infusions
Verapamil	5–10 mg intravenous; can follow with infusion of 3–25 mg/h	1–5/30–60 min	Heart block (first-, second-, and third-degree), especially with concomitant digitalis or beta-blockers; bradycardia
Fenoldopam	0.1–0.3 mg/kg/min intravenous infusion	<5/30 min	Headache, tachycardia, flushing, local phlebitis

Drug	Dose	Onset/Duration	Adverse effects
Hydralazine	10–20 mg as intravenous bolus or 10–40 mg intramuscularly; repeat every 4–6 h	10 min intravenous/>1 h (intravenous); 20–30 min intramuscularly/4–6 h intramuscularly	Tachycardia, headache, vomiting, aggravation of angina pectoris
Enalaprilat	0.625–1.250 mg intravenous every 6 h	15–60 min/12–24 h	Renal failure in patients with bilateral renal artery stenosis; hypotension
Parenteral adrenergic inhibitors			
Labetalol	10–80 mg as intravenous bolus every 10 min; up to 2 mg/min as intravenous infusion	2–5 min/2–4 h	Bronchoconstriction, heart block, orthostatic hypotension
Esmolol	500 µg/kg bolus injection intravenously or 25–100 µg/kg/min by infusion; may repeat bolus after 5 min or increase infusion rate to 300 µg/kg/min	1–5/15–30 min	First-degree heart block, congestive heart failure, asthma

The drugs of choice to treat hypertensive emergencies during pregnancy include hydralazine, methyldopa, and magnesium sulfate. Other commonly used drugs are contraindicated in pregnancy.

Hypertensive crises from pheochromocytomas can occur before or during surgery. Patients require IV treatment with rapidly acting drugs such as nitroprusside, phentolamine, or nicardipine. Of these, sodium nitroprusside is generally preferred due to its rapid onset and short half-life. Oral antihypertensives are too slow acting and their effect on BP is often unpredictable.

PREVENTION

Hypertensive crises are largely preventable. Inadequate management of hypertension, poor adherence to medications, and insufficient access to care are important factors leading to hypertensive crises. Patients often have a history of chronically poorly controlled BP. Aggressive treatment plans are of utmost importance in the effort to prevent hypertensive crises. Patients need to be aware that discontinuation of antihypertensive medications may precipitate a crisis. Timely office visit and telephone calls may help to prevent a crisis.

TIPS TO REMEMBER

- Treatment of severe HTN (hypertensive urgency) without evidence of acute end-organ damage is controversial. No emergent treatment is recommended. Initiation of oral medication may be indicated, with close follow-up.
- A hypertensive emergency is defined as an acute elevation of BP with rapid and progressive end-organ damage.
- Treatment should focus on the organ systems affected.
- Hypertensive crises are largely preventable with good outpatient management.

SUGGESTED READINGS

American College of Physicians. *MKSAP 15 Medical Knowledge Self-Assessment Program, Pulmonary and Critical Care Medicine*. Philadelphia: American College of Physicians; 2009.

Hebert CJ, Vidt DG. Hypertensive crises. *Prim Care*. 2008;35:475–487.

Washington University School of Medicine, Cooper DH, Krainik AJ, Lubner SJ, Reno HEL. *The Washington Manual of Medical Therapeutics*. 32nd ed. Philadelphia: Lippincott Williams & Wilkins; 2007.

An 89-year-old Man With Acute Respiratory Failure Requiring Intubation

Zak Gurnsey, MD, FACP

Mr Daniels is an 89-year-old male with a history of COPD, hypertension, and coronary artery disease. He is admitted to the ICU for acute respiratory failure due to exacerbation of his COPD. He requires intubation and mechanical ventilation. The day after admission, his wife presents evidence of a universal DNR order form. After discussing this with the health care team, it is decided to maintain the current treatment plan of intubation and mechanical ventilation. The patient's son, who was previously appointed the patient's health care power of attorney, disagrees with this decision. He would like the patient to be extubated, removed from mechanical ventilation, and allowed to pass away from natural causes. Before a treatment plan decision is ultimately reached, the patient suffers cardiac arrest and is unable to be revived. The patient is pronounced dead by his attending physician.

1. Was the code status clearly determined?

2. Who is allowed to make health care decisions for this patient?

3. Who may pronounce this patient dead?

Answers

1. This case is an example of common scenarios that arise when taking care of critically ill patients and dealing with end-of-life decisions. The patient's previous wishes were stated by the universal DNR order form. This should have been verified at admission, before the patient was initially intubated.

2. Because the patient's son was the health care power of attorney, he had the right to make medical decisions over the patient's wife.

3. The attending physician is allowed to pronounce this patient deceased.

CODE STATUS AND DEATH

This chapter will discuss areas of health care that are tied to laws and regulations. These may differ from state to state. It is important to understand the rules of the state in which one practices medicine. Unless otherwise stated, general comments in this chapter will be based on reference to Illinois law.

Code Status

All patients interacting with the health care system should ideally have their code status determined. It is important to determine this prior to a cardiopulmonary arrest situation so that the patient's wishes may be fulfilled during a catastrophic event. Performing CPR and life-sustaining measures on a patient who has previously decided against these may be grounds for criminal consequences.

One should approach code status determination as "all-or-none." It is not generally recommended to provide the different treatment options during a code situation as individual decision points. Certain patient scenarios will make the "all-or-none" stance more difficult. For instance, a patient with COPD who has previously been intubated may feel very strongly about never being intubated again. On the other hand, the patient may elect for full cardiac resuscitation during a potentially fatal heart attack. It is extremely important to have candid and upfront conversations with all patients regarding code situations.

DNR stands for do-not-resuscitate. DNI stands for do-not-intubate. The view of vasopressor medications as life-prolonging measures will differ among physicians and health care institutions.

If a patient elects for DNR code status, a universal DNR order form should be filled out. Copies should be kept with the patient, that patient's physicians, and at relevant health care institutions.

Advanced Directives

Advanced directives will vary in their form and their power. The original advanced directive developed was a living will (Figure 18-1). This simply states that the patient does not want life prolonged when death is imminent. It is rather vague and does not give any decisional direction prior to a possibly deadly event.

The universal DNR order form is also considered an advanced directive (Figure 18-2).

Having a previously determined advanced directive is one part of the process. The other important step is determining who will carry out those decisions or help make new decisions. To this end, governments have developed acts that regulate who may make decisions. In Illinois, it is called the Healthcare Surrogacy Act (Figure 18-3). This spells out the steps to use to determine a decision maker, based on that person's relationship with the patient. The surrogate must agree to be the decision maker in order for the act to be completed.

A predetermined decision maker is commonly revealed through health care power of attorney paperwork. This allows a preselected person to make health care–related decisions for the patient any time that the patient is not able to do so. This form takes precedence over the surrogate form. Thus, a patient's best friend may be allowed to make decisions over the patient's spouse or child.

Pronouncing Death

In general, death is determined by means of cardiac or brain death. There are specific protocols for determining brain death. They are beyond the scope of the discussion here. Any licensed physician is allowed to determine cardiac death.

❧Living Will❧
DECLARATION

This declaration is made this _____ day of_____ (month, year).

I, _____, born on _____, being of sound mind, willfully and voluntarily make known my desires that my moment of death shall not be artificially postponed.

If at any time I should have an incurable and irreversible injury, disease, or illness judged to be a terminal condition by my attending physician who has personally examined me and has determined that my death is imminent except for death delaying procedures, I direct that such procedures which would only prolong the dying process be withheld or withdrawn, and that I be permitted to die naturally with only the administration of medication, sustenance, or the performance of any medical procedure deemed necessary by my attending physician to provide me with comfort care.

In the absence of my ability to give directions regarding the use of such death delaying procedures, it is my intention that this declaration shall be honored by my family and physician as the final expression of my legal right to refuse medical or surgical treatment and accept the consequences from such refusal.

Signed_____

City, County and State of Residence_____

The declarant is personally known to me and I believe him or her to be of sound mind. I saw the declarant sign the declaration in my presence (or the declarant acknowledged in my presence that he or she had signed the declaration) and I signed the declaration as a witness in the presence of the declarant. I did not sign the declarant's signature above for or at the direction of the declarant. At the date of this instrument, I am not entitled to any portion of the estate of the declarant according to the laws of intestate succession or, to the best of my knowledge and belief, under any will of declarant or other instrument taking effect at declarant's death, or directly financially responsible for declarant's medical care.

Witness _____

Witness _____

History
(Source: P.A. 85-1209.)
Annotations
Note. This section was Ill.Rev.Stat., Ch. 110 1/2, Para. 703.

Rev 5/2012

Figure 18-1. Sample living will declaration.

DO-NOT-RESUSCITATE • DNR • DO-NOT-RESUSCITATE • DNR • DO-NOT-RESUSCITATE • DNR

(Page 1 of 2)

Illinois Department of Public Health
UNIFORM DO-NOT-RESUSCITATE (DNR) ADVANCE DIRECTIVE

Patient Directive

I, _____, born on _____, hereby direct the following in the event of:
   (print full name)   (birth date)

1. **FULL CARDIOPULMONARY ARREST (When both breathing and heartbeat stop):**

   ☒ **Do Not Attempt Cardiopulmonary Resuscitation (CPR)**
   (Measures to promote patient comfort and dignity will be provided.)

2. **PRE-ARREST EMERGENCY (When breathing is labored or stopped, and heart is still beating):**

   SELECT ONE

   ❑ **Do Attempt Cardiopulmonary Resuscitation (CPR) -OR-**

   ❑ **Do Not Attempt Cardiopulmonary Resuscitation (CPR)**
   (Measures to promote patient comfort and dignity will be provided.)

   Other Instructions _____
   _____

Patient Directive Authorization and Consent to DNR Order (Required to be a valid DNR Order)
   I understand and authorize the above Patient Directive, and consent to a physician DNR Order implementing this Patient Directive.

Printed name of individual	Signature of individual	Date

-OR-

Printed name of (circle appropriate title):	Signature of legal representative	Date
legal guardian		
OR agent under health care power of attorney		
OR healthcare surrogate decision maker		

Witness to Consent (Required to have a witness to be a valid DNR Order)
   I am 18 years of age or older and acknowledge the above person has had an opportunity to read this form and have witnessed the giving of consent by the above person or the above person has acknowledged his/her signature or mark on this form in my presence.

Printed name of witness	Signature of witness	Date

Physician Signature (Required to be a valid DNR Order)

   I hereby execute this DNR Order on _____.
                         Today's date

Signature of attending physician	Printed Name of attending physician	Physician's telephone number

◆ *Send this form or a copy of both sides with the individual upon transfer or discharge.* ◆

DNR • DO-NOT-RESUSCITATE • DNR • DO-NOT-RESUSCITATE • DNR • DO-NOT-RESUSCITATE

Figure 18-2. Uniform do-not-resuscitate (DNR) advance directive form.

DO-NOT-RESUSCITATE · DNR · DO-NOT-RESUSCITATE · DNR · DO-NOT-RESUSCITATE · DNR

Illinois Department of Public Health   (Page 2 of 2)
UNIFORM DO-NOT-RESUSCITATE (DNR) ADVANCE DIRECTIVE

Patient's name _____

Summarize medical condition:

When This Form Should Be Reviewed

This DNR order, in effect until revoked, should be reviewed periodically, particularly if –

- The patient/resident is transferred from one care setting or care level to another, or
- There is a substantial change in patient/resident health status, or
- The patient/resident treatment preferences change.

How to Complete the Form Review

1. Review the other side of this form.
2. Complete the following section.
   If this form is to be voided, write "VOID" in large letters on the other side of the form.
   After voiding the form, a new form may be completed.

Date   **Reviewer**   **Location of review**   **Outcome of Review**
❑ No change
❑ FORM VOIDED; new form completed
❑ FORM VOIDED; **no** new form completed

Date   **Reviewer**   **Location of review**   **Outcome of Review**
❑ No change
❑ FORM VOIDED; new form completed
❑ FORM VOIDED; **no** new form completed

Date   **Reviewer**   **Location of review**   **Outcome of Review**
❑ No change
❑ FORM VOIDED; new form completed
❑ FORM VOIDED; **no** new form completed

Advance Directives

I also have the following advance directives: **Contact person** (name and phone number)

❑ Health Care Power of Attorney   _____

❑ Living Will   _____

❑ Mental Health Treatment   _____
   Preference Declaration

◆ *Send this form or a copy of both sides with the individual upon transfer or discharge.* ◆

IOCI 0741-10

DNR · DO-NOT-RESUSCITATE · DNR · DO-NOT-RESUSCITATE · DNR · DO-NOT-RESUSCITATE

Figure 18-2. (*Continued*)

755 ILCS 40/25. Surrogate decision making:

Sec. 25. Surrogate decision making. (a) When a patient lacks decisional capacity, the health care provider must make a reasonable inquiry as to the availability and authority of a health care agent under the Powers of Attorney for Health Care Law [755 ILCS 45/4-1 et seq.]. When no health care agent is authorized and available, the health care provider must make a reasonable inquiry as to the availability of possible surrogates listed in items (1) to (4) of this subsection. The surrogate decision makers, as identified by the attending physician, are then authorized to make decisions as follows: (i) for patients who lack decisional capacity and do not have a qualifying condition, medical treatment decisions may be made in accordance with subsection (b-5) of Section 20 [755 ILCS 40/20]; and (ii) for patients who lack decisional capacity and have a qualifying condition, medical treatment decisions including whether to forgo life-sustaining treatment on behalf of the patient may be made without court order or judicial involvement in the following order of priority:

(1) the patient's guardian of the person

(2) the patient's spouse

(3) any adult son or daughter of the patient

(4) either parent of the patient

(5) any adult brother or sister of the patient

(6) any adult grandchild of the patient

(7) a close friend of the patient

(8) the patient's guardian of the estate

The health care provider shall have the right to rely on any of the above surrogates if the provider believes after reasonable inquiry that neither a health care agent under the Powers of Attorney for Health Care Law [755 ILCS 45/4-1 et seq.] nor a surrogate of higher priority is available.

Where there are multiple surrogate decision makers at the same priority level in the hierarchy, it shall be the responsibility of those surrogates to make reasonable efforts to reach a consensus as to their decision on behalf of the patient regarding the forgoing of life-sustaining treatment. If 2 or more surrogates who are in the same category and have equal priority indicate to the attending physician that they disagree about the health care matter at issue, a majority of the available persons in that category (or the parent with custodial rights) shall control, unless the minority (or the parent without custodial rights) initiates guardianship proceedings in accordance with the Probate Act of 1975 [755 ILCS 5/1-1 et seq.]. No health care provider or other person is required to seek appointment of a guardian.

(b) After a surrogate has been identified, the name, address, telephone number, and relationship of that person to the patient shall be recorded in the patient's medical record.

(c) Any surrogate who becomes unavailable for any reason may be replaced by applying the provisions of Section 25 [755 ILCS 40/25] in the same manner as for the initial choice of surrogate.

(d) In the event an individual of a higher priority to an identified surrogate becomes available and willing to be the surrogate, the individual with higher priority may be identified as the surrogate. In the event an individual in a higher, a lower, or the same priority level or a health care provider seeks to challenge the priority of or the life-sustaining treatment decision of the recognized surrogate decision maker, the challenging party may initiate guardianship proceedings in accordance with the Probate Act of 1975 [755 ILCS 5/1-1 et seq.].

(e) The surrogate decision maker shall have the same right as the patient to receive medical information and medical records and to consent to disclosure.

Figure 18-3. Except from Illinois Healthcare Surrogacy Act.

Health care institutions will usually have a policy that allows nonphysicians to pronounce death as well. For instance, 2 licensed registered nurses (RNs) may be allowed to pronounce death.

Death Summary

The death summary should have the same format as the discharge summary. Listed items should include admission and death dates, admission diagnosis, presumed cause of death, physicians/consultants on the case, important procedures and imaging, important lab and test results, a summary of the hospital course, and the events ultimately leading to the patient's death.

Other items to consider may include code status, details of prior discussions with the patient and/or family, autopsy request, and organ donor status.

TIPS TO REMEMBER

- Code status should be determined on all patients, especially the elderly and those with chronic medical conditions. This should be reviewed at regular intervals.
- Using advanced directives will help determine a decision maker during times in which the patient is unable to make decisions him/herself.

COMPREHENSION QUESTIONS

1. A patient is admitted to the hospital with pneumonia. He has a history of COPD. The patient gives his nurse a copy of a universal DNR order form that he filled out with his primary care physician 6 months ago. His wishes for DNR code status are confirmed at this time. The patient becomes lethargic and minimally arousable. His respiratory status worsens, and the health care team determines that intubation and mechanical ventilation may be helpful. What should they do?
    - A. Intubate the patient. He has a treatable condition and he may fully recover.
    - B. Intubate the patient. The physician should always do something. Allowing a patient to die is unacceptable.
    - C. Do not intubate the patient. The patient has clearly stated what his wishes are.

2. A comatose patient in the ICU cannot make his own decisions. A decision maker needs to be determined. A health care power of attorney has not been previously determined. The patient's wife, mother, and 2 sons are all willing to be the decision maker. Who is the decision maker?
    - A. Wife
    - B. Mother
    - C. Oldest son
    - D. Youngest son

3. A patient who was admitted yesterday after an acute myocardial infarction suffers ventricular fibrillation and is unable to be resuscitated. Which of these individuals is *not* allowed to pronounce the patient as dead?

    A. The attending physician

    B. The ICU resident

    C. The patient's daughter, who is an attorney

    D. Two ICU nurses

Answers

1. C. This patient should not be intubated. The universal DNR order form indicates how to treat this patient in this situation. Do not confuse DNR with "do-not-treat." This patient's pneumonia, COPD, and respiratory failure should be aggressively treated with any indicated medications and treatments, including noninvasive positive pressure ventilation. The treatment plan must stop, though, before it reaches intubation and mechanical ventilation.

2. A. Following the steps in the surrogate act, the patient's wife is appointed his decision maker. If the wife was not willing or able to be the decision maker, the next person in line would be the patient's mother.

3. C. The patient's daughter, regardless of her advanced degree, is not allowed to pronounce someone dead. The other listed individuals all have the authority to do so.

SUGGESTED READINGS

IDPH Online [Internet]. Illinois Department of Public Health Home Page; c2010 [updated April 9, 2012]. http://www.idph.state.il.us/.

Illinois General Assembly [Internet]. Illinois General Assembly Home Page [updated April 9, 2012]. http://www.ilga.gov/.

Illinois Guardianship & Advocacy Commission [Internet]. Welcome to the Illinois Guardianship & Advocacy Commission; c2002-11 [updated April 9, 2012]. http://gac.state.il.us/hcsa.html.

Living Will ID [Internet]. Living Will Forms by State; c2007. http://www.livingwillid.com/state.html.

Longo DL, Fauci AS, Kasper DL, Hauser SL, Jameson JL, Loscalzo J, eds. *Harrison's Principles of Internal Medicine*. 18th ed. New York: McGraw-Hill; 2012.

Rabow MW, Pantilat SZ. Palliative care and pain management. In: McPhee SJ, Papadakis MA, eds. *Current Medical Diagnosis & Treatment 2012*. New York: McGraw-Hill; 2012: [chapter 5].

Washington University School of Medicine, Krainik AJ, Lubner SJ, Reno HEL. *The Washington Manual of Medical Therapeutics*. 32nd ed. Philadelphia: Lippincott Williams & Wilkins; 2007.

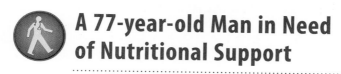

A 77-year-old Man in Need of Nutritional Support

Vajeeha Tabassum, MD, FACP

A 77-year-old man is admitted to the hospital after a cardiac arrest. He suffered a massive anterior wall myocardial infarction. The patient underwent an intra-aortic balloon pump and is now in an intensive care unit requiring mechanical ventilation. He has a history of well-controlled hypertension and hyperlipidemia. There is no history of diabetes mellitus, kidney disease, or stroke. He was a former smoker (1 PPD × 15 years, quit about 35 years ago), does not consume alcohol, and has no allergies. He takes metoprolol 50 mg po twice daily, simvastatin 20 mg po daily, aspirin 81 mg po daily, and lisinopril 10 mg po daily. Prior to this admission, he had lived independently with his wife and was able to perform his daily activities without difficulty. He managed his own finances and was driving.

Physical examination reveals a 5-ft, 48-kg (body mass index [BMI] 21 kg/m²) elderly male on mechanical ventilation on a propofol drip. Per the patient's wife, his weight is about 12% less than what he had weighed about a year ago. Pulse is 120/min regular, BP 100/60 mm Hg, respiration is 24/min, and temperature is 38.9°C. His skin is warm and dry with good capillary refill. Chest is clear to auscultation bilaterally with poor inspiratory support. Cardiac examination reveals tachycardia with occasional skipped beats. S1 and S2 are noted without murmurs. Abdomen has normal bowel sounds. Extremities show good pulses with 1+ pedal edema. The patient is restless and anxious. He is not aggressive but has vigorous movements.

Lab work reveals albumin 2.8 g/dL, BUN 28 mg/dL, creatinine 0.7 mg/dL, hemoglobin 9.6 g/dL, and serum cholesterol 115 mg/dL. Additional lab tests are unremarkable. Nursing reports that the patient had a large bowel movement a day ago.

On day 4, the patient continues to be in the intensive care unit with response to painful stimulus. He opens his eyes to verbal commands and nods appropriately to yes/no questions. It has been difficult to wean him off ventilator support and he continues to remain on mechanical ventilation. The patient's family is concerned about the patient's nutritional status and wants to start nutrition on him; they confirm that the patient continues to be a full code.

1. How would you approach the nutritional assessment in this patient?

2. What are the possible routes for nutritional support in this patient?

3. What are the potential complications associated with the above approach?

Answers

1. In acute care settings, anorexia, various disease processes, test procedures, and medications can compromise dietary intake. Under such circumstances, the goal is to identify and avoid inadequate intake and assure appropriate alimentation. The objective is to gather enough information to establish the likelihood of malnutrition due to poor dietary intake or other causes to assess whether nutritional therapy is indicated. The following indices are helpful with that objective in mind:

A. Anthropometrics: Includes measures of weight and height.

BMI = weight (kg)/height (m^2). The BMI ranges shown are for adults and are not exact for predicting healthy and unhealthy weights. Even within the healthy BMI range, weight gains may carry health risks for adults. BMI is useful as a general guideline to monitor trends in the population, but by itself is not diagnostic of an individual's health status.

   Healthy weight: BMI from 18.5 to 25

   Overweight: BMI from 25 to 30

   Obese: BMI of 30 or higher

BMI can be calculated by using the following formula: BMI = weight (kg)/height (m^2) (metric) or weight (lb)/height (in^2) × 705 (English).

B. Dietary intake assessment: This should be based on information from observed values, medical records, history, clinical examination and anthropometrics, and biochemical and functional status. Inadequate nutritional intake has been defined as the average intake of food groups, nutrients, or energy 25% to 50% below the threshold level of the recommended daily allowance. A weight loss of 5% in 1 month or 10% in 6 months is a useful indicator of nutritional risk and morbidity.

C. Laboratory tests: Abnormal biochemical values (serum albumin levels <3.5 mg/dL; serum cholesterol <150 mg/dL) are nonspecific but may indicate a need for further nutritional assessment.

2. Our patient does not seem to have any signs of GI obstruction or ileus based on the physical examination findings. However, given the ventilator use, he will be unable to take in food orally. Hence, when the gut works and oral intake is not possible, the practical approach to artificial nutrition is administration of tube feeding. Routes of administration can include nasogastric, orogastric, postpyloric, G-tube, or J-tube.

3. Aspiration is the most serious common complication; it occurs in 23% to 58% of patients with percutaneous endoscopic gastrostomy (PEG) tubes. The selection of formula depends on multiple factors. If patients do not tolerate the tube feedings well, they may develop diarrhea.

CASE REVIEW: NUTRITIONAL SUPPORT IN THE HOSPITALIZED PATIENT

Diagnosis

Inadequate nutrition impairs the body's ability to heal and to support normal immune function. The 3 major sources of energy are proteins (amino acids) (15%), carbohydrates (35%–65%), and fats (25%–50%).

Metabolic states can be classified as hypermetabolic (stressed from injury, infections, chronic inflammatory conditions, sepsis) or hypometabolic (unstressed but chronically starved). In both cases nutritional support is important.

In a hypometabolic state there is relatively less stress but ongoing catabolism. The secretion of insulin declines, and secretions of glucagon, growth hormone, and catecholamine increase. This leads to accelerated glucose utilization. Gluconeogenesis continues and eventually proteolysis is initiated to provide energy. Lipids are broken down to ketones and a large amount of proteins is broken down as well. Patients in chronic hypometabolic states will develop cachexia/marasmus over time.

In a hypermetabolic state there is ongoing stress (trauma, sepsis, etc) activating the sympathetic nervous system. Utilization of carbohydrates is inhibited, leading to hyperglycemia. Insulin secretion declines. Blood levels of glucagon, growth hormones, ACTH, thyroid hormones, and catecholamines increase. Lipolysis is activated; proteolysis and gluconeogenesis provide energy. Patients in a hypermetabolic state develop protein calorie malnutrition/kwashiorkor if nutritional needs are not met and/or the illness does not resolve quickly.

These 2 states are distinguished by differing in the rates at which proteolysis, lipolysis, and gluconeogenesis occur. These differences are mediated by proinflammatory cytokines and counterregulatory hormones that are relatively reduced in hypometabolic states and increased in hypermetabolic states.

Metabolic rate

In starvation and semi-starvation, the resting metabolic rate falls between 10% and 30% as an adaptive response to energy restriction, slowing the rate of weight loss. By contrast, in hypermetabolic states the resting metabolic rate may increase by about 10% in elective surgery, 20% to 30% after bone fractures, 30% to 60% with severe infections, and about 100% to 110% after major burns. In such situations, if the energy requirement is not matched to the energy intake, weight loss results. Losses of more than 10% of body mass in an acutely ill hypermetabolic patient may be associated with rapid deterioration in body function.

1. Estimating energy needs:

    A. Calculated:

        i. Calorie/kilogram body weight:

            1. Permissive underfeeding if obese, respiratory failure, use 20 to 25 kcal/kg per day

2. Maintenance for surgery, mild infection, use 25 to 30 kcal/kg per day

3. Repletion/hypermetabolism, if fracture, hemodialysis, severe infection, COPD, cancer, use 30 to 35 kcal/kg per day

  ii. Mifflin-St. Jeor calculation for resting energy needs, where weight (W) is in kilograms, height (H) is in centimeters, and age (A) is in years:

1. Men: $(9.99 \times W) + (6.25 \times H) - (4.92 \times A) + 5$

2. Women: $(9.99 \times W) + (6.25 \times H) - (4.92 \times A) - 161$

B. Measured energy or indirect calorimetry ("metabolic cart"):

  iii. Completed by respiratory therapy.

  iv. Must be on ventilator or room air:

1. Suggested FiO_2 <50%

  v. Patient must be at rest for at least 10 minutes during test in order to be accurate.

  vi. NPO × 8 hours prior to test:

1. Do not hold if continuous tube feeding

  vii. Report provides:

1. Measured energy expenditure (MEE):
   - Multiply by 1.1 to 1.3 for actual calorie needs.

2. Respiratory quotient (RQ):
   - <0.7 may indicate underfeeding or hypoventilation.
   - >1 may indicate overfeeding, hyperventilation, or inaccurate gas collection.

Protein catabolism

During uncomplicated energy deprivation, the rate of protein breakdown falls. After about 10 days of total starvation, an unstressed individual loses about 12 to 18 g per day of protein. In contrast, in stressful states (sepsis, trauma) protein breakdown accelerates in proportion to the degree of stress, reaching 30 to 60 g per day after elective surgery, 60 to 90 g per day with infection, 100 to 130 g per day with severe sepsis or skeletal trauma, and >175 g per day with major burns. These losses are reflected by a proportional increase in the excretion of urea nitrogen, the major by-product of protein breakdown.

    A hypometabolic patient is adapted to starvation and conserves body mass by reducing the metabolic rate and using fat as the primary fuel (rather than glucose and its precursor amino acids). A hypermetabolic patient also uses fat as a fuel but rapidly breaks down body protein to produce glucose, causing loss of muscle and organ tissue and endangering vital body functions.

Calculating protein needs:

A. Needs range from 0.6 to 2 g/kg per day.

B. Body will break down lean body mass if there is inadequate protein intake.

C. Studies indicate the body cannot metabolize greater than 2 to 3 g of protein/kg per day.

Micronutrient malnutrition

Deficiencies of nutrients that are stored in small amounts are lost through external secretions. Table 19-1 provides a reference for the physical signs of deficiencies:

Table 19-1. Vitamin and Mineral Deficiencies

Vitamin or Mineral	Physical Signs of Deficiency
Vitamin A	Hair follicle blockage with a permanent "goose-bump" appearance
	Dry, rough, skin
	Small, grayish, foamy deposits on the conjunctiva adjacent to the cornea
	Drying of the eyes and mucous membranes
Vitamin K	Small hemorrhages in the skin or mucous membranes
Thiamine	Weight loss
	Muscular wasting
	Sometimes edema (wet beriberi)
	Malaise
	Tense calf muscles
	Distended neck veins
	Jerky movement of eyes
	Staggering gait and difficulty walking
	Infants may develop cyanosis
	Round, swollen (moon) face
	Foot and wrist drop
Riboflavin	Tearing, burning, and itching of the eyes with fissuring in the corners of the eyes
	Soreness and burning of the lips, mouth, and tongue with fissuring and/or cracking of the lips and corners of the mouth
	Purple swollen tongue
	Seborrhea of the skin in the nasolabial folds, scrotum, or vulva
	Capillary overgrowth around the corneas

(continued)

Table 19-1. Vitamin and Mineral Deficiencies (*Continued*)

Vitamin or Mineral	Physical Signs of Deficiency
Niacin	Dermatitis or skin eruptions Tremors Sore tongue Skin that is exposed to sunlight will develop cracks and a scaly form of dermatitis with pigmentation May also show signs of riboflavin deficiency
Vitamin B$_6$	Tongue inflammation Inflammation of the lining of the mouth Fissures in the corners of the mouth
Folate	Weakness, fatigue, and depression Pallor Dermatologic lesions
Vitamin B$_{12}$	Lemon-yellow tint to the skin and eyes Smooth, red, thickened tongue
Vitamin C	Impaired wound healing Edema Swollen, bleeding, and/or retracted gums or tooth loss; mottled teeth; enamel erosion Lethargy and fatigue Skin lesions Small red or purplish pinpoint discolorations on the skin or mucous membranes (petechiae) Darkened skin around the hair follicles Corkscrew hair or unemerged, coiled hair
Magnesium	Tremors, muscle spasms, and tetany Personality changes
Iron	Skin pallor Pale conjunctiva Fatigue Thin, concave nails with raised edges
Zinc	Delayed wound healing Hair loss Skin lesions Eye lesions Nasolabial seborrhea Decubitus ulcers

(continued)

Table 19-1. Vitamin and Mineral Deficiencies (*Continued*)

Vitamin or Mineral	Physical Signs of Deficiency
Copper	Hair and skin depigmentation
	Pallor
Iodine	Goiter
Chromium	Corneal lesions

Nutritional assessment

The nutritional evaluation of a patient requires an integration of the history, physical examination, anthropometrics, and laboratory studies. This approach helps both to detect nutritional problems and to confirm the findings when nutritional deficiencies are suspected. In complicated patients, a nutrition care plan should be developed using an interdisciplinary team approach involving the patient and the nutrition support team, the patients' physician, dietitian, and appropriate health care personnel.

One needs to create a nutritional plan of care, including patient-specific goals. Nutrition education should be provided on topics such as diabetes, cardiac, gluten-free, low sodium, renal, weight management, fiber, and others as needed.

Nutrition care and the administration of nutrition support therapy then proceeds according to a series of steps with feedback loops (see Figure 19-1).

There are many patients at risk for nutritional problems during their hospital stay. One needs to be aware of high-risk patients so one can ensure adequate nutrition during their hospitalization. These include:

- Patients with poor oral intake due to problems such as anorexia, cognitive dysfunction, and major depression. Patients who have been made NPO for more than 5 days are also at risk.
- Patients with protracted nutrient losses from malabsorption, enteric fistulas, and draining abscesses and wounds.
- Patients in hypermetabolic states such as sepsis, trauma, and extensive burns.
- Patients who abuse alcohol.
- Patients on catabolic drugs such as steroids, immunosuppressants, and antitumor chemotherapy.
- Patients who are underweight and chronically malnourished due to poverty, advanced dementia, social isolation, advanced age, and other functional limitations.
- Underweight (body mass index <18.5) and/or recent loss of more than 10% of usual body mass.

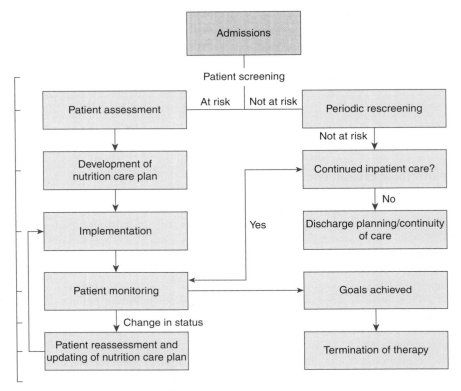

Figure 19-1. Patient nutritional assessment screening.

One should be aware of common drug–vitamin and nutrient interactions as these can unintentionally precipitate nutritional deficiencies that may be avoided with prophylactic vitamin and nutrient supplementation. Important ones to remember are:

- Alcohol interacts with the absorption of zinc, vitamins A, B_1, B_2, B_6, and B_{12}, and folate, thus making them less available. Patients who drink alcohol are often deficient in these vitamins.
- Antacids impair the absorption of vitamin B_{12}, folate, and iron.
- Broad-spectrum antibiotics used for prolonged periods of time may facilitate a deficiency of vitamin K.
- Diuretic use chronically may lead to deficiencies of vitamin B_6, potassium, copper, zinc, and magnesium.
- Laxative use leads to deficiencies of water-soluble vitamins such as vitamins D, E, A, and K, as well as of calcium and vitamin B_{12}.

- Chronic phenytoin use may impair absorption of vitamin D and folate.
- Salicylates may cause vitamin C and folate deficiencies.

Routes of feeding

The enteral route is more physiologic and safe. If the gut works, use it! Ways to deliver enteral nutrition include using nasogastric tube, orogastric tube, gastrostomy tube, and jejunal tube. Caloric, protein, and fluid needs are required to be estimated to help determine which tube feed to choose and the rate and run time. In general, when initiating tube feeds, begin with a continuous rate of 20 to 40 mL/h and advance as tolerated. The general standard is to increase by 10 mL/h every 4 hours. It is suggested to check residuals every 4 hours for adults. If greater than 250 mL for more than 2 hours, tube feeds may need to be held. Checking residuals is not required for patients with small bowel feedings. Some patients with tube feeds may develop diarrhea. Before changing the tube feeding in a patient who has developed diarrhea, answer the following questions:

- Is the patient receiving any elixir medications containing sorbitol?
- Is this secretory diarrhea?
- Is the patient receiving magnesium antacids, potassium elixir, laxatives, stool softeners, or lactulose?
- Is the patient impacted?
- Is the patient on antibiotics?
- Does the patient need fiber?
- Could it be c-diff?

If none of these is present, a change in formula may be indicated.

Parenteral route options include peripheral parenteral nutrition (PPN) or total parenteral nutrition (TPN). These are intravenous therapies that provide prescribed amounts of carbohydrates, protein, lipids, electrolytes, fluids, vitamins, and minerals and are indicated whenever nutritional support is needed and the enteral route is unavailable, or when adequate nutrition cannot be achieved through the GI tract. TPN requires access via a central line, such as a PICC line, and is used when expected length of use is >10 days. PPN can be given through a peripheral line for short term (7–10 days) or if unable to achieve central access.

Refeeding syndrome

This is a series of metabolic events precipitated by the provision of nutrients, primarily carbohydrate, to a patient in a nutritionally compromised state. It is associated with severe electrolyte abnormalities and fluid retention, and low potassium, magnesium, and phosphorus levels. It is seen most commonly with TPN, but is also seen with EN and oral nutrition. Those at risk for refeeding syndrome include patients with anorexia nervosa, chronic alcoholism, cancer, postoperative states, depression in the elderly, uncontrolled DM (DKA), chronic malnutrition, prolonged fasting, high-stress patients not fed for >7 days, or those with prolonged hypocaloric feeding.

Treatment

Initiate nutritional support at 50% of estimated needs. Supplement with a multi-vitamin/mineral once daily and thiamine 100 mg daily. Restrict glucose infusion to 150 to 200 mg per day or 2 mg/kg/min initially. Monitor potassium, phosphorus, and magnesium levels every 6 hours, 12 hours, or daily for 3 days to 1 week. Replete electrolytes as indicated. Gradually increase intake to goal over several days once electrolytes are stable and in the normal range.

Obesity is considered a nutritional syndrome where the BMI >30 kg/m^2. It is associated with comorbid conditions such as hypertension, diabetes mellitus, cardiovascular disease, and osteoarthritis. Adverse outcomes include impaired functional status, increased health care resource use, and increased mortality. Its prevalence has increased in all age groups in the United States. For frail, obese older adults, emphasize preservation of strength and flexibility rather than weight reduction. Treatment includes dietary modifications, behavioral modifications, and exercise.

TIPS TO REMEMBER

- Impaired nutrition impairs the body's ability to heal wounds and to support normal immune function.
- Providing adequate and proper nutrients to support the metabolism of the body helps to maintain the function and structures of the organs, and to accelerate recovery.
- Malnutrition is a common problem in older adults at hospital admission.
- The consequences of malnutrition impact on quality of life, increase length of stay in the hospital, and increase the risk of unsuccessful treatment outcomes.

COMPREHENSION QUESTIONS

1. A 67-year-old, well-controlled diabetic patient on metformin 1000 mg po twice daily complains of new onset of a red thickened tongue and yellowish tinge to her skin. You explain to her that the most likely cause of her presentation is due to deficiency of which one of the following?

    A. Vitamin A
    B. Vitamin B$_{12}$
    C. Folate
    D. Iron

2. An 86-year-old man is evaluated because he has been unable to take oral nutrition since hip surgery 1 week ago due to a fall. With encouragement he can take oral medications. Formal speech and swallow assessment finds mild oral pharyngeal dysphagia. He lives at home with his wife, and has a history of advanced dementia. He has lost approximately 15 lb over the last year. Physical examination is unremarkable. Laboratory results show albumin 2.8 g/dL, BUN 28 mg/dL, creatinine 0.7 mg/dL, hemoglobin 10.7 g/dL, and total cholesterol 115 mg/dL. Which of the following is the most appropriate next step?
    A. Arrange for placement of a percutaneous gastrostomy tube.
    B. Determine the patient's goals of medical care and preferences.
    C. Refer to hospice care.
    D. Prescribe nutritional supplements and multivitamins.

Answers

1. **B.** The patient is experiencing a drug–nutrient interaction. Metformin reduces the availability of vitamin B_{12}, which when uncorrected for a long time may cause a patient to present with symptoms of the nutrient deficiency. In this case the patient presents with vitamin B_{12} deficiency that includes a red thickened tongue and yellow tint to the skin and eyes.

2. **B.** Prior to proceeding with any form of artificial nutrition, it is extremely important to consider the patient's wishes after discussing the benefits and risks with the patient and surrogates. Patients and surrogates should have appropriate counseling of the consequences of various options for care. Artificial feeding may be withheld or terminated in accordance with a patient's wishes, with careful consideration of additional comorbidities and futility. In patients whose decision making is impaired, every effort should be made to determine if (s)he had previously made wishes known to the surrogate. If not, assistance with decision making should be sought (eg, hospital ethics consultation).

SUGGESTED READINGS

Academy of Nutrition and Dietetics. *ADA Evidence Analysis Library*. <www.adaevidencelibrary.com>; Accessed March 6, 2012.

American Geriatrics Society. Malnutrition. In: *Geriatric Review Syllabus*. 7th ed. New York: American Geriatrics Society; 2010 [chapter 26]. Accessed March 15, 2012.

Dwyer J. Nutrient requirements and dietary assessment. In: Longo DL, Fauci AS, Kasper DL, Hauser SL, Jameson JL, Loscalzo J, eds. *Harrison's Online Principles of Internal Medicine*. 18th ed. New York: McGraw-Hill; 2011 [chapter 73]. Accessed March 7, 2012.

Escott-Stump S. *Nutrition and Diagnosis-Related Care*. 5th ed. Philadelphia, PA: Williams & Wilkins; 2002.

Heimburger DC. Malnutrition and nutritional assessment. In: Longo DL, Fauci AS, Kasper DL, Hauser SL, Jameson JL, Loscalzo J, eds. *Harrison's Online Principles of Internal Medicine*. 18th ed. New York: McGraw-Hill; 2011 [chapter 75]. Accessed March 7, 2012.

Mahan L, Escott-Stump S, Raymond J. *Krause's Food and the Nutrition Care Process.* 13th ed. Philadelphia, PA: Saunders; 2011.

Piland C, Adams S, eds. *Pocket Resource for Nutrition Assessment.* Chicago, IL: Consultant Dietitians in Health Care Communities, Academy of Nutrition and Dietetics; 2009.

Shikora SA, Martindale RG, Schwaitzberg SB, Lane RJ, American Society for Parenteral & Enteral Nutrition, eds. *Nutritional Considerations in the Intensive Care Unit; Science, Rationale and Practice.* Dubuque, IA: Kendall Hunt Publishing; 2002.

Ukleja A, Freeman KL, Gilbert K, et al. Standards for nutrition support: adult hospitalized patients. *Nutr Clin Pract.* 2010;25(4):403–414.

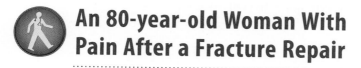

An 80-year-old Woman With Pain After a Fracture Repair

Alan J. Deckard, MD, FACP

An 80-year-old female is admitted to the hospital following a fall on an icy sidewalk. She suffered a left intertrochanteric hip fracture. There was no loss of consciousness or other injury. She was promptly transported to the ED for evaluation. Her primary physician admits her, completes a preoperative risk assessment, and consults the orthopedic surgery service after finding her to be suitable to undergo the risk of an orthopedic procedure. She has a history of well-controlled hypertension. She has no history of diabetes mellitus, coronary artery disease, kidney disease, congestive heart failure, or stroke. She is a nonsmoker, does not consume alcohol, and has no allergies. She takes hydrochlorothiazide 25 mg daily and atenolol 50 mg daily. She had an appendectomy 40 years ago without complication. She is widowed, lives independently, and completes her activities of daily living, including light housework and climbing 1 flight of stairs, independently. She drives and manages her own finances.

The orthopedic surgery service surgically repaired the fracture with an open reduction and internal fixation. She tolerated the procedure well with spinal anesthesia. She is now on the medical-surgical floor. You are called by the orthopedic surgery resident, who asks that you manage her pain and hypertension. She is otherwise following routine postoperative orthopedic protocol for venous thromboembolism (VTE) prophylaxis, activity, diet, and wound care. The patient states her pain is rated at 8 out of 10 in severity during your evaluation.

Physical examination reveals a 5-ft 2-in, 52-kg (BMI 21) elderly Caucasian female in moderate distress from pain. Her pulse is 100 bpm and regular, BP is 150/90 mm Hg, RR is 20/min, and temperature is 37°C. Her skin is warm and dry and with good capillary refill. Chest is clear to auscultation bilaterally with good inspiratory effort. Cardiac examination reveals tachycardia with a regular rhythm. S1 and S2 are noted without murmurs. Abdomen has normal bowel sounds and is nontender to palpation. Extremities show good pulses in all extremities with no edema. The left hip surgical dressing is intact and dry. The patient is oriented to person, place, and time. She has intact sensation and spontaneously moves all extremities, with significant pain noted in the left hip following any movement. Her pulse oximeter is 95% on room air. Postoperative hemoglobin is 9.8 g/dL.

1. How would you describe the type of pain this patient is experiencing?

2. How would you approach the ongoing assessment and management of the patient's pain?

3. What are potential adverse effects of her pain treatment?

Answers

Summary: A healthy 80-year-old female in the immediate orthopedic postoperative period needs a pain management approach to safely and effectively provide analgesia for her musculoskeletal pain. Control of the pain will lessen physical stress and allow more rapid rehabilitation. Safety concerns are especially noteworthy in patients with advanced age or comorbid conditions that affect analgesic metabolism and increase the likelihood of adverse effects.

1. Type of pain this patient is experiencing: acute somatic.

2. Pain assessment and control may be accomplished by the use of any of several patient pain-reporting scales and physical findings. A multimodal analgesic approach of NSAIDs, IV narcotic agents, and local ice compresses would serve as an effective initial strategy.

3. Potential side effects include constipation, ileus, nausea, delirium, somnolence, allergic reactions, respiratory depression, hypotension, acute renal failure, and others, depending on the agent.

CASE REVIEW

The elderly patient in this clinical scenario has fracture-related and postoperative tissue injury pain consistent with somatic (nociceptive) pain. Pain scales, pulse rate, blood pressure, and observation of general comfort can be used to assess the severity of the pain and adequacy of treatment. Multimodal pain therapy may be appropriate in this situation. Nonsteroidal anti-inflammatory drugs or COX-2 inhibitors are effective for acute musculoskeletal pain and inflammation. They can be given with IV narcotics and local cold therapy to the postoperative site. Multimodal therapy is a way to optimize analgesia with the lowest possible dose of each agent. A short-term patient-controlled IV narcotic delivery system is an effective way to deliver relief rapidly and safely. With improvement of pain in the subsequent postoperative days, narcotics may be changed to oral form in combination with acetaminophen.

Acute adverse reactions to narcotic analgesic agents include allergic reactions, neurologic depression and delirium, hypotension, respiratory depression, nausea, and others. Constipation is a subacute side effect that can be prevented with use of fiber-rich foods or fiber supplements and stool softeners. NSAIDs may cause GI upset, peptic ulcer disease, or acute renal failure.

PAIN MANAGEMENT IN THE HOSPITAL

Diagnosis

Pain, specifically acute pain, is one of the most common symptoms encountered in the inpatient setting. It is a source of patient suffering, anxiety, physical stress, and metabolic demand. It is an important diagnostic clue in many disease processes and conditions. The etiology of pain should be understood as it is treated, so that its underlying cause can be appropriately addressed. The emotional and physical well-being of the patient requires that pain be effectively treated.

Nociceptive pain is a response to strong mechanical, thermal, or chemical stimuli generated by nociceptors. These stimuli are transmitted as nerve impulses that are interpreted as pain. Tissue injury induces inflammatory mediators that contribute to this response. Nociceptive pain can be categorized as either somatic (related to skin, muscles, bone, and other tissue of somatic embryologic origin) or visceral (related to internal organs). Neuropathic pain refers to peripheral or central nerve injury or dysfunction. Nociceptive pain responds favorably to local therapy, acetaminophen, NSAIDs, and narcotic analgesics, while neuropathic pain is more responsive to nontraditional therapy such as antidepressants, anticonvulsants, and lidocaine.

Pain is always subjective. It is defined by the International Association for the Study of Pain as an unpleasant sensory and emotional experience, most often associated with actual or potential tissue damage. There is no test to verify or quantify the severity of the pain except for the patient's word and physical response to the pain. An individual's response to pain is as unique as is the response to analgesics. A thorough history on all patients should include quantification, localization, temporal features, aggravating and alleviating factors, previous use of analgesics, and previous alcohol or drug dependence. Physical examination should note the patient response to pain and localize it. Clues to etiology can also be determined by the examination, such as CVA pain, rebound tenderness, reproducible chest pain, and others.

Pain scales should be used to quantify pain initially and to measure ongoing analgesic effectiveness. Scales may be self-assessment tools used by the patient to report to caregivers, or pain observation scales that target patients with cognitive impairments or communication challenges. The simplest self-assessment scales have the patient rate the pain on a 0 to 10 scale, with 10 being the most severe pain, or a 0 to 9 face scale, with a neutral face indicating no pain to a crying face meaning severe pain. Any scale may be used as long as it is patient appropriate and used consistently. A reasonable goal for a conscious patient is a pain rating of 3 or less out of 10 (Figure 20-1).

Wong-Baker FACES pain rating scale
See Figure 20-2.

Brief word instructions Point to each face using the words to describe the pain intensity. Ask the child to choose face that best describes own pain and record the appropriate number.

Original instructions Explain to the person that each face is for a person who feels happy because he has no pain (hurt) or sad because he has some or a lot of pain. *Face 0* is very happy because he doesn't hurt at all. *Face 1* hurts just a little bit. *Face 2* hurts a little more. *Face 3* hurts even more. *Face 4* hurts a whole lot. *Face 5* hurts as

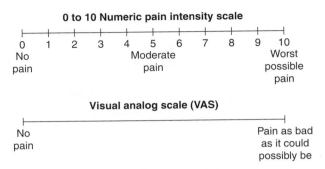

Figure 20-1. Examples of visual pain intensity assessment scales. (Reproduced with permission from Hockenberry MJ, Wilson D. *Wong's Essentials of Pediatric Nursing.* 8th ed. St. Louis: Mosby; 2009.)

much as you can imagine, although you don't have to be crying to feel this bad. Ask the person to choose the face that best describes how he is feeling.

Rating scale is recommended for persons aged 3 years and older.

Treatment

Methods of treating acute pain include relaxation techniques, hypnosis, acupuncture, transcutaneous electrical neural stimulation (TENS), massage therapy, heat and cold topical treatments, and pharmaceutical analgesic agents. Pharmaceutical agents include acetaminophen, NSAIDs, corticosteroids, opioids, ketamine, clonidine, and topical anesthetic agents. They may be administered locally, such as in intra-articular or regional blockade, orally, parenterally, or via epidural route.

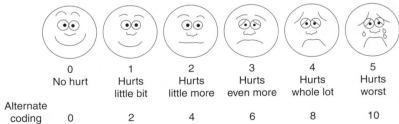

Figure 20-2. Wong-Baker FACES pain rating scale. (Reproduced with permission from Hockenberry MJ, Wilson D. *Wong's Essentials of Pediatric Nursing.* 8th ed. St. Louis: Mosby; 2009. Copyright Mosby.)

This discussion will focus on oral and parenteral agents used by most internal medicine residents. It is worthwhile to be aware of other modalities and the other medical professionals available to help with challenging patients.

Analgesics reduce the sensation of pain by altering perception of pain in the CNS, inhibiting local pain and inflammatory mediator production, or interrupting the neural impulse in the spinal cord, such as with a neuraxial block. One should pick the lowest effective dose of analgesic agent, taking into account metabolic pathways, comorbid illnesses, medication interactions, and potential side effects. Always have dosing references for specific agents available that include opioid equivalent dosing information.

Acetaminophen and NSAIDs, including COX-2 inhibitors, are step 1 agents in the WHO analgesic ladder. They are for pain on the low end of the severity scale. Acetaminophen may be used at 325 to 1000 mg per dose up to 4 g daily. It has antipyretic and analgesic properties. It can potentiate warfarin at higher dosing and may cause acute liver failure in overdoses. It does not have antiplatelet effects. Aspirin and NSAIDs, including COX-2 inhibitors, have anti-inflammatory, antipyretic, and analgesic effects. They have a variable effect on platelet function, may induce gastrointestinal bleeding, should be used with caution in patients with hepatic and renal disease, and should be avoided in patients with an aspirin allergy. They may be used in conjunction with opioid agents.

Step 2 agents include tramadol, and the opioids codeine, hydrocodone, and meperidine. Meperidine is not recommended due to the potential for accumulation of metabolites and risk of seizures. These agents reach a dose-response plateau unlike step 3 agents. Tramadol is a nonopiate with serotonin reuptake inhibiting properties. It binds to opioid receptors. Tramadol is dosed at 50 to 100 mg every 6 hours prn. Dosing reduction is recommended for the elderly and those with renal or liver dysfunction. See Table 20-1 for other dosing comparisons of step 2 agents.

Step 3 agents are morphine, hydromorphone, oxycodone, fentanyl, and methadone (see Table 20-1). Morphine is the standard to which the other agents are compared. Opioid-naive patients should be started with lower doses than opioid-tolerant patients. There is no ceiling to the analgesic effect of these agents. Some are used in patient-controlled analgesia (PCA) regimens. Most institutions will have order sets that specify a patient-controlled dose, a lockout interval between doses, and a maximum dose per specific period of time. A basal rate of constant infusion may be given along with the patient-triggered doses. All the opioid agents may cause nausea, constipation, and neurologic of respiratory suppression. The onset and duration of the agent helps to determine the appropriate dosing interval and route of administration. Transdermal preparations of fentanyl should only be given for chronic pain of moderate or severe intensity. Bowel regimens such as a stool softener plus a mild stimulant agent (eg, senna) should be considered. Antiemetics may be used as needed. Dosages should be adjusted with hepatic impairment and used cautiously with lung disease, malnutrition,

Table 20-1. Equianalgesic Doses of Opioid Analgesics

Medication	Onset	Duration	Parenteral Dosing (mg)	Enteral Dosing	Comments
Fentanyl	Rapid (<10 min)	Short (1–2 h)	0.1 mg IM/IV/SC	Not available orally	Also available in patch form
Hydromorphone	Quick (15–30 min)	Moderate (4–5 h)	1.0–2.0 mg IM/IV/SC	7.5 mg	
Methadone	Slow (45–60 min)	Long (6–8 h)	10 mg IM/IV/SC	20 mg	Commonly used for chronic pain
Morphine	Quick (15–30 min)	Moderate (4–6 h)	10 mg IM/IV/SC	60 mg	
Oxycodone	Quick (15–30 min)	Moderate (4–6 h)	Not available parenterally	30 mg	
Meperidine	Variable (10–45 min)	Short (2–4 h)	75 mg IM/IV/SC	300 mg	Typically not recommended due to efficacy studies
Codeine	Quick (15–30 min)	Moderate (4–6 h)	120 mg IM/IV/SC	200 mg	Most commonly given orally

Note: For comparative reference only. Consult therapeutic sources for individual patient dosing.

endocrine disease, and other psychotropic or sedative agents. Urinary retention may be caused by increased bladder, ureteral, and urethral sphincter tone.

Intraspinal administration of opioids may be given with the assistance of the anesthesiology clinicians. Coordination of dosing after acute intraspinal analgesia requires timely and clear communication.

Naloxone may be given to reverse the effect of opioids. It should be used with caution in chronic opioid users. It can precipitate agitation, anxiety, nausea, and seizures.

TIPS TO REMEMBER

- The cause of acute pain should be determined prior to, or in conjunction with, treatment of the pain.
- Pain scales should be used to determine severity of pain and effectiveness of treatment.
- Multimodal analgesic therapy should be used when possible.
- Concurrent medications, comorbid medical conditions, age, and previous exposure to narcotic agents should be considered in opioid dosing decisions.
- Bowel regimens should be anticipatory therapy on all patients taking opioids.

COMPREHENSION QUESTIONS

1. A 24-year-old female is hospitalized with a kidney stone and pyelonephritis. She is started on appropriate intravenous antibiotics and fluid therapy. She has no allergies and has never had opioids in the past. Her weight is 48 kg. Her colicky pain is rated at 7 to 8 out of 10 in severity at admission, with significant nausea and occasional vomiting. She has not passed the stone. What is/are reasonable analgesic option(s)?

    A. Fentanyl transdermal 12 µg/h patch every 3 days
    B. Acetaminophen 1000 mg orally every 8 hours as needed
    C. Naloxone 0.4 mg IV every 8 hours as needed
    D. Hydromorphone 0.6 mg IV every 3 hours as needed

2. A 65-year-old man is on his third postoperative day following a knee replacement. He is progressing as expected but is limited in physical therapy due to pain. He is only on intravenous morphine every 3 hours. He is allergic to aspirin that caused hives and dyspnea. What agent should be avoided?

    A. Naproxen
    B. Acetaminophen/hydrocodone
    C. Oxycodone
    D. Clonidine

3. Which of the following agents is not commonly administered via PCA?
   A. Fentanyl
   B. Morphine
   C. Oxycodone
   D. Hydromorphone

Answers

1. **D.** Transdermal fentanyl should be used only with opioid-tolerant patients with moderate to severe chronic pain requiring continuous analgesic dosing. Acetaminophen is likely not potent enough to control this moderate to severe pain, and may not be absorbed well orally due to the potential for vomiting. Naloxone is used to reverse the effects of opioids. Hydromorphone at this dose is appropriate for an opioid-naive patient.

2. **A.** Naproxen should be avoided with a known allergy to aspirin. There is a potential for similar reactions. The others have no cross-reactivity to aspirin or other NSAIDs.

3. **C.** Oxycodone has no intravenous preparation, therefore cannot be used in PCA systems.

SUGGESTED READINGS

Helfand M, Freeman M. *Assessment and Management of Acute Pain in Adult Medical Inpatients: A Systematic Review* [Internet]. Washington, DC: US Department of Veterans Affairs; 2008.
Hockenberry MJ, Wilson D. *Wong's Essentials of Pediatric Nursing.* 8th ed. St. Louis: Mosby; 2009.
Wachter RM, Goldman L, Hollander H. *Hospital Medicine.* Philadelphia: Lippincott Williams & Wilkins; 2000.
Washington University School of Medicine Department of Medicine, Green GB, Harris IA, Lin GA, Moylan KC. *The Washington Manual of Medical Therapeutics.* 31st ed. Philadelphia: Lippincott Williams & Wilkins; 2004.

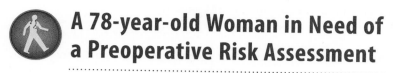

A 78-year-old Woman in Need of a Preoperative Risk Assessment

Robert Robinson, MD, MS, FACP

You are asked to perform a preoperative risk assessment on a 78-year-old female with a traumatic femur fracture after slipping on ice. The patient takes no medications, has no known medical problems, has no cardiac symptoms, has no problems with easy bruising or prolonged bleeding, and is usually able to climb several flights of stairs. The patient does have a 50 pack-year smoking history, but quit smoking about 10 years ago.

Physical examination is unremarkable except for evidence of the femur fracture.

Preoperative tests show a normal sinus rhythm on ECG, hyperinflation of the lungs on chest x-ray, and unremarkable electrolytes and CBC. The surgical resident indicates that the surgery will take about 3 hours and require general anesthesia.

1. **What additional tests are needed to assess this patient's risk of surgical complications?**

2. **What are this patient's risk factors for postoperative pulmonary complications?**

3. **What actions should be taken postoperatively to reduce the patient's risk of complications?**

Answers

1. No additional tests will influence the decision as to whether the patient is appropriate for this urgent surgery. The patient does not appear to have any active cardiac issues and has good exercise tolerance. The *ACC/AHA Guidelines on Perioperative Evaluation and Care for Noncardiac Surgery* indicate that it is reasonable to proceed to surgery under these circumstances. Pulmonary function tests are not strong predictors of perioperative pulmonary complications, and checking a PT and PTT is not needed because the patient has no history of bleeding disorders.

2. Age (over 60 years) and the prospect of a prolonged surgery under general anesthesia are known risk factors for postoperative pulmonary complications. Cigarette smoking is not a risk factor because the patient quit smoking about 10 years ago. The patient may have COPD based on her smoking history and hyperinflation of the lungs. If the patient does have COPD, it is an additional risk factor for postoperative pulmonary complications.

3. This patient would benefit from DVT prophylaxis in the postoperative time frame. Due to the nature of the injury and surgery, the patient is at increased risk of DVT. In addition, monitoring for evidence of bleeding should be routine after a surgical procedure.

CASE REVIEW

This patient has no known medical problems, good functional status (>4 METS), and no active cardiac issues. Using the *ACC/AHA Guidelines on Perioperative Evaluation and Care for Noncardiac Surgery* criteria, this patient can go to surgery without further cardiac testing or the initiation of a beta-blocker or other drug therapy. Additional testing, though commonly performed, is unlikely to alter the decision regarding the patient's stability for surgery.

Part of a preoperative examination is to also identify potential postoperative risks. This patient is at increased risk of pulmonary and thrombotic complications. Recommending DVT prophylaxis and incentive spirometry is appropriate.

PERIOPERATIVE MEDICINE

Cardiac Risk Factors

The ACC/AHA guidelines identify 6 risk factors for cardiac complications of surgery: high-risk surgery, history of ischemic heart disease, heart failure, cerebrovascular disease, diabetes treated with insulin, and a serum creatinine >2 mg/dL.

The risk of cardiac complications rises with the number of risk factors: 1% for 1 risk factor, 5% for 2 risk factors, and 10% for 3 or more risk factors (Figure 21-1; Table 21-1).

Cardiac Risk Reduction

Cardiac risk reduction for noncardiac surgery is an area of active research. Recent studies have called into question the utility of strategies using revascularization and beta-blockers for this purpose (Table 21-2).

Pulmonary Risk Factors

Pulmonary complications of surgery are common; however, few studies have focused on risk assessment for pulmonary complications of surgery. The ACP guidelines indicate that the type of surgery and duration of surgery are the most powerful, but nonmodifiable, predictors of postoperative pulmonary complications (Table 21-3).

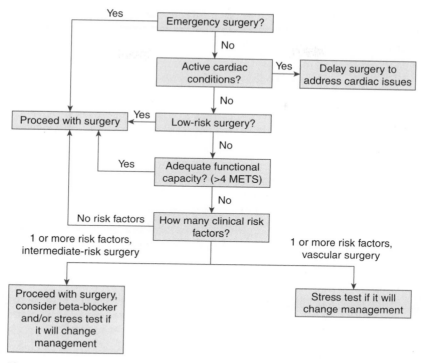

Figure 21-1. Perioperative cardiac evaluation.

Table 21-1. Surgery-specific Risks for Postoperative Cardiac Complications

Low Risk	Intermediate Risk	High Risk
Endoscopy	Intraperitoneal surgery	Aortic surgery
Superficial surgery	Intrathoracic surgery	Peripheral vascular surgery
Breast surgery	Endovascular repair of aorta	
Cataract surgery	Carotid endarterectomy	
Ambulatory surgery	Head/neck surgery	
	Orthopedic surgery	
	Prostate surgery	

Table 21-2. Cardiac Risk Reduction Strategies for Noncardiac Surgery

Intervention	Clinical Trial/Results
Revascularization	CASS trial—CABG 4–6 years before surgery reduced risk of perioperative cardiac complications for high- and intermediate-risk surgeries
	CARP trial—CABG showed mortality benefit in patients with angina, left main disease, an EF less than 20%, or aortic stenosis when undergoing vascular surgery
	PCI guidelines (several trials)—ACC/AHA recommends the use of a bare metal stent and delaying surgery by at least 4 weeks post-PCI. If a drug-eluting stent is used, surgery should be delayed for at least 1 year
Beta-blockers	ACC/AHA now recommends beta-blockers for patients with reversible ischemia on stress testing or patients with 3 or more cardiac risk factors
	POISE trial—patients receiving a beta-blocker had a decreased risk of MI, but had an increased risk of stroke or death

Pulmonary Risk Reduction

The ACP guidelines indicate several interventions that may reduce the risk of postoperative pulmonary complications. Patients with known lung disease should have the underlying condition appropriately treated before and after surgery (Table 21-4).

Table 21-3. Risk Factors for Pulmonary Complications

Unmodifiable	Modifiable
Age >60 years	Current smoking
COPD	Malnutrition
ASA Class II or higher	Functional dependence[a]
Heart failure	
Obstructive sleep apnea	

[a]Possibly modifiable.

Table 21-4. Risk Reduction Strategies for Pulmonary Complications

Good Evidence to Support Use	Fair Evidence to Support Use
Incentive spirometry	Selective nasogastric tube decompression
	Use of short-acting neuromuscular blockers
	Smoking cessation >8 weeks before surgery

DVT and PE Prevention

DVT and PE can be prevented with several strategies including heparin, low-molecular-weight heparin, and mechanical devices. A DVT prevention strategy should be implemented in all hospitalized patients with 1 or more risk factors for DVT.

Inferior vena cava (IVC) filters are DVT prevention options in patients with clear risk factors for DVT with contraindications for anticoagulation. The use of IVC filters for DVT prevention is most commonly seen in neurological trauma patients (Table 21-5).

HIGH-RISK MEDICATIONS

There are medications that should be adjusted prior to surgery in order to help to minimize complications. These may include those listed in Table 21-6.

Table 21-5. Prevention Options for DVT

Method	Dosing
Unfractionated heparin (UFH)	5000 U subcutaneously every 8–12 h
Low-molecular-weight heparin (LMWH)	Varies by drug selected
Fondaparinux	2.5 mg subcutaneously every day
Warfarin	Adjust to target INR of 2–3
Pneumatic compression devices	While in bed or immobile
Inferior vena cava filter	

Table 21-6. Perioperative Medication Management

Medication	Management
Warfarin	Discontinue 3–5 days before surgery. Consider heparin bridge if patient is at high risk of thrombosis
Clopidogrel	Discontinue 3–7 days before surgery. Delay surgery and do not discontinue clopidogrel if patient has had drug-eluting stent placed in the past year due to risk of stent thrombosis
Insulin	Discontinue short-acting insulin. Administer one third or two thirds of usual morning dose of intermediate- to long-acting insulin. Monitor blood glucose carefully
Oral hypoglycemic agents	Discontinue the morning of surgery. Monitor blood glucose carefully
ACE inhibitors or angiotensin receptor blockers	Consider discontinuing the morning of surgery if large fluid shifts or blood volume loss is anticipated
Diuretics	Consider discontinuing the morning of surgery if large fluid shifts or blood volume loss is anticipated
Corticosteroids	Continue at current dose. Consider stress dosing for intermediate- or high-risk surgeries

TIPS TO REMEMBER

- Evaluate and document patient risk factors and the risk factors of the proposed surgery.
- Testing should be selective and focused on the identification of problems that may impact surgical planning.
- High-risk medications (anticoagulants, hypoglycemic agents, and steroids) require careful attention in the perioperative period.
- Surgical patients should be started on therapy to prevent DVTs.
- Beta-blockers should only be started in high-risk patients with clear indications for beta-blocker therapy.

COMPREHENSION QUESTIONS

1. You are evaluating the cardiac risk for a right total knee replacement in a 59-year-old male with diabetes (treated with insulin) and diabetic nephropathy (serum creatinine 1.5 mg/dL). The patient has difficulty walking due to severe osteoarthritis, and is scheduled for surgery in 1 week. The patient denies cardiac symptoms, and is able to climb 2 flights of stairs. His only limitation on mobility is knee pain at this time.

What additional information is needed to assess this patient's risk of surgical complications?

    A. A cardiac stress test due to the presence of 2 risk factors (diabetes treated with insulin and renal disease)

    B. An echocardiogram

    C. A CBC, BMP, chest x-ray, and 12-lead ECG

    D. None of the above

2. You are evaluating the cardiac risk for a right total knee replacement in a 59-year-old male with diabetes (treated with insulin), diabetic nephropathy (serum creatinine 1.5 mg/dL), and a history of myocardial infarction 6 months ago. The patient had left main coronary artery disease and underwent a CABG.

The patient has difficulty walking due to severe osteoarthritis, and is scheduled for surgery in 1 week. The patient denies cardiac symptoms, and is able to climb 2 flights of stairs. His only limitation on mobility is knee pain at this time. The patient is taking a beta-blocker for his CAD and has a resting pulse rate of 70 beats/min.

What additional information is needed to assess this patient's risk of surgical complications?

    A. A cardiac stress test

    B. An echocardiogram

    C. A CBC, BMP, chest x-ray, and 12-lead ECG

    D. None of the above

3. You are evaluating the cardiac risk for a right total knee replacement in a 77-year-old female with hypertension and a history of myocardial infarction 6 months ago. The patient underwent PCI at that time, but is unsure if a stent was placed. The patient is on clopidogrel and a beta-blocker.

The patient has difficulty walking due to severe osteoarthritis, and is scheduled for surgery in 1 week. She denies cardiac symptoms, and is able to climb 2 flights of stairs. Her only limitation on mobility is knee pain at this time.

What additional information is needed to assess this patient's risk of surgical complications?

    A. A cardiac stress test

    B. An echocardiogram

C. A CBC, BMP, chest x-ray, and 12-lead ECG

D. Information regarding the patient's PCI 6 months ago

E. None of the above

4. The case in Question 3 continues: Review of records from the patient's cardiologist shows that a drug-eluting stent was placed 6 months ago. How should this patient be managed?

A. Discontinue clopidogrel 3 to 7 days before surgery.

B. Delay surgery for 12 months.

C. Delay surgery for 6 months.

D. Discontinue clopidogrel 3 to 7 days before surgery; start patient on IV heparin for full anticoagulation before surgery.

Answers

1. **D.** The patient has no active cardiac issues and exercise tolerance >4 METS, so it is reasonable to proceed with surgery without additional testing. The patient has just 1 risk factor—diabetes treated with insulin. The patient's renal insufficiency is not severe enough to qualify as a risk factor.

2. **D.** No additional testing is indicated at this time. He has had a recent CABG and has no active cardiovascular symptoms. This patient is low risk for cardiovascular complications from surgery.

3. **D.** It is essential to know if the patient had a stent placed at the time of PCI, and also to know what type of stent was placed.

4. **C.** Delay the surgery for at least 6 more months (12 months from the time of stent placement) to reduce the risk of stent thrombosis when the clopidogrel is discontinued.

SUGGESTED READINGS

Fleisher LA, Beckman JA, Brown KA, et al. ACC/AHA 2007 guidelines on perioperative cardiovascular evaluation and care for noncardiac surgery: executive summary: a report of the American College of Cardiology/American Heart Association Task Force on Practice Guidelines (Writing Committee to Revise the 2002 Guidelines on Perioperative Cardiovascular Evaluation for Noncardiac Surgery) developed in collaboration with the American Society of Echocardiography, American Society of Nuclear Cardiology, Heart Rhythm Society, Society of Cardiovascular Anesthesiologists, Society for Cardiovascular Angiography and Interventions, Society for Vascular Medicine and Biology, and Society for Vascular Surgery. *J Am Coll Cardiol.* 2007;50(17):1707–1732.

Killip T, Passamani E, Davis K. Coronary artery surgery study (CASS): a randomized trial of coronary bypass surgery. Eight years follow-up and survival in patients with reduced ejection fraction. *Circulation.* 1985;72(6 pt 2):V102–V109.

Lawrence VA, Cornell JE, Smetana GW, American College of Physicians. Clinical guidelines: strategies to reduce postoperative pulmonary complications after noncardiothoracic surgery: systematic review for the American College of Physicians. *Ann Intern Med.* 2006;144:596–608.

McFalls EO, Ward HB, Moritz TE, et al. Predictors and outcomes of a perioperative myocardial infarction following elective vascular surgery in patients with documented coronary artery disease: results of the CARP trial. *Eur Heart J.* 2008;29(3):394–401.

POISE Study Group, Devereaux PJ, Yang H, et al. Effects of extended-release metoprolol succinate in patients undergoing non-cardiac surgery (POISE trial): a randomised controlled trial. *Lancet.* 2008;371(9627):1839–1847.

A 72-year-old Man With Pneumonia

Robert Robinson, MD, MS, FACP

You are called by the emergency department and told of a 72-year-old male non-smoker with a history of diabetes, coronary artery disease, and hypertension who presents with pneumonia and needs to be admitted to the hospital. The patient is febrile and tachypneic, has a blood pressure of 145/65, and has an oxygen saturation of 95% on room air. Physical examination is significant for rhonchi in the right lower lung fields, and a chest x-ray shows a right lower lobe infiltrate. Laboratory studies show a white blood cell count of 14,000 and no evidence of acute renal failure. Blood cultures have been obtained and an unknown antibiotic has been started in the emergency department.

1. Should this patient be admitted to the hospital?
2. What historical information is needed to make a treatment decision for this patient?
3. What is the best initial treatment if this patient has no antibiotic allergies and no significant contact with the health care system?
4. What would be the best initial treatment if this patient has no antibiotic allergies and is a resident of a long-term care facility?
5. What additional steps need to be taken to ensure compliance with the pneumonia core measures?

Answers

1. Yes, to a non-ICU setting. This patient is hemodynamically stable and has a CURB-65 score (an easy-to-use risk assessment method for community-acquired pneumonia [CAP] described below) of 2 (age, tachypnea), so it is reasonable to manage the patient out of the ICU.

2. A history of medication allergies, particularly antibiotic allergies, is essential for the development of a safe treatment plan. Additionally, because initial antimicrobial therapy is selected primarily based on the type of pneumonia a patient has, risk factors for health care–associated pneumonia (HCAP) and other respiratory infections should be considered.

3. Ceftriaxone and azithromycin, ampicillin/sulbactam, and azithromycin or levofloxacin are all appropriate choices for this patient for first-line therapy in a hospitalized patient with CAP.

4. This patient likely has HCAP, and is at risk of infection with bacteria commonly seen in patients with CAP, but is also at risk of infection with MRSA

and *Pseudomonas*. Levofloxacin will be effective against most causes of CAP, vancomycin is for potential MRSA, and piperacillin/tazobactam is useful for the treatment of *Pseudomonas*.

5. Pneumonia vaccine before discharge is the last remaining quality measure. The patient has had blood cultures drawn, rapid initiation of antibiotic therapy, selection of appropriate antibiotics for an immunocompetent patient not requiring ICU admission, and evaluation of his oxygenation status with a pulse oximeter. As a nonsmoker, the patient does not need smoking cessation counseling, but documentation of the patient's smoking status is required. *Note*: Use of a standard order set increases the likelihood that all relevant quality measures will be met.

CASE REVIEW

This patient appears to have pneumonia that requires hospital admission based on his CURB-65 score. Hemodynamic stability and a low CURB-65 score indicate that the patient is appropriate for admission to a non-ICU level of care.

Insufficient data are provided to determine if the patient has CAP, HCAP, or another type of respiratory illness. Additional history is needed to better assess risk factors for other pneumonias. A history of recent travel should raise concern for avian influenza, SARS, parasites, lung flukes, fungi, etc. Exposure to others who are symptomatic for a respiratory illness should raise concern for *Bordetella*, mycobacteria, *Legionella*, etc. A history of high-risk sexual behavior, injectable drug use, long-term steroid use, or a history of malignancy should raise concern for an immunocompromised status, and the differential diagnosis should include viral infections (ie, HIV, cytomegalovirus, varicella, and herpes), mycobacterial infections, fungal infections (including *Pneumocystis*), and atypical bacterial infections (ie, *Nocardia*, *Actinomyces*, etc).

PNEUMONIA

Diagnosis

Pneumonia is suggested by a history that contains 1 or more symptoms of pneumonia such as cough, fever, pleuritic chest pain, dyspnea, and/or sputum production. The history is insensitive for the diagnosis of pneumonia, but is essential for eliciting risk factors for immunocompetent status, and the likely type of pneumonia (CAP, hospital-acquired pneumonia [HAP], HCAP, other).

Physical examination may reveal fever, tachycardia, tachypnea, rales, and evidence of pulmonary consolidation (egophony and dullness to percussion). However, physical examination has not been shown to be sensitive for the diagnosis of pneumonia either.

Table 22-1. Differential Diagnosis for Pulmonary Infiltrates

Acute Infiltrate	Chronic or Nonresolving Infiltrate
Pneumonia	Nonresolving infection
Pulmonary edema	ARDS
Aspiration pneumonitis	Lung abscess
Hemorrhage	Mycobacterial infection
Contusion	*Pneumocystis jiroveci*
Pulmonary infarction	Fungal infection
Postobstructive pneumonia	Chronic aspiration
Inhalation injury	Hypersensitivity pneumonitis
Radiation pneumonitis	Lipoid pneumonia
ARDS	Eosinophilic lung disease
	Malignancy
	Sarcoidosis
	Rheumatologic conditions
	Vasculitis
	Radiation pneumonitis
	Fibrosis
	Pulmonary alveolar proteinosis
	Parasites
	Pneumoconiosis
	Inhalation injury
	Cryptogenic organizing pneumonia

A CBC, BMP, and blood cultures should be obtained on all patients with suspected pneumonia. The value of sputum cultures is controversial. Urine antigen testing (*Legionella* and *Streptococcus pneumoniae*) and viral testing (influenza and others) may also be helpful.

Chest radiography showing a new infiltrate with a compatible history and examination is considered the gold standard for the diagnosis of pneumonia. A chest x-ray should be ordered on all patients with suspected pneumonia. Comparison with prior radiographs (if available) should be made (Table 22-1).

Risk stratification with CURB-65

The CURB-65 criteria are an easy-to-use risk assessment method for CAP, and they are useful for determining which patients can be managed as outpatients (Table 22-2).

Table 22-2. CURB-65 Criteria

Criteria	Treatment Location
Confusion	0–1 criteria → outpatient
Uremia	2 criteria → inpatient
Respiratory rate >30	3 or more criteria → ICU
Systolic blood pressure ≤90	
Age ≥65	

Microbiology

The microbiology of pneumonia differs considerably based on patient risk factors for exposure to multidrug-resistant bacteria, leading to 2 major classifications of pneumonia: CAP and health care–related pneumonias.

Community-acquired pneumonia

CAP is further subclassified as being caused by typical or atypical bacterial organisms. More than 100 organisms (bacteria, viruses, fungi, and parasites) have been identified as causative agents for CAP, but the vast majority of cases are caused by a short list of microbes (Tables 22-3 and 22-4).

Health care–related pneumonias

Health care–related pneumonias are important causes of increased morbidity and mortality, and are often caused by drug-resistant organisms. The major classifications of health care–related pneumonia are HAP, ventilator-associated pneumonia (VAP), and HCAP (Tables 22-5 and 22-6).

Treatment

The initial treatment of patients with pneumonia is driven by the classification of pneumonia. Duration of antibiotic therapy remains controversial. Duration ranges from 5 to 14 days (Table 22-7).

Table 22-3. Common Bacterial Causes of Community-acquired Pneumonia

Typical Bacteria	Atypical Bacteria
Streptococcus pneumoniae	Mycoplasma pneumoniae
Haemophilus influenzae	Chlamydophila pneumoniae
Moraxella catarrhalis	Legionella pneumophila

Table 22-4. Nonbacterial Causes of Community-acquired Pneumonia

Viruses	Fungal
Influenza	*Cryptococcus*
Coronavirus	*Histoplasma*
Rhinovirus	*Coccidioides*
Varicella	*Blastomyces*

Table 22-5. Definitions of Heath Care–related Pneumonias

Hospital-acquired pneumonia	Occurs 48 h or more after admission
	Did not appear to be incubating at time of admission
Ventilator-associated pneumonia	Occurs 48 h or more after endotracheal intubation
Health care–associated pneumonia	Extensive health care contact
	Within 30 days
	IV therapy (antibiotics, chemotherapy, or other)
	Wound care
	Hospital visit
	Dialysis
	Within 90 days
	Hospital stay of 2 or more days
	Long-term care facility residence

Table 22-6. Microbiology of HAP, VAP, and HCAP

	HAP (%)	VAP (%)	HCAP (%)
MSSA	13	9	
MRSA	20	18	27
Pseudomonas aeruginosa	9	18	25
Stenotrophomonas maltophilia	1	7	
Acinetobacter spp.	3	8	

Table 22-7. Treatment Recommendations From 2007 IDSA Guidelines

CAP (non-ICU status)	Respiratory fluoroquinolone alone
	Or
	One of the following:
	Third- or fourth-generation cephalosporin
	Ertapenem
	Ampicillin/sulbactam
	Macrolide or doxycycline
CAP (ICU status)	Antipneumococcal beta-lactam
	And
	Respiratory fluoroquinolone *or* a macrolide
	Add antipseudomonal coverage for patients with risk factors for *Pseudomonas* infection
HAP/VAP/HCAP (initial therapy)	One of the following:
	Antipseudomonal cephalosporin
	Antipseudomonal carbapenem
	Piperacillin/tazobactam
	Respiratory fluoroquinolone *or* aminoglycoside
	Linezolid *or* vancomycin

Consider de-escalation of antibiotic therapy 48 to 72 hours after initiation of antibiotics, depending on culture results and the clinical status of the patient.

Fungal pneumonia
Fungi causing respiratory infection are ubiquitous, and symptoms are often mild and nonspecific. Risk factors for severe fungal pneumonia include immunosuppression, abnormal pulmonary parenchyma (bronchiectasis, emphysema, and pulmonary fibrosis), and chronic lung disease. It is important to remember that exposures to large fungal loads can overwhelm an immunocompetent person's ability to adequately respond as well (Table 22-8).

Table 22-8. Fungal Causes of Pneumonia, Diagnostic Methods, and Treatment Options

Fungus	Diagnostic Tests	Initial Treatment
Aspergillus	CT of chest Bronchoscopy Culture Fungal antigen testing (1-3)-β-D-Glucan assay	Voriconazole or amphotericin B
Cryptococcus	Culture Fungal antigen testing PCR Bronchoscopy	Amphotericin B (until CNS disease is excluded)
Histoplasma	Urine antigen Culture	Amphotericin B
Blastomyces	Culture	Amphotericin B
Coccidioides	Antibody titers Culture	Amphotericin B or ketoconazole or fluconazole or itraconazole

Viral pneumonia

Viral respiratory tract infections are extremely common; however, the vast majority of patients do not require hospitalization for these infections. Serious cases of viral pneumonia do require hospital admission and supportive care. Some viral respiratory tract infections have antiviral treatment options (Table 22-9).

Of note, influenza pneumonia is a risk factor for development of MRSA pneumonia.

Table 22-9. Selected Treatable Causes of Viral Pneumonia

Virus	Diagnosis	Treatment
Influenza	Rapid antigen test Culture	Zanamivir or oseltamivir plus rimantadine
Varicella	Culture	Acyclovir

Table 22-10. Selected Bioterrorism Agents

Bioterrorism Agent	Diagnosis	Treatment
Anthrax	Widened mediastinum and/or pleural effusions on CXR Culture, Gram stain	Ciprofloxacin or doxycycline
Pneumonic plague	Culture	Streptomycin or doxycycline or ciprofloxacin Respiratory isolation
Tularemia	Culture	Doxycycline or ciprofloxacin

Bioterrorism agents

Bioterrorism is a public health concern worldwide. Prompt reporting, proper identification, and early treatment are essential in limiting the impact of a bioterrorism agent on the public. Several potential bioterrorism agents can present as pneumonia (Table 22-10).

Health care quality

Due to the frequency of hospital admissions with pneumonia, it is a target of national quality improvement efforts. Statistics for each hospital's quality measures are published online by the Department of Health and Human Services (hospitalcompare.hhs.gov).

Pneumonia core quality measures:

- Oxygenation assessment (by pulse oximetry or ABG)
- Blood cultures, preferably before antibiotics are started
- Pneumococcal vaccine before discharge
- Influenza vaccine before discharge (October–February)
- Smoking cessation
- Initial antibiotic therapy within 6 hours
- Appropriate antibiotic selection

The use of a standardized hospital pneumonia protocol can help insure all these quality measures are met.

Health care costs

Antibiotic selection is one of the largest costs associated with the treatment of a patient with pneumonia. When possible, select a less expensive alternative drug.

Table 22-11. Cost-effective Treatments

Drug	Less Expensive Alternatives
Antipseudomonal carbapenem	Antipseudomonal cephalosporin or piperacillin/tazobactam
Linezolid	Vancomycin
Third-generation cephalosporin + macrolide	Respiratory fluoroquinolone
Ertapenem + macrolide	Respiratory fluoroquinolone

Antipseudomonal carbapenems (meropenem, doripenem) are quite expensive, often costing several hundred dollars per dose (Table 22-11).

TIPS TO REMEMBER

- A detailed history is essential for determining appropriate treatment, focusing on risk factors for multidrug-resistant bacterial infection.

- HAP occurs 48 hours or more after hospital admission. Pneumonia diagnosed on hospital day 2 may be CAP, aspiration pneumonia, or an alternative diagnosis.

- Deterioration or slow clinical improvement warrants further investigation. Causes may include inadequate antibiotics, an alternative diagnosis, or a complication of pneumonia.

- Key health care quality measures related to pneumonia are oxygenation assessment, drawing blood cultures before starting antibiotics, starting antibiotics promptly, selecting appropriate antibiotics, counseling smokers about smoking cessation, and providing pneumococcal and influenza vaccination before discharge.

COMPREHENSION QUESTIONS

1. While on night call, you are called to urgently evaluate a cross-cover patient. The patient is an 81-year-old female admitted 3 days prior for CAP, who was started on levofloxacin and unfractionated heparin for DVT prophylaxis. Blood and sputum cultures are thus far negative. The patient reports the sudden onset of dyspnea. She has no other chronic medical problems, and is unable to recall any triggering events. The patient has a respiratory rate of 30, and her oxygen saturation is 85% on room air. Her examination is significant for rales in all lung fields, and she has

no lower extremity edema, calf tenderness, or JVD. What is your differential diagnosis for the patient's dyspnea and hypoxia?

2. What should be done to evaluate the cause or causes of the patient's dyspnea and hypoxia?

3. What initial management is appropriate for this patient?

4. You are consulted by the orthopedic service to evaluate a patient with postoperative confusion. The patient is a 57-year-old male who underwent elective right knee replacement 5 days ago. The patient has no chronic medical problems and has been on DVT prophylaxis during the postoperative period. The patient is unable to provide a useful history, and physical examination is unrevealing. The patient is afebrile and his vital signs are stable.

Diagnostic studies reveal an elevated white blood cell count of 18,000, a hemoglobin of 8.5, and a right upper lobe infiltrate on chest x-ray that was not present in his preoperative chest x-ray.

What is your differential diagnosis for the right upper lobe infiltrate?

5. What is the most appropriate treatment for this patient?

6. You are called by the emergency department to admit a patient with pneumonia. The patient is a 61-year-old male smoker with no significant past medical history or contact with the health care system, who presented to the emergency department with a 4-day history of worsening cough, dyspnea, and fever. The emergency department physician has ordered blood and sputum cultures, obtained a chest x-ray, CBC, and BMP, and started intravenous levofloxacin. The hospital pneumonia order set has also been activated.

Examination of the patient reveals rhonchi and moderate respiratory distress. The patient has an elevated white blood cell count. No other laboratory studies are abnormal.

Chest x-ray shows a cavitary lung lesion.

What other orders should be written for this patient?

Answers

1. The differential diagnosis for this patient is broad.

    a. Treatment failure of pneumonia due to antibiotic choice:

- MRSA
- *Pseudomonas*
- Viral pneumonia
- Fungal pneumonia
- Mycobacteria

  b. A complication of pneumonia:

  - ARDS

  - Pleural effusions

  - Myocardial ischemia/infarction

  - CHF

  - Acute renal failure with volume overload

  - Acute exacerbation of COPD

  c. Aspiration event

  d. Pulmonary embolus

  e. Mucus plug

  f. Allergic response to the antibiotics

2. Consider ordering a chest x-ray, ECG, blood cultures, CBC, BMP, BNP, and cardiac enzymes urgently. An arterial blood gas may be needed if the patient's respiratory status does not rapidly improve with supplemental oxygen.

3. Remember your ABCs (airway, breathing, circulation). Provide adequate supplemental oxygen to increase the patient's oxygen saturation to 90% or better, order diagnostic studies, establish resuscitation status of the patient, and notify the attending. If the patient deteriorates, or does not improve rapidly, transfer to the ICU may be appropriate for management of the patient's acute respiratory failure. Further management will depend on the results of the initial diagnostic studies.

4. The differential diagnosis for this patient includes HAP, aspiration pneumonia, mucus plugging, and acute mitral regurgitation causing focal pulmonary edema.

5. After excluding acute mitral regurgitation, initiate antibiotic therapy for HAP. Postoperative patients receiving pain medications are at increased risk of aspiration pneumonia and mucus plugging secondary to low tidal volumes. Ensure that the head of the bed is elevated ≥45°, sedating medications are minimized, and an appropriate respiratory hygiene protocol is initiated. If aspiration pneumonia is suspected, a speech therapy evaluation can determine if the patient has swallowing defects, such as poor muscle tone or vocal cord dysfunction.

6. This patient should be placed in respiratory isolation until tuberculosis can be excluded. Sputum should be sent for Gram stain, AFB, and fungal culture. An interferon gamma release assay and/or a tuberculin skin test should be placed as well. A CT scan of the chest will assist in better characterization of the cavitary lung lesion noted on the CXR.

SUGGESTED READINGS

American Thoracic Society, Infectious Diseases Society of America. Guidelines for the management of adults with hospital-acquired, ventilator-associated, and healthcare-associated pneumonia. *Am J Respir Crit Care Med.* 2005;171(4):388.

Kollef MH, Shorr A, Tabak YP, Gupta V, Liu LZ, Johannes RS. Epidemiology and outcomes of health-care-associated pneumonia: results from a large US database of culture-positive pneumonia. *Chest.* 2005;128(6):3854.

Metlay JP, Fine MJ. Testing strategies in the initial management of patients with community-acquired pneumonia. *Ann Intern Med.* 2003;138(2):109.

Metlay JP, Kapoor WN, Fine MJ. Does this patient have community-acquired pneumonia? Diagnosing pneumonia by history and physical examination. *JAMA.* 1997;278(17):1440.

Weber DJ, Rutala WA, Sickbert-Bennett EE, Samsa GP, Brown V, Niederman MS. Microbiology of ventilator-associated pneumonia compared with that of hospital-acquired pneumonia. *Infect Control Hosp Epidemiol.* 2007;28(7):825.

Respiratory Failure

Christine I. Todd, MD, FACP, FHM

A 72-year-old Man With Acute Respiratory Failure

Mr Cantrall is a 72-year-old man with no known pulmonary history admitted to the hospital with *E. coli* sepsis due to cholecystitis. He receives antibiotics, fluids, and narcotic analgesia. On hospital day 3, he gets out of bed to go to the bathroom and becomes "winded." When you arrive to see him, he is sitting on the edge of his bed with his elbows on his knees, breathing at 30 breaths/min. He states he cannot catch his breath. His pulse ox registers an SaO_2 of 87%.

1. What is your differential diagnosis for Mr Cantrall's acute respiratory failure (ARF)?

Answer

1. There are quite a few entities that could explain Mr Cantrall's acute dyspnea and hypoxia. Since he is in the postoperative period, a DVT with pulmonary embolism should be on your differential, as should a hospital-acquired or aspiration-type pneumonia. Cardiac causes include fluid overload or CHF (patients commonly exhibit reduced ejection fractions after sepsis). In patients with kyphoscoliosis, which is relatively common in the geriatric population, the addition of narcotic analgesia can result in a reduction of their vital capacity to the point where normal activity causes hypoxia. Another problem that could cause shallow ventilation would be the development of peritonitis from his infected gallbladder.

A 64-year-old Woman Found Unresponsive in the Hospital After a Knee Replacement

Ms Golden is a 64-year-old chronic smoker hospitalized for a knee replacement. As part of the orthopedic care protocol, she receives 2 L O$_2$ per nasal cannula and a patient-controlled analgesia pump with morphine postoperatively. Although she initially does well, a rapid response call is made on her on her second postoperative day when the nurses find her unresponsive. Vital signs are normal, as is a blood glucose check done at bedside.

1. What would be your next evaluative step?

Answer

1. You should obtain an arterial blood gas in order to evaluate this patient's ability to ventilate and exchange gases adequately. Her history suggests that she could have chronic COPD and undiagnosed chronic, mild hypoxia. With the addition of sedating analgesics, her ventilatory capacity could be reduced and cause her to retain CO$_2$, accounting for her unresponsive state. Alternatively in a patient with undiagnosed COPD, the addition of supplemental oxygen could have reduced her hypoxic drive leading to CO$_2$ retention and unresponsiveness.

ACUTE RESPIRATORY FAILURE

Diagnosis

ARF is defined as a sudden (minutes to hours) inability of the lungs to maintain normal respiratory function, resulting in abnormal arterial oxygen or carbon dioxide levels. Whether classified as Type 1 (hypoxemic) or Type 2 (hypercarbic), ARF represents a major immediate threat to homeostasis and is a medical emergency. Work to diagnose the initiating problem as well as augmentation of the patient's ability to exchange gases must proceed quickly, and in parallel. An initial workup including a cardiac and pulmonary examination, chest x-ray, ABG, and EKG should point you in the right direction by helping to classify the ARF and generate a differential diagnosis as to the cause.

Patients with Type 1 ARF have hypoxemia as their predominant blood gas abnormality. Typically, these patients are anxious and intensely focused on relieving their dyspnea. When you attempt to obtain their history, they may not be able to cooperate, repeating phrases like "I can't breathe" or "Help me." You may note use of accessory muscles of respiration and, in severe cases, cyanosis. The patient may exhibit unstable vital signs as well. Your differential should include parenchymal and interstitial disease (pneumonia, aspiration, COPD or CHF exacerbation, ARDS) as well as diseases that can cause an acute right-to-left shunt (pulmonary embolism).

Patients with Type 2 ARF have high pco_2 levels as their predominant blood gas problem. They may be hypoxemic as well. These patients can exhibit a "narcosis," appearing confused, intoxicated, or unresponsive. On physical examination, you may find a tremor or asterixis, peripheral vasodilation with pink nail beds, and significant bradycardia or sinus pauses. Your differential should include disease states that can induce a shallow or inadequate respiratory effort such as asthma or COPD exacerbation in a patient who has "tired out," neuromuscular issues such as Guillain-Barré syndrome, oversedation with narcotic medications, strokes or brain stem lesions, and structural issues such as severe kyphoscoliosis. In the hospital setting, a few of these issues can combine to turn a chronic condition into an acute problem. For instance, a patient with morbid obesity and resultant sleep apnea who is then hospitalized for a knee replacement and given narcotics for pain control could develop significant hypercarbia due to an acute worsening of the sleep apnea from the sedating effects of the analgesics.

Treatment

Treatment for both Type 1 and Type 2 ARF is aimed at stabilizing and reversing the derangements in the patient's ability to properly exchange gases in the lung. Diagnosing and treating the underlying issue is important, but acute strategies to augment oxygenation and support the ventilatory release of CO_2 must also be utilized to relieve the patient's symptoms and prevent organ failure.

In patients with Type 1 ARF, providing supplemental oxygen is key. This can be done most easily through a nasal cannula, the use of which allows patients to continue to eat, drink, and speak easily. Unfortunately, since much of the oxygen supplied is lost to the air around the patient, oxygen by nasal cannula is only useful for patients who require low flow rates (2–5 L) to support their oxygen levels. Patients who require higher flow rates of oxygen require venturi masks, which can deliver FiO_2s of up to 50% or non-rebreather masks, which have a 1-way valve that prevents exhaled gases from diluting the delivered oxygen, resulting in 80% to 90% O_2 concentrations. All of these methods of increased oxygen delivery should be used cautiously in patients with chronic lung disease, in whom an increased po_2 can result in the loss of their hypoxic drive and subsequent retention of pco_2. Although these patients may initially present as Type 1 ARF, they may need treatment strategies more in line with Type 2 ARF patients, as described below. Patients exhibiting severe levels of hypoxia, unstable vital signs, mental status changes that make them unable to protect their airway, or stridor should proceed immediately to intubation and mechanical ventilation.

Patients with Type 2 ARF require ventilatory support so that they can "blow off" their excess CO_2. They may also need supplemental oxygen. As above, patients who are hemodynamically unstable or unable to protect their airway should be intubated and ventilated. In more stable patients, a course of noninvasive ventilation can be very helpful. Two types of noninvasive ventilation are commonly used—continuous positive airway pressure (CPAP) masks and bilevel positive airway pressure (BiPAP) masks.

CPAP masks are tight-fitting apparati that support the patient's ventilatory effort by adding a few centimeters of pressure to the air they breathe. This decreases the workload of breathing and gives patients some rest so that they can improve their ventilatory effort. Supplemental levels of oxygen can be given through the mask if needed. BiPAP masks provide heavier pressure with inhalation and a lower level of pressure with exhalation. This decreases the workload of breathing and improves gas exchange by preventing alveolar collapse on exhalation.

It is important to remember that noninvasive methods of supporting ventilation are only for temporary use while the underlying cause of ARF is diagnosed and treated. Patients who are on CPAP or BiPAP therapy for ARF should be reassessed with an ABG 1 hour after beginning treatment. If significant improvement in their pco_2 and po_2 levels is not seen after this period of time, patients should be intubated and mechanically ventilated.

TIPS TO REMEMBER

- Novice clinicians sometimes avoid obtaining ABGs on patients, having heard that they are very painful. In fact, patients rate them less painful than many other common procedures (nasogastric tube placement, Foley catheter placement). ABGs are essential for the correct diagnosis and treatment of ARF, and doctors should not hesitate to order them when appropriate.

- Do not hesitate to intubate and mechanically ventilate a patient with ARF who is not appropriate for or not responding to noninvasive ventilation. A calm, organized intubation is much safer and results in better clinical outcomes than an emergent intubation done after a patient has become unstable or suffered a cardiopulmonary arrest.

- Many patients have undiagnosed chronic hypoxia with few clinical signs or symptoms. When hospitalized, the addition of supplemental oxygen, sedating medications, or the stress of an acute illness can cause hypercarbic ARF, which often manifests clinically as altered mental status or delirium.

COMPREHENSION QUESTIONS

1. Your patient, Ms August, is hospitalized for severe necrotizing pancreatitis. Her main complaints are severe abdominal pain, nausea, and vomiting. You have been very concerned about her pulmonary status, as increasing hypoxia and fluffy bilateral infiltrates on her chest x-ray suggest the development of ARDS. What would be the best way to support this patient's pulmonary function if it continues to decline?

2. Mr Paul is a patient in the emergency room whom you have met many times before. He has Class 3 systolic left-sided CHF and due to financial issues, frequently

skips his medications, leading to CHF exacerbations that necessitate admission to the hospital. He reports a similar story this time, and presents with respiratory distress. He cannot speak in full sentences due to dyspnea, and is sitting straight up in bed with clearly elevated JVD and loud rales in both lung bases. His ABG shows a mildly decreased po_2 and a low pco_2. What would be the best strategy to support Mr Paul's pulmonary status?

Answers

1. This patient may need ventilatory support beyond oxygen delivered by nasal cannula or mask, as patients with ARDS can develop Type 2 or hypercarbic ARF. If so, the use of noninvasive ventilation would be *inappropriate* in this patient due to her nausea and vomiting. CPAP and BiPAP masks form a tight seal to the patient's face, and require time and dexterity to remove. There is a risk that the patient could have an episode of emesis while wearing the mask, which can result in massive aspiration of gastric contents, a devastating clinical event. Using an NG tube to help prevent vomiting would also preclude the use of the CPAP or BiPAP masks, as the presence of the tube prevents the masks from making the tight seal necessary for their function. If this patient's pulmonary status continues to decline, intubation and mechanical ventilation would be the next step in management.

2. Although Mr Paul's severe dyspnea may lead you to consider intubation and mechanical ventilation, he could be an excellent candidate for noninvasive forms of ventilation. Using a CPAP or BiPAP mask for an hour while waiting for a stat furosemide dose to have its effect on his CHF exacerbation could allow you to avoid intubating this patient. Intubation and positive pressure ventilation can have a negative effect on patients with CHF, as the changes in the cardiac cycle produced by intubation decrease cardiac output.

SUGGESTED READINGS

Bordow RA, Moser KM, eds. *Manual of Clinical Problems in Pulmonary Medicine.* 3rd ed. Boston: Little Brown and Company; 1991.

Brochard L, Mancebo J, Wysocki M, et al. Noninvasive ventilation for acute exacerbations of chronic obstructive pulmonary disease. *N Engl J Med.* 1995;333(13):817–822.

Gallagher EJ. Nasogastric tubes: hard to swallow. *Ann Emerg Med.* 2004;44(2):138–141.

George RB, Light RW, Matthay MA, Matthay RA. *Chest Medicine: Essentials of Pulmonary and Critical Care Medicine.* 5th ed. Philadelphia: Lippincott Williams & Wilkins; 2006.

Loscalzo J, Fauci A. *Harrison's Manual of Medicine.* 17th ed. New York: McGraw-Hill; 2009.

Washington University School of Medicine, Cooper DH, Krainik AJ, Lubner SJ, Reno HEL. *The Washington Manual of Medicine Therapeutics.* 32nd ed. Philadelphia: Lippincott Williams & Wilkins; 2007.

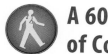

A 60-year-old Woman With Loss of Consciousness

Edgard Cumpa, MD

A 60-year-old woman is admitted to the hospital after a loss of consciousness. She had a "strange feeling" before losing consciousness. Her husband stated that she fell to the ground and had generalized stiffening and then shaking. She was unresponsive for approximately 1 minute, had urinary incontinence, and was confused for a few minutes after regaining consciousness. She had a similar episode 2 months ago; evaluation at that time, which included electrocardiography, stress electrocardiography, and a continuous-loop event electrocardiographic recorder, revealed no abnormal findings. The patient takes no medications.

Physical examination including a full neurologic examination is normal.

MRI of the brain and electroencephalogram (EEG) during waking and sleeping are also normal.

1. What is the most likely diagnosis?

Answer

1. The patient likely had a seizure. Seizure is classified according to the history and physical examination. Diagnostic testing is used to confirm or clarify the suspected cause. When a patient has loss of consciousness with urinary incontinence and stiffening and shaking lasting 1 to 2 minutes, seizure should always be considered as the cause until proven otherwise. When there is a high clinical suspicion of epilepsy, normal MRI of the brain and EEG do not rule out that diagnosis.

SEIZURES

The first step in evaluating a patient with a suspected seizure is to rule out other conditions, such as syncope or a transient ischemic attack. As is most often the case, a complete history and physical examination are essential. Based on the results of those examinations, one pursues appropriate diagnostic testing. If a seizure is suspected, the next step is to distinguish between provoked (secondary) and unprovoked (primary) seizure. Acute symptomatic seizures are usually secondary to an acute neurologic event or to a metabolic problem.

Appropriate management should be aimed at correcting the underlying cause. Antiseizure medication is reserved for refractory seizures or primary seizures (epilepsy) only. Epilepsy is a condition of at least 2 or more unprovoked seizures. It is appropriate to get a neurology consult when the diagnosis is unclear or when medication choice is difficult. Otherwise neurology consultation is often unnecessary.

253

In the majority of patients with epilepsy, no reversible cause of the seizures is found. Elderly patients more commonly have an identified etiology. Cerebrovascular disease is responsible for approximately 30% of seizures in older patients.

Diagnosis

Seizures are classified into 2 types: generalized and partial. Generalized seizures affect both sides of the brain and are not usually associated with a cerebral lesion. Partial seizures arise from a localized area and may indicate the possibility of an underlying lesion.

Seizures may be accompanied by loss of consciousness. Three seizure types include a loss of consciousness: complex partial seizures, absence seizures, and generalized tonic-clonic seizures. Since patients have lost consciousness during these seizures, they do not remember what happened.

Complex partial seizures, also known as temporal lobe seizures, are the most common type of seizures in adults with epilepsy. They usually last less than 3 minutes. After a complex partial seizure, patients generally are confused, somnolent, and complain of a headache.

Absence seizures are characterized by the sudden onset of staring along with impaired consciousness. They usually last between 5 and 10 seconds and may be associated with hyperventilation. They usually start in childhood, and most patients have a spontaneous remission before adulthood.

Generalized tonic-clonic seizures, also known as grand mal seizures, are a subtype of generalized seizures. These may begin with a loud scream. The extremities stiffen, and then the patient falls to the ground. After approximately 60 to 90 seconds, the extremities begin jerking, which generally lasts 1 to 2 minutes. There is typically a postictal period during which the patient appears to be asleep or sleepy. The patient wakes up gradually over the course of minutes to hours. Patients commonly subsequently complain of a severe headache after the seizure.

Etiology

The most common causes of secondary seizures are cerebrovascular disease, developmental brain disorders, remote head trauma, brain tumors, and neurodegenerative conditions. In epilepsy, seizure triggers include sleep deprivation, alcohol, flashing lights, and menstruation. Medications, including quinolone antibiotics, antipsychotic agents, and antidepressants, may lower seizure threshold, thus precipitating a seizure.

There are many conditions that may mimic seizures, including cardiac syncope, arrhythmias, TIA, migraine, metabolic problems, intoxication, and vertigo.

Psychogenic nonepileptic spells (PNES) are seizure-like episodes that are seen in patients with a conversion disorder. They mimic an epileptic seizure, but do not have the EEG findings associated with seizures. They used to be called pseudoseizures. Features commonly seen in PNES are biting the tip of the tongue, seizures lasting more than 2 minutes, seizures having a gradual onset, eyes being closed during a seizure, and side-to-side head movements. Features that are unusual in PNES are severe tongue biting, biting the inside of the mouth, and urinary and/or fecal incontinence.

Additional diagnostic testing may be needed to confirm or clarify the underlying cause or precipitant of the seizure. Evaluation for metabolic problems, cardiac disease, cerebrovascular disorders, or vestibular dysfunction may be needed based on your history and physical examination. Laboratory investigations may include a complete blood count, serum electrolyte, plasma glucose levels, and a toxicology screen.

A lumbar puncture is usually indicated if there are signs or symptoms suggesting an underlying infection of the brain or if the patient is immuno-compromised. Electroencephalography (EEG) is the standard of the diagnostic workup. EEGs are done not only to formally diagnose seizures but also to classify the seizure type. When a routine EEG is negative and seizure is still suspected, ambulatory EEG monitoring or an inpatient continuous video EEG monitor should be considered.

For adults, neuroimaging is done to rule out underlying conditions, such as stroke, intracerebral hemorrhage, or malignancy, which may require emergency intervention. MRI is superior to CT for detection of epileptogenic lesions, except for acute intracerebral bleeding.

All adult patients with a new-onset seizure should get a brain MRI, unless there is evidence from the history, an EEG confirming a primary seizure disorder, or if there is a contraindication to MRI.

Treatment

Patients diagnosed with epilepsy should be treated with single-agent pharmacotherapy. Monotherapy is better tolerated, less expensive, and associated with better medication adherence. If seizures persist, the monotherapy regimen should be changed to a different drug, again choosing a single-drug regimen. Valproic acid and lamotrigine are first-line drugs for generalized seizures, whereas carbamazepine and lamotrigine are first choices for partial seizures. Phenobarbital, phenytoin, carbamazepine, and oxcarbazepine all induce hepatic cytochrome P450 enzymes, and valproic acid inhibits them. In patients with suspected drug interactions or underlying liver disease, gabapentin, pregabalin, and levetiracetam should be considered. Chronic use of first-generation antiepileptic drugs has been linked with an increased risk of osteoporosis and vitamin D deficiency; therefore, calcium and vitamin D should be started.

TIPS TO REMEMBER

- The first step in evaluating a patient with a suspected seizure is to rule out other conditions, such as syncope or transient ischemic attack, by taking a complete history and physical examination, and obtaining appropriate diagnostic testing.

- Partial seizures arise from a localized area and may indicate the possibility of an underlying lesion.
- Depending on the history, evaluation for metabolic problems, cardiac disease, cerebrovascular disorders, or vestibular dysfunction may be appropriate.
- A lumbar puncture is generally only indicated if there are signs or symptoms suggesting an underlying infection of the brain or if the patient is immunocompromised.
- All patients with a seizure should have a brain MRI, unless there is evidence from the history, an EEG of a primary epilepsy, or if there is a contraindication to MRI.
- Newly diagnosed epilepsy should be treated with single-agent pharmacotherapy. Monotherapy is better tolerated, less expensive, and associated with better adherence.

COMPREHENSION QUESTIONS

1. A 30-year-old woman is admitted with new onset of seizures. She had a witnessed generalized tonic-clonic seizure and was evaluated in the emergency department, where results of physical examination, complete blood count, measurement of serum electrolyte levels, and urine toxicology screen were all normal. She is otherwise healthy, has no significant personal or family medical history, and takes no medications. Repeat physical examination is also normal. In addition to EEG, which of the following diagnostic tests should be performed next?
    A. CT of the head
    B. LP
    C. MRI of the brain
    D. PET

2. A 50-year-old man is admitted to the hospital after having 2 generalized tonic-clonic seizures in a 24-hour period. He has had seizures in the past, which were always attributed to alcohol withdrawal. He has end-stage liver disease secondary to alcoholic cirrhosis and is awaiting a liver transplant. His kidney function is normal. His current medications include propranolol, spironolactone, and furosemide. On physical examination, the patient is awake and alert, and vital signs are normal. Neurologic examination findings are normal. The general physical examination shows jaundice and ascites. The creatinine level is 0.6 mg/dL and blood alcohol level is nondetectable. Electrolyte levels are normal. An MRI of the brain is normal. An EEG is negative.
    Which of the following is the best treatment for this patient?
    A. Levetiracetam
    B. Oxcarbazepine
    C. Phenytoin
    D. Valproic acid

Answers

1. **C.** Evaluate a new-onset seizure with EEG and MRI. For patients with new onset of a seizure and no provocative cause, an EEG and MRI of the brain should be obtained. These tests will help to confirm the diagnosis, predict the risk of recurrence, and rule out any underlying condition (such as a brain tumor). MRI has been shown to be clearly superior to CT in detecting potentially epileptogenic lesions.

2. **A.** Levetiracetam, gabapentin, and pregabalin are preferred in patients with significant liver disease, because there is no significant hepatic metabolism and low protein binding.

SUGGESTED READINGS

American College of Physicians, Dodick DW. *MKSAP 15 Medical Knowledge Self-Assessment Program 15: Neurology.* Philadelphia: American College of Physicians; 2009.

Krumholz A, Wiebe S, Gronseth G, et al. Practice parameter: evaluating an apparent unprovoked first seizure in adults (an evidence-based review): report of the Quality Standards Subcommittee of the American Academy of Neurology and the American Epilepsy Society. *Neurology.* 2007;69(21):1996–2007.

Schachter SC. Seizures disorders. *Med Clin North Am.* 2009;93(2):343–351.

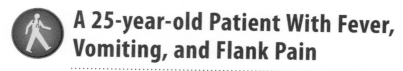

A 25-year-old Patient With Fever, Vomiting, and Flank Pain

Tiffany Leung, MD, MPH

A 25-year-old female presents to the emergency department with fever, nausea, vomiting, and flank pain. She has had dysuria for the past 2 days, with progressively worsening flank pain. She has not been able to tolerate oral intake for the past 2 days. She has no prior medical history. On examination, she has a fever of 103.1°F, blood pressure of 85/40, heart rate of 125 bpm, respiratory rate of 24/min, and pulse oximetry of 89% on room air. She appears diaphoretic, tachypneic, and in severe pain. She has crackles at the lung bases bilaterally, and on cardiac examination she is tachycardic but has no murmurs, gallops, or rubs. She has tenderness to palpation of both costovertebral angles. Laboratory evaluation demonstrates WBC of 16,000 cells/mm³. Chest x-ray demonstrates small bibasilar pleural effusions. Urinalysis shows large leukocyte esterase and nitrites, with 50 WBCs/hpf and 10 RBCs/hpf. Additional labs are in process, including an arterial blood gas, serum lactic acid level, liver function tests, urine culture, and blood cultures.

1. What is the clinical syndrome presented?

2. What is the next appropriate step in management?

Answers

1. This patient meets criteria for systemic inflammatory response syndrome (SIRS) based on the presence of fever, tachycardia, leukocytosis, and hypoxia, which meets all 4 of the SIRS criteria. Additionally, because the patient has a suspected source of infection, she meets the definition for sepsis. It is not yet known whether she has severe sepsis or septic shock, as there is insufficient detail provided at this point.

2. The next appropriate step in management is aggressive intravascular volume resuscitation. Additional steps to consider immediately thereafter include ordering appropriately directed laboratory and imaging studies to guide infection source identification, and initiating empiric broad-spectrum antimicrobial therapy. Appropriate consultation and evaluation by the intensive care unit (ICU) medical team may be necessary to help determine if critical care in the ICU is indicated.

CASE REVIEW

The case provides limited but adequate detail to determine this patient's current clinical status. She is acutely ill based on the presence of signs and symptoms indicative of sepsis. More data will be needed before determining if this patient has severe sepsis or septic shock. Laboratory data may reveal end-organ damage, which would suggest the presence of severe sepsis. Because of hypotension, early and aggressive volume resuscitation in this patient is essential for both therapeutic and diagnostic purposes to determine if septic shock is present. In parallel to treatment, efforts to identify the source of infection should begin based on information obtained from the history and physical examination, along with indicated laboratory testing, imaging studies, and consultation. Close follow-up of the patient's initial clinical course after initiation of therapy marks an important triage step where the clinical decision must be made about level of care needed for this patient. Lack of clinical response to early and aggressive treatments would suggest the presence of septic shock and intensive care management is indicated.

SEPSIS

There are several definitions used to describe the level of severity of septic patients (see Table 25-1).

Table 25-1. Definitions Used to Describe the Condition of Septic Patients

Systemic inflammatory response syndrome (SIRS)	Four clinical or laboratory criteria. The etiology for SIRS may be *any* systemic inflammatory process, infectious or noninfectious. A patient has SIRS if he or she meets at least 2 of the following: 1. Temperature >38°C or <36°C 2. Heart rate >90 beats/min 3. Respiratory rate >24 breaths/min or P_aCO_2 <32 mm Hg 4. White blood cell count >12,000 or <4000 cells/mm^3 or 10% bands
Sepsis	SIRS *and* a source of infection is identified or suspected
Severe sepsis	Sepsis *and* clinical or laboratory signs of end-organ dysfunction, for example, encephalopathy, or: 1. Hypotension 2. Decreased urine output 3. Respiratory failure 4. Lactic acidosis or unexplained acidosis 5. Troponin elevation
Septic shock	Severe sepsis *and* hypotension refractory to fluid resuscitation

Diagnosis

Pathophysiology

Infection caused by any class of microbiologic pathogen causes the body's immune system to release both proinflammatory and anti-inflammatory mediators. In the setting of sepsis, the balance of these factors favors proinflammatory mediators, particularly TNF-alpha and IL-1. Certain pathogens may also have a direct effect on the host inflammatory response via bacterial cell components or produced toxins. As the inflammatory response escalates, uncontrolled peripheral vasodilation and intravascular volume depletion result from direct endothelial damage, leading to hypotension, tissue hypoperfusion, and organ failure. Tachycardia may occur in response to hypotension and intravascular volume depletion. Tachypnea may occur in response to the metabolic acidosis that results from tissue hypoperfusion and associated elevation in serum lactic acid levels as end-organ damage ensues. If tachypnea persists and cannot adequately compensate for the lactic acidosis from severe sepsis, then respiratory fatigue and subsequently respiratory failure or arrest may occur. The clinical manifestations of acute illness due to the host inflammatory responses can appear at any point on the spectrum from SIRS to septic shock.

History

Fever and symptoms suggestive of infection are often, but not always, the first pieces of history that raise the clinical suspicion of sepsis. In the elderly, fever is frequently absent, and subtle alterations in mental status alone can be the first manifestation of infection. The primary goal of the history is to identify symptoms and risk factors to guide the selection of empiric broad-spectrum antibiotic therapy and subsequent laboratory testing and imaging studies. It is important to identify medication allergies early, as this can also influence the choice of antibiotics.

Certain populations may be more susceptible to opportunistic or more resistant pathogens. Immunocompromised patients may acquire certain opportunistic infections, and also are at increased risk for rapid deterioration, progression from SIRS to septic shock, and poorer outcomes. Immunocompromised hosts include patients receiving chemotherapeutic agents or immunomodulatory medications, and patients with HIV/AIDS, certain hematologic malignancies, and asplenia (Table 25-2). Health care–associated infections may present in patients with frequent or prolonged contact with health care settings, which is important to recognize early to guide appropriate empiric broad-spectrum antibiotics for more resistant infections (Table 25-3). This population commonly includes patients on hemodialysis, nursing home residents, patients who were recently hospitalized, postsurgical patients, and health care workers. Patients who present with sepsis and have indwelling central lines such as a peripherally inserted central catheter (PICC) line or a hemodialysis catheter are at risk for central line–associated bloodstream infections, which often are due to gram-positive

Table 25-2. Immunocompromised States

Impairments of humoral immunity

Congenital

Acquired (eg, hypogammaglobulinemia due to multiple myeloma, chronic lymphocytic leukemia, and asplenia)

Neutropenia (eg, patients with acute leukemia, or after hematopoietic stem cell transplantation or myelosuppressive chemotherapeutic agents)

Impairments of cellular immunity

Use of immunomodulatory or immunosuppressive drugs (includes chemotherapeutic agents and chronic systemic corticosteroids)

Diabetes mellitus

Human immunodeficiency virus (HIV) or autoimmune deficiency syndrome (AIDS)

Lymphoreticular malignancies (eg, Hodgkin disease)

---

pathogens. Long-term instrumentation, such as a tracheostomy tube, percutaneous gastrostomy feeding tube, or indwelling urinary catheter, can also be sites of entry for pathogenic organisms causing sepsis. A history of malfunction or malpositioning of any of these types of instrumentation may warrant appropriate antimicrobial selection.

A detailed social history and travel history can help guide appropriate empiric antibiotic therapy and laboratory evaluation to identify the source of infection. Social history should identify risk factors that may increase the risk for undiagnosed HIV/AIDS. A history of intravenous drug use increases the risk of having HIV/AIDS, but also raises concern about endocarditis as a possible etiology for

Table 25-3. Common Resistant Organisms

Methicillin-resistant *Staphylococcus aureus* (MRSA)

Vancomycin-resistant *Enterococcus faecalis* (VRE)

Extended-spectrum beta-lactamase (ESBL)–producing bacteria, including *Escherichia coli* and *Klebsiella pneumonia* (*K. pneumonia* carbapenemases [KPC])

Carbapenemase-resistant *Acinetobacter baumanii* (CRAB)

Multidrug-resistant (MDR) *Pseudomonas aeruginosa*

---

sepsis. Living conditions, for example, residence in a dormitory or on a military base, can raise suspicion for meningococcal infection in the appropriate clinical settings. Travel history guides empiric coverage of certain pathogens that may be endemic to certain geographic distributions.

Physical examination

The physical examination, particularly in the acutely ill patient, should focus on identifying or confirming possible sources of infection. For example, in a patient complaining of a fever, productive cough, and shortness of breath, auscultating for rhonchi and checking for dullness to percussion, egophony, or tactile fremitus may help to confirm a suspicion of pneumonia as the etiology for sepsis. Cardiac auscultation may identify new murmurs or abnormal heart sounds that suggest endocarditis. Signs of end-organ damage that can manifest clinically, such as mental status changes and delirium, are also important to note. In the severely septic or septic shock patient, signs of intravascular volume depletion and warm, clammy extremities may be present. Appropriate placement, condition, and function of any indwelling tubes or devices should be examined carefully, and their sites of entry should always be examined for induration, erythema, purulent drainage, or other signs of infection.

Laboratory and imaging studies

To identify a pathogen causing sepsis, blood cultures must always be obtained. For blood cultures, obtaining 2 sets of blood cultures from 2 separate venipuncture sites prior to antibiotic initiation can be helpful in order to compare the results of both. If 1 blood culture set is contaminated, then the second blood culture set obtained from a different site remains to identify the causative agent. Often, Gram stains are done within hours of collection of blood or other fluid culture, which can help guide initial antibiotic selections. In patients with indwelling central lines with suspected sepsis, central line–associated bloodstream infections should also be considered and if indicated, the line should be removed or replaced and the tip of the catheter sent for culture as well.

Additional microbiologic data should be collected by sampling tissue or fluid based on clinical history or physical examination findings. Urinalysis and urine culture are often obtained regardless of presence or absence of symptoms reported, as the tests are relatively inexpensive and urinary sources of infection are easily treatable if identified. Urine pregnancy testing is appropriate in reproductive-age females to better guide medical management and choices of imaging studies. If ascites is present, obtaining peritoneal fluid may be appropriate. It should be sent for cell count and differential, total protein, albumin, Gram stain, and culture. If a joint appears to be the septic source, joint aspiration, followed by sending fluid for cell count and differential, Gram stain, and culture, is indicated. Lumbar puncture may be indicated to rule out meningitis. For wound debridement or abscess incision and drainage, purulent drainage or tissue obtained during the procedure should be sent for culture. In less common circumstances, sometimes surgical or interventional consultations may be needed to obtain tissue or fluid for diagnostic purposes.

Imaging studies should be chosen judiciously with the goal of identifying the etiologic agent for sepsis. Often, chest x-rays are done because they are relatively inexpensive and can obviate the need for additional testing. Additional testing may include computed tomography (CT) or magnetic resonance imaging (MRI) scans, or interventional or surgical procedures performed with radiographic guidance. Tests should be ordered based on the clinically suspected source of sepsis.

Treatment

Severity of sepsis must be initially assessed based on the clinical history, physical examination, and initial laboratory findings, in order to direct further therapies. Septic shock necessitates more aggressive and intensive therapies to provide hemodynamic support. Early goal-directed treatment must be initiated promptly, and if response to fluid resuscitation is inadequate, then vasopressor support in an intensive care monitoring setting may be appropriate. Management should include aggressive intravenous resuscitation with specific hemodynamic parameters, including maintaining a central venous pressure of 8 to 12 mm Hg, mean arterial pressure of 65 to 90 mm Hg, and central venous oxygen saturation of 70% (Figure 25-1).

In all cases of sepsis, regardless of severity, the etiologic agent should be identified and empiric broad-spectrum antimicrobial therapy initiated while confirmatory laboratory or radiographic data are in process in order to avoid further complications. Common clinical scenarios to consider are urosepsis, pneumonia (including community-acquired, health care–associated, or aspiration types), colitis including *Clostridium difficile*, and peritonitis. Less common scenarios may also necessitate indication-specific evaluation and management with appropriate antimicrobial therapies.

1. Oxygen supplementation ± ventilatory support
2. Central venous catheterization to monitor CVP and $S_{cv}O2$
3. Arterial catheterization to monitor MAP
4. Resuscitate to hemodynamic goals:
    - CVP 8–12 mm Hg; if <8 mm Hg, then use crystalloid or colloid to achieve goal
    - MAP 65–90 mm Hg; if <65 mm Hg, then use vasopressor agents to achieve goal
    - $S_{cv}O2$ > 70%; if <70%, then transfuse red cells until hematocrit >30% or use inotropic agent to achieve goal
5. Continue care in the Intensive Care Unit

CVP, central venous pressure; ScvO2, central venous oxygen saturation; MAP, mean arterial pressure

Figure 25-1. Early goal-directed therapy.

TIPS TO REMEMBER

- The SIRS is defined by 4 clinical or laboratory criteria.
- Sepsis syndromes are a spectrum of illnesses, from SIRS to sepsis, severe sepsis, and septic shock.
- The clinical history, physical examination, laboratory evaluation, and imaging studies are performed with attention to identifying an etiologic agent to guide narrowing of the antibiotic selection.
- Early volume resuscitation and empiric broad-spectrum antibiotic therapy in the septic patient may be the only treatments that prevent rapid clinical deterioration, morbidity, and mortality.

COMPREHENSION QUESTIONS

1. A 78-year-old woman with dementia is brought to the hospital by her caregiver. The patient has been unable to urinate for the past 24 hours, and has a temperature of 95.1°F and confusion. Her respiratory rate is 16 bpm, blood pressure is 147/63, and laboratory analysis reveals WBC of 11,000 cells/mm³. Her caregiver states that the patient did not recognize her today, which is unusual for her, and that she has become increasingly lethargic. What clinical syndrome best describes this patient's clinical presentation?
    A. SIRS
    B. Sepsis
    C. Severe sepsis
    D. Septic shock

2. A 44-year-old man with diabetes presents with increasing purulent drainage from a left foot ulcer. He recently completed a course of oral antibiotics, but has been experiencing fevers up to 102.1°F. His blood pressure is 168/98 and respiratory rate is 14 bpm. Laboratory analysis demonstrates WBC of 18,500 cells/mm³. What clinical syndrome best describes this patient's clinical presentation?
    A. SIRS
    B. Sepsis
    C. Severe sepsis
    D. Septic shock

3. A 51-year-old woman with a long history of alcohol abuse is brought to the hospital by her spouse with jaundice, confusion, increasing lower extremity edema, and abdominal distension for the past 2 weeks. She has a temperature of 101.6°F, a respiratory rate of 16 bpm, and blood pressure of 98/56. She has flank dullness and a fluid wave on physical examination of her abdomen. She also has asterixis. Laboratory analysis is pending. What is the next best step in management?
    A. Empiric broad-spectrum antibiotic therapy
    B. Paracentesis

C. Early goal-directed volume resuscitation

D. ICU consultation

4. A 23-year-old man with a history of mild persistent asthma presents with cough and fever up to 103.4°F for the past 1 week. His respiratory rate is 32 bpm, blood pressure is 82/45, and heart rate is 135 bpm. Laboratory analysis reveals WBC of 15,000 cells/mm^3. An arterial blood gas was also sent and shows a P_aCO_2 of 30 mm Hg and Po_2 of 75 mm Hg. Serum lactate is 3.0. A chest x-ray reveals a consolidation in the right lower lobe. He is receiving his second bolus of intravenous fluids and continuous nebulizer treatment is being administered. Blood cultures have been sent and empiric broad-spectrum antibiotics initiated. He starts to become more somnolent and less responsive. What is the next best step in management?

A. Start vasopressor therapy.

B. Obtain an arterial blood gas.

C. Consult the ICU.

D. Intubate for respiratory failure.

Answers

1. **C.** This patient meets 2 of 4 SIRS criteria and has a suspected source of infection (urinary tract infection). However, she also has decreased urine output and altered mental status, which can be signs of end-organ dysfunction. She does not have hypotension. Severe sepsis is the best description in this scenario.

2. **B.** This patient meets 2 of 4 SIRS criteria and has a suspected source of infection (diabetic foot ulcer). He has no apparent signs of end-organ dysfunction and does not have hypotension. Sepsis is the best description of this patient's clinical presentation.

3. **B.** This patient currently meets 1 SIRS criterion; however, laboratory analysis is pending and it is possible that she will meet a second with an abnormal white blood cell count. Identifying a source of infection is imperative to guide empiric antimicrobial therapy in this clinical scenario in which the patient presents with signs of end-stage liver disease from suspected alcoholic cirrhosis. She does not appear to be in septic shock, which would require aggressive intravascular volume resuscitation and intensivist consultation. Paracentesis to evaluate for spontaneous bacterial peritonitis would be the next most appropriate step in management.

4. **D.** The patient clinically presents with an acute asthma exacerbation, in the setting of pneumonia, and has severe sepsis with possible development of septic shock. Despite continued hemodynamic support with aggressive fluid resuscitation, he is developing respiratory failure, which is due to respiratory fatigue from asthma exacerbation as well as prolonged compensation for acidosis related to

septic shock. Immediate intubation to provide ventilatory support is lifesaving. ICU consultation can occur in parallel with treatment of the patient or immediately thereafter. It is important to monitor for septic shock that would necessitate vasopressor therapy and to check ABGs after the patient has been intubated; however, these interventions do not treat the patient emergently.

SUGGESTED READINGS

Chin-Hong PV, Guglielmo BJ. Common problems in infectious diseases & antimicrobial therapy. McPhee S, Papadakis M, Rabow MW. *Current Medical Diagnosis and Treatment 2012.* New York: The McGraw-Hill Companies; 2011 [chapter 30].

Dellinger RP, Levy MM, Carlet JM, et al. Surviving Sepsis Campaign: international guidelines for management of severe sepsis and septic shock: 2008. *Intensive Care Med.* 2008;34:17–60.

Munford RS. Severe sepsis and septic shock. Longo D, Fauci A, Kasper D, Hauser S, Jameson J, Loscalzo J. *Harrison's Principles of Internal Medicine.* 18th ed. New York: The McGraw-Hill Companies; 2012 [chapter 271].

Rivers E, Nguyen B, Havstad S, et al. Early goal-directed therapy in the treatment of severe sepsis and septic shock. *N Engl J Med.* 2001;345:1368–1377.

A 78-year-old Woman With Slurred Speech

Zak Gurnsey, MD, FACP

Mrs Oswald is a 78-year-old female who presents to the emergency department with a 2-hour history of slurred speech. She also complains of difficulty with word-finding and right-sided weakness and numbness. She denies any vision changes, headache, fever, trauma, chest pain, or abdominal pain. She has a history of hypertension, hyperlipidemia, and atrial fibrillation. Her medications include hydrochlorothiazide, metoprolol, fish oil, and aspirin. She has not taken warfarin for the last 3 years after an incident of diverticular bleeding. She does not smoke or use alcohol. On examination, she is awake yet anxious, with a blood pressure of 194/102 mm Hg, heart rate of 116 bpm, respiratory rate of 20 breaths/min, and oxygen saturation of 96% on room air. Chest auscultation reveals clear lungs and an irregularly irregular rhythm. Abdominal examination reveals a soft, nontender abdomen and normal bowel sounds. Neurological examination reveals expressive aphasia, left facial droop, right-sided sensory deficits, and right-sided motor strength of 3/5. Left arm and leg sensory and motor examination are normal.

Lab data show hemoglobin 12.6, hematocrit 38, WBCs 10,600, and platelets 186,000. Basic metabolic panel is normal. Point-of-care glucose is 109. CT scan of the head is normal.

1. What is the most likely diagnosis?

2. What is the most likely cause of this new diagnosis?

3. What else should be considered in the differential diagnosis?

Answers

1. This is a 78-year-old with risk factors for stroke (age, hypertension, hyperlipidemia, atrial fibrillation) who presents with sudden stroke-like symptoms. Her vital signs reveal compensatory measures being taken by the body. Her normal head CT scan has ruled out an acute hemorrhage.

2. Her stroke is most likely embolic in nature, related to not being on anticoagulation for the atrial fibrillation.

3. Other potential diagnoses to consider include complex migraine headache, tumor or mass, and toxic-metabolic abnormalities. This case allows for a discussion of acute stroke, including types, presenting signs and symptoms, and management.

STROKE

Strokes are the result of ischemia or hemorrhage of affected brain tissue. They are the leading cause of adult disability in the United States and the second leading cause of death worldwide. Risk factors include elderly age, hypertension, hyperlipidemia, diabetes mellitus, atrial fibrillation, previous stroke or transient ischemic attack, and cigarette smoking.

Ischemic stroke and hemorrhagic stroke are the 2 major categories. Eighty percent to 90% of strokes are ischemic in nature.

Ischemic strokes are due to 4 main causes: arterial thrombosis, embolism, hypoperfusion, and venous thrombosis. Arterial thrombosis is usually in the setting of atherosclerosis, but may also be seen with arterial dissection or vasculitis. Arterial embolism typically arises in the heart, such as in the setting of atrial fibrillation, left ventricular thrombus, or infective endocarditis. Hypoperfusion seen in the setting of such disease states as decompensated congestive heart failure and septic shock may lead to inadequate blood flow to areas of the brain, causing a stroke. Cerebral venous sinus thrombosis causes stroke due to increased local pressures.

Hemorrhagic strokes are further classified based on the location of the bleed. These include intraparenchymal hemorrhage, intraventricular hemorrhage, epidural hematoma, subdural hematoma, and subarachnoid hemorrhage. Potential causes include vascular malformations, amyloidosis, trauma, bleeding disorders, illicit drug use, and secondary conversion of an ischemic stroke.

Diagnosis

The World Health Organization has defined stroke as a neurological deficit of cerebrovascular cause that persists beyond 24 hours or is interrupted by death within 24 hours. Stroke is suspected clinically and is typically confirmed by subsequent imaging techniques. CT scan without contrast is the preferred initial imaging modality in determining ischemia versus hemorrhage. This distinction is important because management will be different. CT scan is preferred over MRI scan because it is cheaper and faster, with the same sensitivity for identifying hemorrhage. Acute ischemic strokes are unlikely to show up on CT scan.

Further workup focuses on potential causes. Imaging of the carotid arteries is used to detect stenosis or dissection. Echocardiogram is used to identify intracardiac thrombosis. Electrocardiogram and telemetry are used to detect arrhythmias, such as atrial fibrillation. Fasting cholesterol panel is ordered to look for hyperlipidemia. For younger patients and those who cause a high clinical suspicion, a workup for a hypercoagulable state is indicated. These states may include sickle cell anemia, protein C or S deficiency, factor V Leiden, and antiphospholipid syndrome, among others.

Location, location, location

The involved intracranial artery in stroke patients will usually lead to typical symptom presentations. Understanding these anatomic relationships can assist one in the management of a stroke patient. One may pay closer attention to certain areas on imaging techniques, explain particular signs and symptoms to patients and families, and better define goals for rehabilitation services.

Anterior cerebral artery strokes may present with motor and/or sensory deficits, grasp and sucking reflexes, abulia, and gait apraxia.

Middle cerebral artery strokes present differently, depending on which hemisphere is involved. Dominant hemisphere signs include aphasia, motor and sensory deficits, and homonymous hemianopia. Nondominant hemisphere signs include neglect, anosognosia, motor and sensory deficits, and homonymous hemianopia.

Posterior cerebral artery strokes may present with homonymous hemianopia, alexia without agraphia, and visual disturbances.

Vertebrobasilar artery strokes may present with cranial nerve palsies, diplopia, dizziness, nausea, dysarthria, dysphagia, gait ataxia, and even coma.

Differential diagnosis

The differential diagnosis list for patients presenting with stroke-like symptoms should include the following:

- Complex migraine headache
- Head trauma
- Brain tumor
- Todd's palsy
- Conversion disorder
- Systemic infection/meningitis/encephalitis
- Toxic-metabolic abnormalities (hypoglycemia, renal failure, liver failure, illicit drug use)

Treatment

Management focuses both on the acute event and on secondary prevention. It differs between ischemic strokes and hemorrhagic strokes. For ischemic strokes, antithrombotic medications, such as aspirin, clopidogrel, and dipyridamole, are used to prevent further platelet aggregation. Statin drugs are indicated as a means to stabilize atherosclerotic plaques. Thrombolytic medications, such as tissue plasminogen activator (tPA), are recommended within 3 hours of stroke-symptom onset. Contraindications for tPA include recent stroke, recent major surgery, recent myocardial infarction, resolving stroke symptoms, intracranial hemorrhage, blood pressure of 185/110 mm Hg or higher, platelets <100,000, serum glucose <50, and INR >1.7. Blood pressure management typically revolves around a goal systolic blood pressure of 160 to 180 mm Hg, so as to maintain adequate perfusion to viable brain tissue immediately surrounding the area of ischemia without increasing the risk for hemorrhagic conversion.

For hemorrhagic strokes, the acute management phase involves neurosurgical evaluation and hemodynamic stability. Antithrombotic and thrombolytic medications are contraindicated. Blood pressure should be kept within normal ranges, so as to avoid worsening of the hemorrhage.

Subsequent treatment focuses on rehabilitation services, including physical therapy, occupational therapy, and speech therapy. Patients will often need these services even after discharge from the hospital. Social worker and counseling support should be provided to the patient and family, as this is often a life-altering event.

Secondary prevention focuses on risk factors for subsequent strokes. Blood pressure, blood glucose, and cholesterol levels should be maintained within normal ranges. Smoking cessation counseling should be provided. Long-term anticoagulation medications are indicated for patients with atrial fibrillation (atrial fibrillation carries a 5% yearly risk of stroke). Patients who have carotid artery stenosis should be considered for carotid endarterectomy or carotid angioplasty. Statin medications and antithrombotic medications should be considered for lifelong usage.

TIPS TO REMEMBER

- Consider thrombolytic medications, such as tPA, for stroke patients presenting within 3 hours of symptom onset. Be aware of tPA contraindications.
- Understand the differences in blood pressure management between hemorrhagic strokes and ischemic strokes.
- Determine and treat underlying causes of stroke. For instance, statin medications for hyperlipidemia, cessation counseling for smokers, anticoagulation for atrial fibrillation, and carotid endarterectomy for carotid artery stenosis.

COMPREHENSION QUESTIONS

1. For Mrs Oswald presented at the beginning of the chapter, which medication listed is not obviously indicated?
    A. Warfarin
    B. Simvastatin
    C. Lisinopril

2. A 64-year-old male suffered an ischemic stroke 4 weeks ago. The determined cause of his stroke was left internal carotid artery stenosis. He has residual deficits of minimal right hand weakness. He has stopped smoking. His medications include aspirin, atorvastatin, ramipril, and metoprolol. His vital signs are normal. What is the next step for the secondary prevention of stroke?
    A. Add clopidogrel.
    B. Add warfarin.

C. Maintain current medication and rehabilitation regimen.

D. Refer for carotid endarterectomy.

3. A 71-year-old female has been diagnosed with a hemorrhagic stroke due to intraparenchymal hemorrhage. Her vital signs include a blood pressure of 166/98 mm Hg. What is the next step in managing this patient's blood pressure?

A. Do nothing. Her blood pressure is at an ideal range to maintain cerebral perfusion.

B. Start intravenous fluids. Her intravascular volume should be increased so as to raise the systolic blood pressure to 180 mm Hg.

C. Start intravenous labetolol. The goal systolic blood pressure is <140 mm Hg.

Answers

1. **C.** All patients with a diagnosis of stroke should be treated with a statin medication. The LDL should be lowered to a goal of <100. Because of her atrial fibrillation and subsequent increased stroke risk, this patient should be placed on anticoagulation with warfarin. Lisinopril may be a helpful addition for controlling the blood pressure, but does not in itself have a role for acute stroke management or secondary prevention.

2. **D.** This patient should be referred for carotid endarterectomy. Doing nothing allows the continued stenosis and presumed atherosclerotic disease to place this patient at a high risk for another stroke. The patient is already on aspirin, so clopidogrel does not necessarily need to be added. Some sources will argue that the aspirin should be changed to clopidogrel or dipyridamole. There is no mention of atrial fibrillation, so warfarin is not indicated.

3. **C.** Blood pressure management differs in the setting of hemorrhagic stroke versus ischemic stroke. For patients with hemorrhagic stroke, the blood pressure should be normalized as soon as possible so as to potentially avoid worsening the area of hemorrhage. Maintaining the current blood pressure, or adding measures that may increase it, will put the patient at a higher risk for worsening stroke symptoms.

SUGGESTED READINGS

Aminoff MJ, Kerchner GA. Nervous system disorders. In: McPhee SJ, Papadakis MA, eds. *Current Medical Diagnosis & Treatment*. New York: McGraw-Hill; 2012: [chapter 24].

Dobkin BH. Rehabilitation after stroke. *N Engl J Med*. 2005;352:1677–1684.

Hwang DY, Maheshwari A, Rinne ML, Greer DM. Neurology. In: Sabatine M, ed. *Pocket Medicine: The Massachusetts General Hospital Handbook of Internal Medicine*. 2nd ed. Philadelphia: Lippincott Williams & Wilkins; 2004:4–5: [chapter 9].

Longo DL, Fauci AS, Kasper DL, Hauser SL, Jameson JL, Loscalzo J, eds. *Harrison's Principles of Internal Medicine*. 18th ed. New York: McGraw-Hill; 2012.

Van der Worp HB, van Gijn J. Acute ischemic stroke. *N Engl J Med*. 2007;357:572–579.

Washington University School of Medicine, Cooper DH, Krainik AJ, Lubner SJ, Reno HEL. *The Washington Manual of Medical Therapeutics*. 32nd ed. Philadelphia: Lippincott Williams & Wilkins; 2007.

Wechsler LR. Intravenous thrombolytic therapy for acute ischemic stroke. *N Engl J Med*. 2011;364: 2138–2146.

A 21-year-old Female With Loss of Consciousness

Muralidhar Papireddy, MD,
Se Young Han, MD, and
Susan Thompson Hingle, MD

A 21-year-old college student was brought to the emergency department by EMS following an episode of loss of consciousness on a hot summer afternoon. She is accompanied by her friends who witnessed the episode. She is awake and alert, and claims to be in her usual state of health now. She was in the cheer team and she lost consciousness just before the half time. She felt light-headed and weak prior to the episode with vague abdominal pain and nausea. She has no recollection after that and the next thing she can remember is that her friends were calling her name when she was lying on the floor. As per the friends, she looked pale initially and had shaky movements of the limbs for a few seconds. She was unconscious for less than a minute. After that her color returned and regained consciousness spontaneously. She was in her usual state of health until a few seconds prior to the episode. She never lost consciousness in the past. She has negative review of systems and takes oral contraceptive pills for birth control. Patient denies tobacco, alcohol, or illicit drug use. No significant family history. Vitals signs including orthostatic blood pressure are normal. Examination including neurological examination is unremarkable. EKG is normal. Urine pregnancy test is negative.

1. What is the diagnosis and next step of action?

Answer

1. Neurocardiogenic syncope. Discharge from the emergency department with patient education and precautions to take if she suffers another episode.

CASE REVIEW

Patient in this case description is a young college student cheering for her team on a hot summer day. She had the warning signs with presyncopal symptoms, but she remained up on her feet that led to an episode of brief loss of consciousness followed by rapid spontaneous recovery. This is a classical description for neurocardiogenic syncope, also known as vasovagal syncope. It is not uncommon to have a few shakes during the syncope, usually less than 15 seconds. It is not a seizure as the episode was not long enough and she did not have postictal phase. Neurocardiogenic syncope is the most common type and carries a good prognosis. Description of the episode is diagnostic, and there is role for further investigation. Reassure and educate the patient on syncope and precautions to take to prevent

275

recurrence. "Always position an unconscious patient in a recovery position, and never make him or her sit in the chair or hold him or her in upright position" as this will not help improve the circulation and regain consciousness.

DEFINITION OF SYNCOPE

Syncope is a sudden transient loss of consciousness with loss of postural tone and complete spontaneous recovery. It is a result of transient global cerebral hypoperfusion (Figure 27-1).

Presyncope is the prodromal symptom of near faintness without loss of consciousness. It is more prevalent than syncope, and the symptoms may last for seconds to minutes with light-headedness, warmth, nausea, and blurring of vision. Presyncope and syncope are spectrum of presentations from the same underlying pathophysiology, so the following discussion applies to both conditions.

Syncope is a clinical diagnosis. We do not need further investigations to diagnose this condition. The first and foremost challenge in the history is to differentiate syncope from the other causes of loss of consciousness. Syncope must have the following characteristics: (1) transient loss of consciousness, (2) loss of postural tone, and (3) complete immediate spontaneous recovery. Patients with syncope may have tonic–clonic movements that are brief (<15 seconds) and nonrhythmic, and start after the loss of consciousness. Tongue bite is not common, if happens; it is usually in the front.

Syncope must be differentiated from a seizure. Seizure patients may have aura and longer duration of unconsciousness with coarse movements that start at the time of loss of consciousness and last approximately 1 minute. Tongue bite is common and usually happens on lateral aspect. Postictal phase is longer with confusion and sore muscles.

In metabolic causes (hypoglycemia, hypoxia, and panic attacks) and intoxication, loss of consciousness is not due to global cerebral hypoperfusion. Symptoms may last longer unless intervened early; there will be a pre-event history and associated symptoms suggestive of these conditions.

In neurogenic syncope from vertebrobasilar TIA or stroke and basilar migraine, loss of consciousness is from brain stem ischemia but not due to global hypoperfusion. Syncope is associated with neurological deficits or headaches, and patients do not return to the baseline health status immediately. Because of the mentioned reasons, neurogenic syncope is not considered as a true syncope.

In patients with sudden cardiac death (SCD; cardiac arrest), recovery is not spontaneous. They may need advanced cardiac life support (ACLS) to resuscitate them, and the prognosis is much worse compared with syncope. Coma is a prolonged state of impaired responsiveness to external stimuli with severely diminished level of alertness. It is not a transient condition with spontaneous recovery.

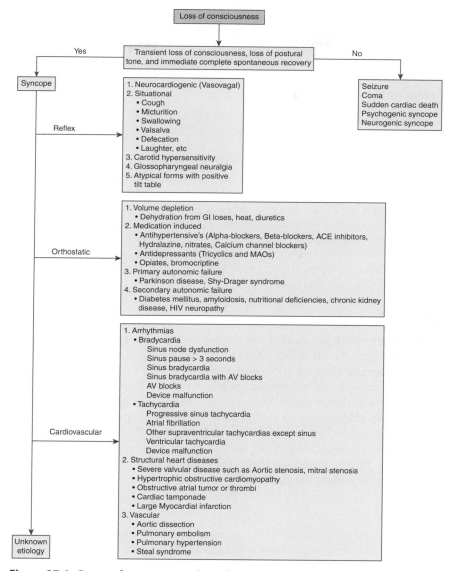

Figure 27-1. Causes of non-traumatic loss of consciousness with etiological classification of syncope.

Diagnosing syncope can be challenging and even more difficult if the presentation is presyncope. Most patients describe their presyncope symptoms as dizziness, which is rather a vague term and may mean different things to different people. So to get a better understanding, ask the patient to describe his or her symptoms without using the word dizzy or dizziness. Most times it helps, but may frustrate the patient at times, so be prepared for his or her frustration. One must pay attention to every detail. History should focus on the events prior to the episode, during the episode, and following the episode.

Pre-event

For the pre-episode events, pay attention to the hydration status in the days to weeks prior to the episode: access to fluids, fluid loss from a new-onset diabetes, diuretics, diabetes insipidus (neurosurgery, head trauma, or medications), and gastrointestinal losses from vomiting or diarrhea. Acute severe bleeding can cause severe hypovolemia and orthostatic syncope. Inquire about taking new medications that may contribute to syncope, such as a new antihypertensive, diuretic, antidepressant, antipsychotics that prolong QT interval, or CNS depressants. Inquire about location, position, situation, and activity engaged prior to the event. Inquire about associated symptoms such as nausea, vomiting, pain, palpitations, or shortness of breath. Patients with psychogenic syncope may provide a positive history for a loss in the family or job or worsening stress leading to exacerbation of their mental health problems.

Event

If there were eyewitnesses, find out the rescue measures they carried out. It is not surprising to hear that they made their dear ones sit in a chair or held them up in the upright position until the ambulance arrived or brought them to the emergency department by bringing them in a seated position in the car. As this will prevent reperfusion of the brain, patient may have longer duration of symptoms and possible complications including watershed infarcts, extensive battery of investigations, and hospital stay. Also find out about the duration of the event, any movements, color changes, and bladder or bowel incontinence. Pay attention to the point of impact if patients had a fall from loss of postural tone, as this may assist with your assessment and plan.

Postevent

Postevent recovery is fast and complete in syncope. If it is prolonged, think about other conditions that might have led to this event. Inquire about the bowel and bladder incontinence and tongue bites patients noted.

PATHOPHYSIOLOGY

Systemic blood pressure is determined by the cardiac output and peripheral vascular resistance. To maintain continuous blood supply to the brain regardless of the position, a harmonious function of baroreceptors, autonomic nervous system, cardiac function, blood volume, and patent blood vessels to the brain is needed. Baroreceptors are located in carotid body and aortic arch to detect sudden decrease in blood pressure, which leads to increased activity of sympathetic nervous system and simultaneous inhibition of parasympathetic nerve system. Consequently, this drives peripheral blood vessels, especially in lower extremities, to constrict, increases venous return, and increases heart rate and contractility. Finally, this blood flow runs through blood vessels to the brain. Syncope is a result of interruption of any of these tightly coordinated mechanisms, leading to a fall in systemic blood pressure and decrease in global cerebral blood flow.

Based on the underlying pathophysiology, syncope is broadly differentiated into reflex syncope, orthostatic hypotension syncope, cardiovascular syncope, and syncope of unknown etiology. We will discuss the approach to diagnose etiology of syncope and then will discuss them in detail.

APPROACH TO SYNCOPE

Once the diagnosis of syncope is made, it is important to risk stratify the patients to determine further management strategy. Patients with short-term high-risk features should be admitted to the hospital for evaluation and treatment. Based on the history, physical examination, EKG findings, electrolytes, and hematocrit, patients are risk stratified. High-risk patients (Table 27-1) have an increased short-term mortality, and they should be evaluated in the hospital immediately. Patients with history suggesting fatal conditions such as massive pulmonary embolism, subarachnoid hemorrhage, acute severe hemorrhage, acute aortic dissection, acute coronary syndromes, malignant arrhythmias, and severe structural heart diseases, as a cause of the syncope, fall into the high-risk category.

Once these are ruled out, investigate further to understand the etiology of syncope as this will determine further management. History, physical examination, EKG, hematocrit, and electrolytes should be checked at the time of presentation.

Now we will spend some time discussing key points from the history, physical examination, and EKG that may lead us to the diagnosis of syncope.

History

History is the most important tool in the diagnosis of syncope. Be prepared to spend a significant amount of time with the patient obtaining a medical history as there is no better sophisticated technique to assist with diagnosis.

Reflex syncope
- Prolonged standing in hot crowded areas, any stressful situations such as pain, fear or intense emotion, or exertion can lead to vasovagal syncope.
- Prodromal symptoms are common with reflex syncope, and patients usually complain of a feeling of warmth, nausea, vomiting, diaphoresis, or vague abdominal pain.

Table 27-1. High-risk Features Requiring Admission to the Hospital for Further Evaluation and Treatment

History, Physical Examination, and Basic Laboratory Work	EKG Findings
History	Sinus bradycardia <50 beats/min or sinoatrial block, A-V nodal block in the absence of nodal blocking agents
Exertion syncope	
Syncope in supine position	QRS duration >120 ms
Palpitation at the time of syncope	Bifascicular block
Acute blood loss	Prolonged or short QT interval
Acute shortness of breath	Nonsustained ventricular tachycardia
Acute sharp tearing or ripping chest pain with radiation	Preexcitation syndromes such as Wolff-Parkinson-White syndrome
Sudden severe worst headache	Brugada pattern with RBBB with ST elevation in the anterior leads
Physical examination	
Severe hypotension	Arrhythmogenic right ventricular dysplasia (ARVD) findings with epsilon wave, inverted T waves, and S-wave upstroke >55 ms in the anterior precordial leads
Severe hypoxemia	
Pulse deficit	
Past medical history	
Congestive heart failure	
Systolic dysfunction	
Myocardial infarction or coronary artery disease	
Valvular or obstructive cardiac abnormalities or history of arrhythmias	
Family history	
Family history of sudden cardiac death	
Basic laboratory work	
Severe anemia	
Severe electrolyte abnormalities	

- Situation or activity involved in prior to the episode gives a clue about the cause of reflex syncope.
- If the syncope occurred in patients above 40 years of age while shaving, turning head, wearing a tight neck collar or necktie, neck massage, or carotid ultrasound, think about carotid hypersensitivity.

- During a meal or postprandial.
- Long history of recurrent syncope in the absence of heart disease.

Orthostatic hypotension
- Sudden upright posture leading to syncope: think about orthostatic hypotension
- Recent initiation of medication such as antihypertensives, antidepressants, or diuretics
- History of Parkinson disease
- History of long-standing diabetes, renal insufficiency, or presence of peripheral neuropathy from any cause

Cardiovascular syncope
- Abrupt syncope without any associated symptoms suggests cardiovascular etiology.
- Palpitations at any time during the syncope.
- Syncope in supine position: think about arrhythmias.
- Exertion syncope: think obstructive cardiac output causes and ischemia.
- Chest pain and dyspnea may suggest acute coronary syndrome, pulmonary embolism, severe anemia from hemorrhage, acute ascending aortic dissection, tachyarrhythmias or severe structural heart diseases such as severe aortic stenosis, hypertrophic cardiomyopathy, obstructive atrial tumor, or thrombus and cardiac tamponade.
- Family history of syncope and SCD: think about cardiomyopathy, familial long QT syndrome, and Brugada syndrome.
- Sudden "worst headache": think about subarachnoid hemorrhage.
- Vertebrobasilar TIA or stroke leaves a patient with neurological deficits or posterior stroke symptoms. It is a rare presentation of the posterior stroke and as there is no complete spontaneous recovery, we will not discuss this under syncope.
- If the syncope is provoked by upper extremity activity and the patient has a history of brain stem symptoms and has syncope, think about subclavian steal syndrome.

Physical Examination

Physical examination as important as history in the evaluation of syncope. Following are some of the signs that may help to diagnose the cause of syncope.

- Orthostatic hypotension is defined as a drop in systolic blood pressure of 20 mm Hg or diastolic blood pressure by 10 mm Hg or a systolic blood pressure of <90 mm Hg when the blood pressure is taken after 3 minutes of standing. This is a diagnostic exam for orthostatic hypotension syncope.

- With tachypnea and/or hypoxemia, think about pulmonary embolism and congestive heart failure.
- With tachycardia and/or hypotension, think about hypovolemia, pulmonary embolism, aortic dissection, myocardial infarction, arrhythmias, and pulmonary hypertension.
- Look for signs/symptoms of Parkinson disease in the elderly patients who present with orthostatic syncope.
- Feel for a displaced and diffuse point of cardiac maximum impulse and listen for an S3, in systolic heart failure patients who are at high risk for arrhythmia-related syncope.
- Listen for any abnormal heart rhythm.
- Listen for severe aortic stenotic murmur that is characterized by long ejection systolic murmur with late peaking radiating to carotids.
- In hypertrophic obstructive cardiomyopathy patients, a systolic murmur is accentuated with a Valsalva maneuver.
- A "tumor plop" is heard with an atrial myxoma.
- Rectal examination is important in hypotensive patients to assess for gastrointestinal bleeding.
- A thorough neurological examination is indicated in patients presenting with symptoms suggestive of a posterior stroke.

Electrocardiogram

Electrocardiogram is an important tool in the evaluation process. Please refer to Table 27-1 for the high-risk EKG abnormalities that are suggestive of cardiovascular syncope. We will discuss the diagnostic EKG changes in the later part of the chapter.

Every effort should be made to identify a cause from history and physical examination, as they yield the most vital information to assist in reaching a diagnosis. EKG alone has a diagnostic yield of only around 5%, but, when added to the history and physical examination, the diagnostic yield can be up to 50%. Further investigations should be streamlined based on the available information, comorbid conditions, single episode or recurrent syncope, and presence of structural heart disease and high-risk features. A cause is still not found in nearly one third of the patients presenting with syncope.

Reflex Syncope

Reflex syncope is the most common cause of syncope. This is an abrupt loss of normal cardiovascular reflexes from a trigger, causing bradycardia or hypotension or both, leading to global cerebral hypoperfusion and syncope.

Reflex syncope is classified based on the most involved efferent pathway:

1. *Vasodepressor type*: If the hypotension predominates
2. *Cardioinhibitory type*: If bradycardia or asystole predominates
3. *Mixed type*: If both mechanisms are involved

Based on the trigger incident, reflex syncope is differentiated into neurocardiogenic (vasovagal), situational, carotid hypersensitivity, and atypical form.

1. *Neurocardiogenic syncope* has a classical description of vagal hyperactivity with nausea, vomiting, cold sweats, and vague abdominal pain prior to passing out. It is precipitated from emotional stressors such as acute stress, fear, or pain or orthostatic stressor from prolonged standing in a crowded warm place.

2. *Situational syncope* occurs during or immediately after a specific trigger action, for example, micturition syncope.

3. *Carotid hypersensitivity* is from accentuated vagal response to carotid sinus massage. Elderly patients are common victims of this condition. Any situation that causes carotid sinus massage leads to syncope.

4. *Atypical reflex syncope* presents without an apparent trigger. Patients with this presentation should be ruled out for structural heart disease prior to considering reflex syncope. Symptoms may be reproduced with tilt-table test for confirmation.

Diagnosis

- Diagnosis of reflex syncope is from history alone. There is no need for further investigations.
- Elderly patients may have a combination of etiologies including vasovagal, carotid hypersensitivity, orthostatic hypotension, polypharmacy, and cardiovascular diseases. This leads to atypical presentation and a need for further investigation.
- Carotid sinus massage if the patient is above 40 years of age.
- More serious potential conditions need to be ruled out with ECHO and stress test. If there is no structural heart disease or no cardiac cause found in structural heart disease, an upright tilt-table test may help differentiate reflex syncope from other causes.

Treatment

- Provide education on the cause, symptom identification, recurrence, precautions to take, and reassurance.
- Physical counterpressure maneuvers.

- Cardiac pacing is an option in patients above 40 years old with syncope from severe cardioinhibitory response with bradycardia and asystole, but not with vasodepressor response.
- Avoid situations that may trigger reflex syncope, such as abrupt standing, prolonged standing, wearing tight neckties, etc.

Orthostatic Syncope

Syncope that occurs on standing up with documented orthostatic hypotension.

On standing up from upright position, significant amount of blood pools in the lower extremities and in the autonomic nervous failure, sympathetic efferent activity is chronically impaired and this leads to decreased vasoconstrictor response and an end result of global cerebral hypoperfusion and syncope/presyncope.

Acute hemorrhage, diarrhea, vomiting, or diuretics can lead to hypovolemia and resultant orthostatic hypotension and syncope. Patients with underlying autonomic failure are more prone to have orthostatic symptoms due to lack of effective vasoconstrictor response. Elderly patients are more prone to orthostatic hypotension possibly due to decreased baroreceptor sensitivity.

Medications such as antihypertensives, antidepressants, and dopamine agonists can cause autonomic dysfunction and orthostatic syncope.

Primary autonomic failure (Parkinson disease and Shy-Drager syndrome) and secondary autonomic failure from chronic conditions such as diabetes, renal failure, or amyloidosis can lead to orthostatic hypotension.

Diagnosis

History and physical examination are sufficient to diagnose orthostatic hypotension. Orthostatic blood pressures should be obtained at rest on lying down for at least 5 minutes and after 3 minutes of active standing.

Orthostatic hypotension is defined as a drop in systolic blood pressure of 20 mm Hg or diastolic blood pressure drop of 10 mm Hg or a drop in systolic blood pressure to <90 mm Hg. No further investigations are required. It is diagnostic if a patient with syncope has documented orthostatic hypotension.

May use head-up tilt-table test at 60° to 70°.

Treatment

- Stop medications leading to hypotension from autonomic failure.
- Maintain adequate hydration and salt intake.
- Fludrocortisone.

- Compression stockings.
- Midodrine, an alpha-agonist, causes vasoconstriction in patients with chronic autonomic failure and improves blood pressure.
- Head-up tilt sleeping to increase fluid volume.

Cardiovascular Syncope

The second common cause of syncope is cardiovascular in origin. Syncope results from abrupt reduction in cardiac output from either an arrhythmia or mechanical obstruction to the outflow. Arrhythmia is the most common cause of syncope, and it should be suspected if the patient had palpitations or suffered syncope while in supine position. Mechanical obstruction is a relatively less common cause, and patients complain of presyncope or syncope on exertion that is most often associated with some chest discomfort.

Initial evaluation is considered diagnostic if there is:

- Ischemic changes with or without myocardial infarction in cardiac ischemia-related syncope
- Severe aortic stenosis, prolapsing atrial tumor, pulmonary hypertension, pulmonary embolism, cardiac tamponade, hypertrophic obstructive cardiomyopathy, or acute aortic dissection
- Persistent bradycardia with heart rate <40/min in an awake patient
- Recurrent sinoatrial block or sinus pause of >3 seconds
- Mobitz II second-degree AV block or complete heart block
- Alternating right and left bundle branch block
- Long or short QT interval
- Nonsustained polymorphic VT
- Rapid paroxysmal supraventricular tachycardia (SVT) or VT
- Pacemaker or implantable cardioverter-defibrillator (ICD) malfunction with pause

Mortality rate is high among patients presenting with cardiovascular syncope and up to nearly one third of them die in the first year. So it is important to identify patients at high risk requiring admission for further evaluation as shown in Table 27-1.

Continuous electrocardiographic monitoring

It is considered diagnostic if the patient experiences symptoms during the time of arrhythmia. Asymptomatic patients experience sinus pause of >3 seconds,

SVT with heart rate more than 160 beats/min for more than 5 seconds or VT, and second-degree AV block and complete heart block in an awake patient who is not a trained athlete, not on nodal blocking agents, or rate controlled for atrial fibrillation.

In-hospital monitoring is appropriate if the patient has high-risk features as in Table 27-1. Diagnostic yield of telemetry is low at 16% in hospitalized patients suspected to have arrhythmia as a cause of syncope. If in such a case the inpatient monitoring is nondiagnostic, Holter may be considered in patients with >1 syncope episode per week. Holter records for up to a week. Diagnostic yield can be very low in unselected patients. For syncopal episodes occurring at intervals <4 weeks, an external loop recorder is an option. Implantable loop recorder that records the rhythm based on the capture criterion or when activated by a magnet is indicated when an extensive evaluation of high-risk patients remains undiagnosed.

Echocardiogram

Echocardiography is indicated in patients suspected to have structural heart disease for diagnosis and risk stratification. Echo is considered diagnostic if there is severe aortic stenosis, obstructive atrial myxoma or thrombi, cardiac tamponade, aortic dissection, or congenital anomalies of coronary artery disease. In patients with low ejection fraction or regional wall motion abnormalities, it helps to guide further management.

Exercise stress testing

It should be considered in patients with exertion syncope who had a nondiagnostic echocardiogram. Exercise testing is considered diagnostic if the symptoms are reproduced with EKG abnormalities or the patient develops severe hypotension. Also, it is considered diagnostic if patients develop second-degree type II or complete heart block in the absence of symptoms as this predicts progression to complete heart block.

Electrophysiological (EP) studies

EP studies should be considered in patients with an abnormal EKG with ischemic heart disease that the cause of syncope remains undiagnosed after an echocardiogram, an exercise stress test, and electrocardiographic monitoring.

Other targeted focused investigations

For suspected subarachnoid hemorrhage, order head imaging (CT scan) to confirm the same. For patients who have an acute anemia and hypotension, workup should be focused to identify the source of bleeding. For suspected pulmonary embolism, acute coronary syndrome, and aortic dissection, see Chapter 7 for an approach to the diagnostic evaluation. In patients with exertion syncope and suspected pulmonary hypertension, an echo provides an estimate of the pulmonary pressures, but right heart catheterization is diagnostic.

Treatment
Arrhythmia
Indications for pacemaker:

- Syncope associated with sinus node dysfunction or any A-V nodal block
- Symptomatic and asymptomatic patients with sinus pause of >3 seconds (except young trained patients, during sleep or nodal blocking agents)
- Symptomatic bradycardia that results from required drug therapy
- Symptomatic chronotropic incompetence
- Syncope of unexplained origin and significant sinus node dysfunction discovered on EP studies
- Syncope with second-degree type II A-V block and complete heart block
- Symptomatic patient with bundle branch block and positive EP study

Indications for ICD:

- Documented VT with structural heart disease
- Sustained monomorphic VT induced with EP studies in patients with previous myocardial infarction
- Documented VT in inherited cardiomyopathies and channelopathies
- Primary prophylaxis from SCD

Catheter ablation is the treatment of choice for VT and SVT associated with syncope.

Antiarrhythmic drugs are indicated for atrial fibrillation and also in VT and SVTs when catheter fails or is not done.

Structural heart diseases: For patients with diagnostic structural heart disease, treatment should be directed at the pathophysiological process.

Syncope of Unknown Etiology

Etiology of syncope remains unknown in nearly one third of the cases after the initial evaluation. Further investigation should be guided by the history, physical examination, and EKG to avoid unnecessary investigation and cost burden.

1. A young patient with no high-risk features but with a single episode of syncope with suspected reflex syncope should be discharged home with education on syncope. No further investigations are warranted.
2. Patients above 40 years of age and suspected to have a reflex syncope should undergo carotid sinus massage for carotid sinus hypersensitivity.

Carotid sinus massage should be avoided if the patient suffered a TIA or stroke in preceding 3 months or has carotid bruit (except if carotid Doppler studies excluded significant stenosis). Carotid sinus massage is considered diagnostic if the syncope is reproduced in the presence of asystole for >3 seconds and/or fall in blood pressure >50 mm Hg.

3. Tilt-table test is indicated after a single episode of unexplained syncope in a high-risk setting, for example, if the patient had a significant physical injury or is at risk for the same and is in a high-risk occupation, such as construction work. It is also indicated with recurrent syncope in the absence of structural heart conditions. Tilt-table testing may also be considered after ruling out other cardiac causes in the presence of structural heart disease.

4. Consider prolonged electrocardiographic monitoring if the carotid sinus massage and tilt-table test are negative in patients with recurrent or severe unexplained syncope.

5. Patients with low-risk features should undergo outpatient evaluation. Most of the times syncope is due to reflex syncope and the mortality is low. In patients suspected to have cardiac syncope, do echocardiography and an exercise stress test. If diagnostic, then treat accordingly. If normal, then consider electrocardiographic monitoring based on the frequency of symptoms. If negative, consider tilt-table testing. Consider psychiatric evaluation if there is concern for psychogenic syncope.

6. In patients with high-risk features admitted to the hospital who did not have a causal etiology diagnosed, consider outpatient electrocardiographic monitoring to look for an arrhythmia. EP testing is indicated in patients with previous myocardial infarction, nondiagnostic sinus bradycardia, bundle branch block, or palpitations associated with syncope.

TIPS TO REMEMBER

- Syncope is defined as sudden transient loss of consciousness with loss of postural tone and complete spontaneous recovery.
- Syncope is a clinical diagnosis. We do not need further investigations to diagnose this condition.
- Do not forget to get the pre-event, event, and postevent history. This will not only help us to differentiate syncope from nonsyncope loss of consciousness but also help to identify the etiology of syncope.
- History, physical examination, and EKG combined has a diagnostic yield up to 50%.
- EKG alone has a diagnostic yield of around 5%.

- Reflex syncope is the most common syncope category. And neurocardiogenic syncope or vasovagal syncope or common faint is the most common cause of syncope.
- Low-risk patients can be evaluated as outpatients.
- Syncope from cardiovascular causes has a high mortality rate, reaching up to 30% in 1 year.
- Arrhythmia is the second most common cause of syncope.
- Carotid sinus hypersensitivity is rare in patients below 40 years of age. It is a disease of the elderly.
- Remember the diagnostic and suggestive EKG findings for cardiovascular syncope.
- First step in the evaluation is risk stratification of the patients, and the high-risk patients should be admitted to the hospital for further management.
- There are several risk stratification scales available, and many high-risk features are given in Table 27-1. If you do not remember anything, then the rule of thumb is an "elderly patient with abnormal EKG and history suggestive of cardiac syncope"—these symptoms denote the patient is at high risk.
- After the initial evaluation, in one third of the patients, etiology remains unknown. Further investigation should be focused based on the available date.
- Exertion syncope, syncope in supine position, and sudden syncope without warning suggest cardiovascular syncope and patients with these symptoms are at high risk.
- Be familiar with the prodromal symptoms with vasovagal syncope, as this suggests a benign cause.
- Remember the dangerous conditions presenting with syncope that need admission to the hospital immediately. They are massive pulmonary embolism, subarachnoid hemorrhage, acute severe hemorrhage, acute aortic dissection, acute coronary syndromes, malignant arrhythmias, and severe structural heart diseases.
- Again, history is the most important part of evaluation.

COMPREHENSION QUESTION

A 72-year-old gentleman presented with syncope on exertion. He had to walk an extra block this morning to buy milk as the store next door was closed. At the end of the block he felt light-headed and was trying to lean against the wall and the next thing he remembers is lying down on the pavement. He was soon picked up by EMS and brought to the ED. There is no eyewitness to describe the episode. He thinks he passed out for a minute and took a few seconds to figure out where he was. He complains of fatigue and increasing dyspnea on exertion. His exercise tolerance is limited to half a block secondary to shortness of breath. He has orthopnea and paroxysmal nocturnal dyspnea. He has no significant past medical history and the last time he saw a physician was 30 years ago. Rest of the history is not significant. On examination, afebrile, BP 102/72 mm Hg, HR of 98/min, RR of 20/min, and saturating 94% on room air. He has a laceration on the left temporal area from the fall. JVD is elevated to the angle of the jaw, ejection systolic murmur with late peaking in the second right intercostal space radiating to the carotids. Lungs show bilateral basal rales and have mild pedal edema. EKG showed left ventricular hypertrophy, biatrial enlargement, and no ischemic ST-T changes. Chest radiograph is significant for cardiomegaly and pulmonary vascular congestion. Basic metabolic profile is normal, and hematocrit is 36.

1. What is the next best step in the evaluation of this patient with syncope and why?
   A. Suture the laceration and discharge as this is the first episode of syncope.
   B. Work up for syncope as outpatient.
   C. Order a tilt-table test as he is elderly and probably had a reflex syncope.
   D. Admit to CCU for further management of syncope.

Answer

1. **D.** Case review: Patient has high-risk features. He has exertional syncope and rest of the history, physical examination, and EKG suggest aortic stenosis. He has a high short-term risk of death. He also has decompensated heart failure with fluid overload. His laceration needs to be taken care of, which should be followed by CT head to rule out intracranial bleed, but he is not a low-risk patient to work up as an outpatient or discharge. Tilt-table test is not an option at this stage with this significant cardiac history.

SUGGESTED READINGS

Brignole M, Hamdan MH. New concepts in the assessment of syncope. *J Am Coll Cardiol*. 2012; 59(18):1583–1591.

Kapoor WN, Karpf M, Wieand S, et al. A prospective evaluation and follow-up of patients with syncope. *N Engl J Med*. 1983;309(4):197–204.

Linzer M, Yang EH, Estes NA 3rd, et al. Diagnosing syncope. Part 1: value of history, physical examination, and electrocardiography. Clinical Efficacy Assessment Project of the American College of Physicians. *Ann Intern Med*. 1997;126(12):989–996.

Moya A, Sutton R, Ammirati F, et al. Task Force for the Diagnosis and Management of Syncope; European Society of Cardiology (ESC). Guidelines for the diagnosis and management of syncope (version 2009). *Eur Heart J*. 2009;30(21):2631–2671.

Strickberger SA, Benson DW, Biaggioni I, et al. AHA/ACCF scientific statement on the evaluation of syncope: from the American Heart Association Councils on Clinical Cardiology, Cardiovascular Nursing, Cardiovascular Disease in the Young, and Stroke, and the Quality of Care and Outcomes Research Interdisciplinary Working Group; and the American College of Cardiology Foundation: in collaboration with the Heart Rhythm Society: endorsed by the American Autonomic Society. *Circulation*. 2006;113(2):316–327.

A 32-year-old Woman With Fever, Chills, and Weakness Status Post a Blood Transfusion

Vajeeha Tabassum, MD, FACP

A 32-year-old woman is evaluated for fever, chills, and weakness. She had a blood transfusion 10 days prior after she underwent an open reduction and internal fixation of the right femur due to a motor vehicle accident. She has had no significant past medical history except for a C-section 2 years ago at which time she successfully received a blood transfusion.

On examination, she has a fever of 100.1°F, blood pressure is 100/64 mm Hg, pulse rate is 110 bpm, and respiration is 20/min. On physical examination, the patient appears uncomfortable and has scleral icterus. The remainder of the examination is unremarkable. There is no evidence of bleeding.

Hemoglobin concentration is 6.2 g/dL compared with a hemoglobin of 8.6 g/dL previously. Platelet and leukocyte count are normal. Direct and indirect Coombs tests are positive. The blood bank identifies a new alloantibody on further testing.

1. What is the most likely diagnosis?

2. What is the next step in management?

Answers

1. Delayed hemolytic transfusion reaction (DHTR).

2. Specific treatment generally is not necessary. Supplemental transfusion of blood lacking the antigen corresponding to the offending antibody may be necessary to compensate for the transfused cells that have been removed from the circulation.

CASE REVIEW

DHTR is an antibody response to previously sensitized RBC alloantigens, which have a negative alloantibody screen due to low antibody levels. This reaction typically occurs in 7 to 14 days following a transfusion. The alloantibody is detectable 1 to 2 weeks following the transfusion, and the posttransfusion direct antiglobulin test may become positive due to circulating donor RBCs coated with antibody or complement. These reactions are detected most commonly in the blood bank when a subsequent patient sample reveals a positive alloantibody or a new alloantibody in a recently transfused recipient. DHTR is associated with jaundice, low-grade fever, and an otherwise unexplained decrease in hemoglobin levels. Many delayed hemolytic reactions will go undetected because the red cell destruction occurs slowly. Any adverse reaction to the transfusion of blood or blood components should be reported to blood bank personnel as soon as possible.

Transfusions

Physiology of anemia

Anemia is defined as a reduction below normal of the number of erythrocytes in the circulation. The World Health Organization defines anemia as a hemoglobin level <13 g/dL in men and <12 g/dL in women. Anemia is the most common indication for RBC transfusion among patients. It results from at least 1 of the following 3 factors:

1. Blood loss related to the primary condition or to the operation
2. Diminished erythropoiesis related to the primary illness
3. Serial blood draws (totaling, on average, approximately 40 mL per day in an ICU setting)

Acute anemia is due to blood loss or hemolysis. If blood loss is mild, enhanced O_2 delivery is achieved through changes in the O_2–hemoglobin dissociation curve mediated by a decreased pH or increased CO_2 (the Bohr effect). With acute blood loss, hypovolemia dominates the clinical picture and the hematocrit and hemoglobin levels do not reflect the volume of blood lost. Signs of vascular instability appear with acute losses of 10% to 15% of the total blood volume. In such patients, the issue is not anemia but hypotension and decreased organ perfusion. When >30% of the blood volume is lost suddenly, patients are unable to compensate with the usual mechanisms of vascular contraction and changes in regional blood flow. The patient will prefer to remain supine and will show postural hypotension and tachycardia. If the volume of blood lost is >40% (ie, >2 L in the average-sized adult), signs of hypovolemic shock including confusion, dyspnea, diaphoresis, hypotension, and tachycardia appear. Such patients have significant deficits in vital organ perfusion and require immediate volume replacement. Symptoms associated with more chronic or progressive anemia depend on the age of the patient and the adequacy of blood supply to critical organs.

With chronic anemia, intracellular levels of 2,3-bisphosphoglycerate rise, shifting the dissociation curve to the right and facilitating O_2 unloading. This compensatory mechanism can only maintain normal tissue O_2 delivery in the face of a 20 to 30 g/L (2–3 g/dL) deficit in hemoglobin concentration. Finally, further protection of O_2 delivery to vital organs is achieved by the shunting of blood away from organs that are relatively rich in blood supply, particularly the kidney, gut, and skin.

Indications for Red Blood Cell Transfusion

Despite extensive physiologic data, indications for RBCs are controversial. Before the 1980s, most of perioperative transfusion protocols used the "10/30 rule," which held that hemoglobin must exceed 10 g/dL and hematocrit should be higher than 30% before major procedures should occur. RBC transfusion is administered most often to surgical and intensive care patients. This recommendation, which was intended for high-risk anesthesia patients, was later applied to all transfusion settings, acute or chronic, and became synonymous with the single hemoglobin value 10 g/dL at which transfusion is indicated (Table 28-1).

Table 28-1. Guidelines for Transfusion and Volume Replacement in Adults

Need based on estimated loss of blood volume			
>40% loss (>2000 mL)	30%–40% loss (1500–2000 mL)	15%–30% loss (800–1500 mL)	<15% blood loss (<750 mL)
Rapid volume replacement RBC transfusion is required	Rapid volume replacement with crystalloids or synthetic colloids RBC transfusion may be required	Volume replacement (crystalloids or synthetic colloids) RBC transfusion unlikely, unless preexisting anemia, ongoing blood loss, reduced cardiovascular reserve	May require volume replacement RBC transfusion is not warranted, unless symptomatic with preexisting anemia, severe cardiac and respiratory distress
Need based on hemoglobin concentration			
Hgb <7 g/dL	Hgb 7–10 g/dL	Hgb >10 g/dL	
RBC transfusion indicated If patient is otherwise stable, should receive 2 U of PRBCs, following which the clinical status and circulating Hgb should be reassessed	Unclear indications Balance of risk versus benefits of transfusion	RBC transfusion not indicated	

High-risk patients: >65 and/or those with cardiovascular or respiratory disease may tolerate anemia poorly. Such patients may be transfused when Hgb <8 g/dL. Data from Murphy MF, Wallington TB, Kelsey P, et al. British Committee for Standards in Hematology, Blood Transfusion Task Force. Guidelines for the clinical use of red cell transfusions. *Br J Haematol* 2001;113:24.

In general, one needs to evaluate the risk-benefit ratio of transfusion. There are no reliable parameters to decide when to transfuse, more so when the hemoglobin is 7 to 10 g/dL. One needs to use clinical judgment and consider the following:

- Ability to compensate for anemia
- Rate of ongoing blood loss
- Likelihood of further blood loss
- Evidence of end-organ compromise
- Risk of ischemia: history of coronary artery disease
- Balance of risk versus benefit of transfusion

Blood Group Antigens and Antibodies

At the beginning of the 20th century, Austrian scientist Karl Landsteiner noted that the RBCs of some individuals were agglutinated by the serum from other individuals. He made a note of the patterns of agglutination and showed that blood could be divided into groups. This marked the discovery of the first blood group system, ABO, and earned Landsteiner a Nobel Prize. Landsteiner explained that the reactions between the RBCs and serum were related to the presence of markers (antigens) on the RBCs and antibodies in the serum. Agglutination occurred when the RBC antigens were bound by the antibodies in the serum. He called the antigens A and B, and depending on which antigen the RBC expressed, blood belonged to either blood group A or blood group B. A third blood group contained RBCs that reacted as if they lacked the properties of A and B, and this group was later called "O" after the German word "Ohne," which means "without." The following year the fourth blood group, AB, was added to the ABO blood group system. These RBCs expressed both A and B antigens (Table 28-2).

Table 28-2. ABO Blood Groups

Blood Group	Antigen(s) (on the RBC)	Antibodies (in the Serum)	Genotype(s)
A	A antigen	Anti-B	AA or AO
B	B antigen	Anti-A	BB or BO
AB (universal recipient)	A antigen and B antigen	None	AB
O (universal donor)	None	Anti-A and anti-B	OO

Rh System

The Rh system is the second most important blood group system in pretransfusion testing. The Rh antigens are found on a 30- to 32-kDa RBC membrane protein that has no defined function. Although >40 different antigens in the Rh system have been described, 5 determinants account for the vast majority of phenotypes. The presence of the D antigen confers Rh "positivity," while persons who lack the D antigen are Rh negative. Two allelic antigen pairs, E/e and C/c, are also found on the Rh protein. The D antigen is a potent alloantigen. About 15% of individuals lack this antigen. Exposure of these Rh-negative people to even small amounts of Rh-positive cells, by either transfusion or pregnancy, can result in the production of anti-D alloantibody.

Blood Components

Blood products intended for transfusion are routinely collected as whole blood (450 mL) in various anticoagulants. Most donated blood is processed into components: PRBCs, platelets, and fresh frozen plasma (FFP) or cryoprecipitate. Whole blood is first separated into PRBCs and platelet-rich plasma by slow centrifugation. The platelet-rich plasma is then centrifuged at high speed to yield 1 U of random donor (RD) platelets and 1 U of FFP. Cryoprecipitate is produced by thawing FFP to precipitate the plasma proteins, and then separated by centrifugation (Table 28-3).

Table 28-3. Characteristics of Selected Blood Components

Component	Volume (mL)	Content	Clinical Response
PRBC	180–200	RBCs with variable leukocyte content and small amount of plasma	Increase Hb by 1 g/dL and hematocrit by 3%
Platelets	50–70	5.5×10^{10}/RD unit	Increase platelet count by 5000–10,000/µL
	200–400	>3×10^{11}/single-donor apheresis product	
FFP	200–250	Plasma protein—coagulation factors, proteins C and S, antithrombin	Increases coagulation factors by 2%

(continued)

Table 28-3. Characteristics of Selected Blood Components (*Continued*)

Component	Volume (mL)	Content	Clinical Response
Cryoprecipitate	10–15	Cold insoluble plasma proteins, fibrinogen, factors VIII, vWF	Topical fibrin glue, also 80 IU factor VIII
Whole blood (not readily available as it is routinely processed into components)	350–450	PRBC, platelets, FFP, cryoprecipitate	

Data from Longo DL, Fauci AS, Kasper DL, Hauser SL, Jameson L, Loscalzo J, eds. *Harrison's Principles of Internal Medicine.* 18th ed. New York: McGraw-Hill; 2012.

Adverse Reactions to Blood Transfusions

Adverse reactions to transfused blood components occur despite multiple tests, inspections, and checks. Fortunately, the most common reactions are not life-threatening, although serious reactions can present with mild symptoms and signs.

Immune-mediated reactions: Immune-mediated reactions are often due to preformed donor or recipient antibody; however, cellular elements may also cause adverse effects (Table 28-4 to 28-6).

Nonimmunologic reactions: Nonimmune causes of reactions are due to the chemical and physical properties of the stored blood component and its additives.

Table 28-4. Transfusion Reactions

Reaction Type	Symptoms	Cause	Treatment/ Prevention
Hypothermia	Chills, cardiac dysrhythmias	Exposing sinoatrial node to cold fluids	Use of an inline warmer
Electrolyte abnormalities	Renal failure, circumoral numbness, and/or tingling sensation of the fingers/toes	Hyperkalemia—RBC leakage during storage	Using fresh or washed RBCs
		Hypocalcemia—citrate, commonly used to anticoagulate blood components, chelates calcium and inhibits coagulation cascade	

(continued)

Table 28-4. Transfusion Reactions (*Continued*)

Reaction Type	Symptoms	Cause	Treatment/ Prevention
Iron overload	Symptoms and signs of iron overload affecting endocrine, hepatic, and cardiac functions are common after about 100 U of RBCs has been transfused	Each unit of RBCs contains 200–250 mg of iron	Deferoxamine and deferasirox. Alternative therapies— erythropoietin— and judicious transfusion are preferable
Hypotensive reactions	Drop of at least 10 mm Hg in the absence of other signs/symptoms of other transfusion reactions	Patients on ACE-I. Since blood products contain bradykinin that is normally degraded by ACE, patients on ACE-I may have increased levels of bradykinin that causes hypotension	Usually does not require any intervention—BP returns to normal

Transfusion-transmitted infections: Transfusion-transmitted viral infections are increasingly rare due to improved screening and testing. Multiple tests performed on donated blood to detect the presence of infectious agents using nucleic acid amplification testing (NAT) or evidence of prior infections by testing for antibodies to pathogens further reduce the risk of transfusion-acquired infections.

Table 28-5. Transfusion-transmitted Infections

Infections	Frequency (United States) (Episodes:Unit)
Hepatitis B	1:220,000
Hepatitis C	1:1,800,000
HIV-1, -2	1:2,300,000
HTLV-I and -II	1:2,993,000
Malaria	1:4,000,000

Infectious agents rarely associated with transfusion, theoretically possible, or of unknown risk include: West Nile virus, hepatitis A virus, parvovirus B19, *Babesia microti*, *Borrelia burgdorferi*, *Anaplasma phagocytophilum*, *Trypanosoma cruzi*, *Treponema pallidum*, and HHV-8.

Table 28-6. Immune Mediated Reaction Types to Blood Transfusion

Reaction Type	Symptoms	Cause	Frequency	Treatment/Prevention
Acute hemolytic reaction	Fever, chills, chest/flank discomfort, tachypnea, tachycardia, hypotension, hemoglobinemia, discomfort at infusion site	ABO incompatibility Clerical errors	1:12,000	Immediately discontinue the transfusion while maintaining venous access for emergency management Treat shock, disseminated intravascular coagulation when appropriate
Delayed hemolytic transfusion reactions	Falling hematocrit and a positive direct Coombs test. Fever, leukocytosis Most commonly occur about 7–14 days following a transfusion, may also develop up to 1 month later	Previous sensitization to RBC alloantigens who have a negative alloantibody screen	1:1000	No specific treatment Supplemental transfusion of RBC lacking the antigen corresponding to the offending antibody
Febrile nonhemolytic transfusion reactions	Fever—rise of 1.0°C from baseline, chills, rigors	Cytokines and antibodies to leukocyte antigens reacting with leukocytes or leukocyte fragments	1–4:100	Non-aspirin antipyretic agents

Allergic reactions	Rash, laryngeal edema, bronchospasm	Foreign plasma protein in transfused components	1–4:100	Stop the transfusion temporarily. Administer antihistamine. Transfusion can be completed after symptoms resolve
Anaphylactic reactions	Dyspnea, stridor, hypotension, cardiac/respiratory arrest, shock	Anti-IgA	1:150,000	Stop transfusion. Maintain vascular access and administer epinephrine. Glucocorticoids for severe cases
Graft versus host reactions	Rash, fever, diarrhea, cytopenia, liver dysfunction 3–4 weeks after transfusion	Donor T lymphocytes recognize host HLA antigens as foreign and mount an immune response in immunodeficient recipients/immunocompetent recipients who share HLA antigens with the donor	Rare	Can be prevented by irradiation of cellular components before transfusion to patients at risk

(continued)

Table 28-6. Immune Mediated Reaction Types to Blood Transfusion (*Continued*)

Reaction Type	Symptoms	Cause	Frequency	Treatment/Prevention
Transfusion-related acute lung injury	Respiratory compromise and symptoms of noncardiogenic pulmonary edema within 6 h of transfusion	Antibodies in donor plasma reactive to recipient leukocyte antigens	1:5000	Immediately discontinue the transfusion while preserving venous access Patients with mild episodes should respond to oxygen administered by nasal catheter or mask If shortness of breath persists after oxygen administration, transfer the patient to an intensive care setting where mechanical ventilation can be administered Supportive. Patient usually recovers without sequelae
Posttransfusion purpura	Purpura. Thrombocytopenia 7–10 days after platelet transfusion	Production of antibodies that react to both donor and recipient platelets	Rare	IV immunoglobulins or plasmapheresis to remove antibodies

TIPS TO REMEMBER

- One needs to evaluate the risk-benefit ratio of transfusions.
- Febrile nonhemolytic transfusion reactions are the most commonly encountered reactions associated with blood transfusion. Non-aspirin antipyretic agents can resolve the symptoms.
- Hyperkalemia and hypocalcemia are some of the most common electrolyte abnormalities involved with transfusion.
- Notify the blood bank if symptoms are suggestive of an adverse reaction due to transfusion.

COMPREHENSION QUESTIONS

1. Which of the following blood levels is considered as an adequate clinical response after 2 U of platelet transfusion?
   A. 1000 to 3000/µL
   B. 5000 to 10,000/µL
   C. 10,000 to 20,000/µL
   D. 20,000 to 25,000/µL

2. An acute hemolytic transfusion reaction occurs due to which of the following?
   A. Presence of an atypical antibody in the recipient that was undetectable in the initial antibody screen
   B. Presence of antibody in the recipient that is directed against HLA antigens on donor leukocytes
   C. ABO mismatch or due to antibodies in the host against the antigens on donor RBCs
   D. Presence of anti-IgA

3. Which of the following electrolyte abnormalities would contribute to circumoral numbness in a patient who has received 4 U of packed red blood cells due to acute blood loss involving a motor vehicle accident?
   A. Hyponatremia
   B. Hypernatremia
   C. Hypomagnesemia
   D. Hypocalcemia

Answers

1. **B.** Platelets are given as either pool preparations from RD or single-donor apheresis platelets. In an unsensitized patient without increased platelet consumption (from splenomegaly, fever, or DIC), 2 U of transfused RD platelets is anticipated to increase the platelet count by approximately 10,000/µL.

2. **C.** Acute hemolytic transfusion reactions may be intravascular (ABO mismatch) or extravascular (due to antibodies in the host against antigens on donor RBCs). Signs and symptoms include hypotension, burning at infusion site, fever, pain in the lower back or chest, DIC, oliguria, and hemoglobinuria. Infusion of ABO-mismatched blood is most commonly the result of human error, in which the patient blood bank identification number is not matched with the number of the unit of blood to be transfused.

3. **D.** Citrate is commonly used to anticoagulate blood components. Citrate chelates calcium and thereby inhibits the coagulation cascade. Hypocalcemia may manifest as circumoral numbness, and tingling sensation of the fingers and toes may result from multiple rapid transfusions. Because citrate is quickly metabolized to bicarbonate, calcium infusion is seldom required in this setting. If calcium is required, it must be given through a separate line.

SUGGESTED READINGS

Dean L. *Blood Groups and Red Cell Antigens*. Bethesda, MD: National Center for Biotechnology Information; 2005.

Klein HG, Spahn DR, Carson JL. Red blood cell transfusion in clinical practice: *Lancet*. 2007;370:415–426.

Longo DL, Fauci AS, Kasper DL, Hauser SL, Jameson L, Loscalzo J, eds. *Harrison's Principles of Internal Medicine*, 18th ed. New York: McGraw-Hill Professional; 2011.

Owings J, Utter G, Gosselin R. *Basic Surgical and Perioperative Considerations: Bleeding and Transfusions*. New York: WebMD Inc; 2006.

University of Michigan. Adverse reactions to transfusions. In: *Blood Bank Manual*. Ann Arbor, MI: University of Michigan; version July 2004, revised 11/12/09.

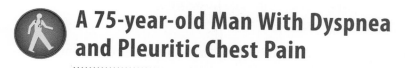

A 75-year-old Man With Dyspnea and Pleuritic Chest Pain

Robert Robinson, MD, MS, FACP

You are called by the emergency department and told of a 75-year-old male non-smoker with a history of coronary artery disease and hypertension who presents with pleuritic chest pain with dyspnea. You are asked to admit this patient to the hospital for a pneumonia seen on chest x-ray. The patient is febrile and tachypneic, and has a blood pressure of 145/65, a pulse of 115, and an oxygen saturation of 87% on room air. Physical examination shows right lower extremity edema with tenderness. Laboratory studies show a white blood cell count of 14,000, no evidence of acute renal failure, and a positive D-dimer. Blood cultures have been obtained and levofloxacin has been started in the emergency department.

1. What is this patient's risk of a coexisting pulmonary embolism?
2. How could you diagnose a pulmonary embolism in this patient?
3. When should treatment start for a suspected PE?
4. What are the initial treatment options for PE in hemodynamically stable patients?
5. Is it worthwhile to evaluate this patient for a DVT?

Answers

1. The patient is at moderate risk for a coexisting pulmonary embolism. The patient's Wells score, a clinical risk stratification for VTE described in Table 29-2, is 4.5 (+3 for signs/symptoms of DVT, +1.5 for tachycardia). Pneumonia can cause a positive D-dimer in the absence of venous thromboembolism.

2. Either a ventilation perfusion (V/Q) scan or a CT angiography of the chest is acceptable for a first-line diagnostic strategy depending on the expertise at your institution. CT angiography is the preferred choice in most settings due to availability, speed, and the ability to evaluate for other potential causes of chest pain and dyspnea. Pulmonary angiography is rarely performed for the diagnosis of PE due to the risk, limited availability, and cost of this procedure. A positive D-dimer alone is not specific for PE.

3. Treatment for suspected PE should be initiated quickly, while waiting for confirmation of the PE in patients with no contraindications for systemic anticoagulation. Treatment can be discontinued if no PE is found. Patients should be evaluated for contraindications to anticoagulation before starting anticoagulation. If a contraindication to anticoagulation is found, an alternative strategy such as an inferior vena cava (IVC) filter will need to be developed.

4. Both intravenous unfractionated heparin and subcutaneous low-molecular-weight heparin (LMWH) are effective treatments for acute PE. Warfarin, for long-term treatment, is often started at the same time. Warfarin will take several days to become effective. Aspirin and Plavix have not been shown to be effective for the treatment of PE. The role of thrombolytic therapy for acute PE is controversial, and is only considered in patients with hemodynamic compromise. No treatment is always an option, and may be the patient's preference after discussing the risks of systemic anticoagulation with the doctor.

5. Yes, if there is no PE. Treatment for DVT differs little from the treatment of a patient with PE, so it is reasonable to forgo an ultrasound of the lower extremities in a patient with a confirmed PE. However, in unstable patients, identifying remaining DVTs may help in the decision-making process about placing an IVC filter. In reality, workup for a DVT and possible PE are often ordered at the same time due to systems-based issues such as availability of testing.

CASE REVIEW

This patient is at moderate risk of a pulmonary embolus given his Wells score of 4.5. Most of his symptoms can be explained by pneumonia, but the unilateral leg swelling and positive D-dimer is suggestive of a deep venous thrombosis. Further investigation is required to determine if the patient has a DVT and/or pulmonary embolus. Ultrasonography is the most common means to evaluate for the presence of DVT. CT angiography of the chest is the most common means to evaluate for the presence of a pulmonary embolus. V/Q scanning is an alternative, and is useful in patients with chronic kidney disease due to the risk of contrast nephropathy from a CT scan. Treatment for a potential pulmonary embolus should start immediately with either LMWH or unfractionated heparin.

VENOUS THROMBOEMBOLISM

Diagnosis

Risk factors

The primary risk factors for DVT and PE are venous stasis, endothelial injury, and hypercoagulable states. Many patients who develop a DVT or PE have more than 1 of these risk factors. See Table 29-1.

Risk stratification

Clinical risk stratification for VTE can be done with the simplified Wells Scoring System (see Table 29-2).

Table 29-1. Risk Factors for VTE

Venous Stasis	Endothelial Injury	Hypercoagulability
Immobility	Prior DVT	Drugs
Surgery	Leg trauma	Genetic predisposition
CHF	Central vascular catheters	Acquired
Venous obstruction		Malignancy
Morbid obesity		Trauma/burns
		Lupus

Add the points for all risk factors to determine the Wells score. A score greater than 6 puts the patient at high risk, 2 to 6 at moderate risk, and a score of less than 2 represents a low risk for VTE.

DVT and PE prevention

DVT and PE can be prevented with several strategies including heparin, LMWH, and mechanical devices. A DVT prevention strategy should be implemented in all hospitalized patients with 1 or more risk factors for DVT.

IVC filters are DVT prevention options for patients with clear risk factors for DVT and contraindications for anticoagulation. The use of IVC filters for DVT prevention is most commonly seen in neurological trauma patients (Table 29-3).

Diagnosis of pulmonary embolism

Clinical and laboratory findings for pulmonary embolism are nonspecific. Imaging studies are required to establish a diagnosis of pulmonary embolism. The test

Table 29-2. The Simplified Wells Scoring System

Risk Factor	Score
Clinical signs/symptoms of DVT	3
No alternative diagnosis other than PE	3
Heart rate >100 beats/min	1.5
Immobilization or surgery within 4 weeks	1.5
History of prior VTE	1.5
Hemoptysis	1
Cancer treated within 6 months	1

Table 29-3. Prevention Options for DVT

Method	Dosing
Unfractionated heparin (UFH)	5000 U subcutaneously every 8–12 h
Low-molecular-weight heparin (LMWH)	Varies by drug selected
Fondaparinux	2.5 mg subcutaneously every day
Warfarin	Adjust to target INR of 2–3
Pneumatic compression devices	While in bed or immobile
Inferior vena cava filter	

characteristics indicate that CT angiography of the chest is the superior method in most situations.

V/Q scanning is a useful alternative to CT angiography in patients with significant contrast allergy or renal failure and a high probability of PE. The major drawback of V/Q scanning is the high frequency of indeterminate scans (27% in 1 study) and the availability of testing.

Pulmonary angiography is considered the gold standard test, but is rarely done due to expense, availability, and the risk of this procedure. In the PIOPED study, the risk of mortality due to pulmonary angiography was 0.5% while the risk of serious injury was 6% (Table 29-4).

Diagnosis of deep venous thrombosis

The majority (90%) of DVTs that lead to clinically significant pulmonary emboli arise from the lower extremities. Thus, DVT diagnosis primarily focuses on the identification of lower extremity DVTs.

Common diagnostic options for DVT diagnosis include ultrasonography, plethysmography, and venography. Due to its widespread and ready availability, ultrasonography has become the first choice in many institutions for the evaluation of potential DVTs. Some CT scanners are capable of combining CT angiography of the chest with lower extremity contrast venography. History,

Table 29-4. Diagnostic Options for PE

Method	Sensitivity	Specificity
CT angiography	83%	96%
V/Q scan	77%	98%
Pulmonary angiography	Gold standard	Gold standard

Table 29-5. Diagnostic Options for DVT

Method	Sensitivity	Specificity
Ultrasonography	>95%	>95%
Impedance plethysmography	91%	96%
Contrast venography	Gold standard	Gold standard
Physical examination	11%	
D-dimer	78%–100%	32%–35%

physical examination, and D-dimer testing lack specificity for the diagnosis of DVT (Table 29-5).

Treatment

DVT and PE are usually treated with unfractionated or LMWH followed by warfarin with a target INR of 2 to 3 for a minimum of 3 months. Long-term therapy with LMWH alone may be considered in patients with malignancy, pregnancy, or other factors that make warfarin unsuitable. Lifelong anticoagulation with LMWH or warfarin should be considered in patients with recurrent DVTs or PEs and patients with a major nonmodifiable risk factor such as malignancy.

Thrombolytic therapy is controversial for the treatment of PE. No clear mortality benefit has been demonstrated in multiple clinical trials, but short-term (1 week) improvement in right ventricular function can be seen when compared with no thrombolytic therapy. The major risk of thrombolytic therapy is life-threatening bleeding, which occurred in 19% of patients in 1 series.

Absolute contraindications for thrombolytic therapy are a history of hemorrhagic stroke, intracranial neoplasm, and intracranial surgery or head trauma within the last 2 months (Table 29-6).

Table 29-6. Initial Treatment Options for VTE

Method	Dosing
Unfractionated heparin (UFH)	Weight-based protocol to reach a target aPTT of 1.5–2.5× normal
Low-molecular-weight heparin (LMWH)	Varies by drug selected
Thrombolytic therapy	Consider in unstable patients with life-threatening PE
Inferior vena cava filter	In patients with contraindications to anticoagulation with significant PE

Health care quality

Hospital core measures for acute stroke require the use of DVT prophylaxis in all patients without contraindications who are admitted with an acute stroke. The use of a standard stroke order set can help increase compliance with this and other core measures.

Health care costs

DVT prophylaxis has been shown to be cost effective, and should be considered in all patients with 1 or more risk factors. The pharmaceutical costs for the treatment or prevention of DVT and PE are dependent on the choice of drug. Unfractionated heparin is the lowest cost option on the basis of drug costs alone. However, the use of unfractionated heparin is associated with higher laboratory and personnel costs than other options. In some health care delivery settings, these expenses may offset the higher cost of LMWH or fondaparinux.

TIPS TO REMEMBER

- Consider DVT prophylaxis for all hospitalized patients.
- Initiate treatment for PE while waiting for diagnostic confirmation.
- CT angiography is the test of choice to diagnose PE in most cases.
- Monitor patients for bleeding and heparin-induced thrombocytopenia (HIT).
- History and physical examination are not sensitive for DVT or PE.

COMPREHENSION QUESTIONS

1. While on duty in the intensive care unit, you receive an unstable patient transferred from the inpatient (non-ICU) internal medicine service. The patient is a 63-year-old female who was admitted for pneumococcal pneumonia 4 days ago. The patient was afebrile and responding well to IV antibiotics. The patient was transferred to the ICU after developing tachycardia, hypotension (BP 94/60), and hypoxia. The inpatient medicine service ordered an ECG, cardiac enzymes, a chest x-ray, CBC, blood cultures, and a metabolic panel before transferring the patient. The ECG shows sinus tachycardia with a rate of 125. The remainder of the studies are pending.

   Your physical examination of the patient is remarkable for tachypnea, hypotension, tachycardia, and hypoxia. No calf tenderness or edema is present. The patient is afebrile. Review of the chart indicates that the patient was on LMWH for DVT prophylaxis during this hospital stay and no documented contraindications for anticoagulation are present. What is this patient's risk of a PE?

   A. Zero. The patient is on LMWH for DVT prophylaxis.
   B. Low.
   C. Moderate.
   D. High.

2. The patient's chest x-ray is completed and is unchanged from the admission chest x-ray. What interventions should be ordered while waiting for lab results?
  A. Supplemental oxygen.
  B. Change antibiotics to cover hospital-acquired pneumonia.
  C. D-dimer assay.
  D. Fluid bolus.
  E. Full-dose LMWH to treat a potential DVT or PE.

3. The laboratory studies are reported for this patient, showing no elevations of cardiac enzymes or the white blood cell count. The patient's serum creatinine is 1 mg/dL. What tests should you order now?
  A. Serial cardiac enzymes to rule out a myocardial infarction
  B. Cardiac stress test
  C. Ultrasonography of the lower extremities to evaluate for DVT
  D. Echocardiogram
  E. CT angiogram of chest to evaluate for PE

4. The patient is found to have bilateral pulmonary emboli on CT angiography of the chest, signs of right ventricular overload on echocardiogram, and multiple large residual clots in the lower extremities. The patient's blood pressure is now 95/60 with a pulse of 90 beats/min. What additional interventions should be considered at this time?
  A. Starting warfarin
  B. Thrombolytic therapy
  C. Placing an IVC filter
  D. A workup for a hypercoagulable state

Answers

1. C. At this time, the patient's Wells score is 3 (tachycardia and immobilization), which is in the moderate risk category. As additional information becomes available, and other alternative diagnoses are excluded, the patient's risk may become higher. DVT prophylaxis, with LMWH or other means, reduces, but does not eliminate, the risk of DVT and PE.

2. **A, D, and E are all appropriate at this time.** Supplemental oxygen may be able to address the hypoxia. A fluid bolus may help with the hypotension. Full-dose LMWH is a reasonable option at this time because of the potential for a significant PE and/or acute coronary syndrome with cardiogenic shock (a differential diagnosis for the patient's presentation to the ICU). With an unchanged chest x-ray, no fever, and clinical improvement on the initial antibiotic regimen, changing antibiotics does not appear warranted at this time. This could change with additional information such as an elevated WBC, evidence of aspiration by history or

examination, or evidence of an infected IV site. A D-dimer assay would not be helpful in this situation, and is likely to be positive due to the patient's pneumonia and immobilization.

3. **A, C, D, and E should be ordered at this time.** Myocardial infarction has not been excluded, so further evaluation for this diagnosis should continue. Echocardiography may be helpful in evaluating the potential of an acute myocardial infarction, acute valve dysfunction, and right ventricular overload. Ultrasonography will determine if the patient has a lower extremity DVT. CT angiography of the chest will evaluate for PE and other potential causes of dyspnea, hypoxia, and hypotension.

4. **A, B, and C.** With hemodynamic compromise and a large PE, emergent thrombolytic therapy should be considered. Starting warfarin for long-term treatment of the patient's DVTs and PE is appropriate at this time if thrombolytic therapy is not started. Consideration can be given to the placement of an IVC filter with signs of right-sided heart strain and a large residual clot burden. A hypercoagulable workup should be postponed at this time.

SUGGESTED READINGS

Chunilal SD, Eikelboom JW, Attia J, et al. Does this patient have pulmonary embolism? *JAMA*. 2003;290(21):2849–2858.

Dong B, Jirong Y, Liu G, Wang Q, Wu T. Thrombolytic therapy for pulmonary embolism. *Cochrane Database Syst Rev*. 2006;(2):CD004437.

Kearon C, Kahn SR, Agnelli G, Goldhaber S, Raskob GE, Comerota AJ, American College of Chest Physicians. Antithrombotic therapy for venous thromboembolic disease: American College of Chest Physicians evidence-based clinical practice guidelines (8th edition). *Chest*. 2008;133(6 suppl):454S.

Luxembourg B, Schwonberg J, Hecking C, et al. Performance of five D-dimer assays for the exclusion of symptomatic distal leg vein thrombosis. *Thromb Haemost*. 2012;107(2):369–378 [Epub ahead of print].

Mattos MA, Londrey GL, Leutz DW, et al. Color-flow duplex scanning for the surveillance and diagnosis of acute deep venous thrombosis. *J Vasc Surg*. 1992;15(2):366.

Robinson KS, Anderson DR, Gross M, et al. Accuracy of screening compression ultrasonography and clinical examination for the diagnosis of deep vein thrombosis after total hip or knee arthroplasty. *Can J Surg*. 1998;41(5):368–373.

Sostman HD, Stein PD, Gottschalk A, Matta F, Hull R, Goodman L. Acute pulmonary embolism: sensitivity and specificity of ventilation-perfusion scintigraphy in PIOPED II study. *Radiology*. 2008;246(3):941–946 [Epub January 14, 2008].

Spencer FA, Emery C, Lessard D, et al. The Worcester Venous Thromboembolism study: a population-based study of the clinical epidemiology of venous thromboembolism. *J Gen Intern Med*. 2006;21(7):722.

Stein PD, Fowler SE, Goodman LR, et al, PIOPED II Investigators. Multidetector computed tomography for acute pulmonary embolism. *N Engl J Med*. 2006;354(22):2317.

Section II.
Outpatient Medicine

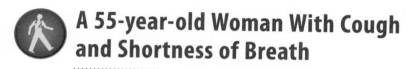

A 55-year-old Woman With Cough and Shortness of Breath

Siegfried W. B. Yu, MD, FACP

A 55-year-old female presents for the first time to the outpatient clinic, complaining of a gradual increase in cough and shortness of breath with wheezing for the past month. Her documented past medical history is notable only for seasonal allergic rhinitis. She notes that previously between attacks of her breathing difficulty, described as shortness of breath with wheezing, she would feel pretty normal. For the past year, she feels her breathing "isn't what it used to be," because episodes have become worse, and symptoms do not seem to fully resolve after attacks. She had been prescribed an albuterol inhaler that helps relieve the symptoms, but this has become a daily problem, and she has run out of her last prescription. She is also obese, and has been smoking 2 packs of cigarettes per day since the age of 16. No pets are in the home, and she denies having any prior or recent exposure to industrial chemicals.

On examination, she is afebrile, with a heart rate of 83 bpm, blood pressure 117/82 mm Hg, respirations of 18/min, and resting oxygen saturation of 92%. She appears to be slightly uncomfortable, and is able to speak in sentences. Her lung examination is notable for mild wheezing that is worse with forced expiration, and no other adventitious sounds are noted on auscultation. A peak expiratory flow rate (PEFR) done in clinic was noted at 76% predicted.

1. In light of her reported intermittent symptoms by history, what is the patient's most likely primary diagnosis?

2. Given her heavy smoking and recent progressive symptoms, what illness is she at risk of having?

3. What diagnostic test would you proceed to next?

Answers

1. A 55-year-old female smoker with a prior history of allergic rhinitis, and intermittent shortness of breath and wheezing, presents with progressive symptoms that have become daily in frequency, and are not fully relieved by frequent bronchodilator use. She demonstrates signs of airflow limitation on examination. In light of her reported intermittent symptoms by history, the patient's most likely primary diagnosis is uncontrolled asthma.

2. Given her heavy smoking and recent progressive symptoms, she is at risk of having chronic obstructive pulmonary disease.

3. The next diagnostic test would be spirometry/pulmonary function testing.

CASE REVIEW

Given the patient's intermittent episodes of shortness of breath and wheezing, separated by essentially normal respiratory function, her history is clinically consistent with a diagnosis of asthma. Her symptom frequency and need for frequent short-acting beta-2 agonist (SABA) use, decreased peak flow, and worsening symptoms with exertion classify her as having uncontrolled asthma (see Table 30-1). Some features of her presentation of concern include the following: (1) she has not been formally diagnosed with having asthma previously and (2) her progressive symptoms and heavy smoking history suggest she may be at risk for developing COPD, if she hasn't already (see Table 30-2). Clinically, she is not in severe respiratory distress, although symptoms aren't controlled well, so she should continue her use of SABAs as needed, while waiting for spirometry to confirm the asthma diagnosis and evaluate her for COPD. Adding an inhaled corticosteroid (ICS), or short course of oral steroids, would be reasonable to consider.

Table 30-1. GINA Classification of Levels of Asthma Control

Characteristics	Controlled (All of the Following)	Partly Controlled (Any Measure Present)	Uncontrolled
Assessment of current clinical control over 4 weeks			
Daytime symptoms	None (twice or less per week)	More than twice per week	Three or more features of partly controlled asthma
Limitations of activities	None	Any	
Nocturnal symptoms or awakening	None	Any	
Need for reliever or rescue treatment	None (twice or less per week)	More than twice per week	
Lung function (PEF or FEV$_1$)	Normal	<80% predicted or personal best (if known)	
Medical management	Maintain lowest dose necessary	Consider stepping up control	Step up control

Data from *Global Strategy for Asthma Management and Prevention*, Global Initiative for Asthma (GINA). <http://www.ginasthma.org/>; 2010 (update).

Table 30-2. GOLD Spirometric Classification for COPD

Stage	FEV_1/FVC	FEV_1
I. Mild	<0.70	≥80% predicted
II. Moderate	<0.70	≥50% predicted, <80% predicted
III. Severe	<0.70	≥30% predicted, <50% predicted
IV. Very severe	<0.70	<30% predicted or <50% with chronic respiratory failure

Data from Global Initiative for Chronic Obstructive Lung Disease (GOLD). *Global Strategy for the Diagnosis, Management, and Prevention of Chronic Obstructive Pulmonary Disease.* Bethesda, MD: Global Initiative for Chronic Obstructive Lung Disease (GOLD); 2011 (update).

ASTHMA AND COPD

Asthma and COPD can be understood as belonging to a larger group of obstructive lung diseases. This group includes emphysema, bronchitis, cystic fibrosis, bronchiolitis, bullous lung disease, and airway stenosis. The most prevalent of these are emphysema, chronic bronchitis, and asthma—affecting 25 to 30 million people in the United States. COPD is characterized by airflow limitation that is not fully reversible. It includes emphysema, anatomically defined by destruction and enlargement of lung alveoli; chronic bronchitis, clinically defined by chronic cough and phlegm; and small airway disease, in which small bronchioles are narrowed. Chronic bronchitis without airflow limitation is not COPD.

Asthma is characterized by airflow limitation, which is considered fully reversible (in its early stages). When exposed to various risk factors, chronically inflamed airways become hyperresponsive, resulting in bronchoconstriction, mucous plugs, and increased inflammation.

Asthma and COPD can coexist.

Asthma is one of the most common chronic diseases globally and affects around 300 million people. The prevalence has risen in affluent countries over the last 30 years, but has stabilized at around 10% to 12% of adults and 15% of children. Bronchial hyperresponsiveness is common to all types of asthma. Allergic asthma is characterized by an immediate-phase reaction of mast cells and basophils, and a late-phase reaction in which eosinophils become prominent. It is thought because of the way TH_2 helper cells produce IL-4, stimulating IgE synthesis and IL-5, producing an intense eosinophilic inflammation, that atopic asthma is caused by a preferential activation of TH_2 lymphocytes. Numerous risk factors have been implicated in asthma, and it is believed to result from an interplay between genetic and environmental risk factors (see Table 30-3).

Table 30-3. Risk Factors and Triggers Involved in Asthma

Endogenous Factors	Environmental Factors	Triggers
Genetic predisposition	Indoor allergens	Allergens
Atopy	Outdoor allergens	Upper respiratory tract viral infections
Airway hyperresponsiveness	Passive smoking	Exercise and hyperventilation
Gender	Respiratory infections	Cold air
		Sulfur dioxide
		Drugs (beta-blockers, aspirin)
		Stress
		Irritants (household sprays, paint fumes)

Data from Fauci AS, Braunwald E, Kasper DL, et al, eds. *Harrison's Principles of Internal Medicine.* 17th ed. New York: McGraw-Hill; 2008.

Diagnosis of Asthma

A diagnosis of asthma can be suspected using the patient's symptoms and medical history. Spirometry, also known as pulmonary function testing, is the preferred method of measuring airflow limitation and reversibility to establish the diagnosis. An increase in the forced expiratory volume at 1 second (FEV_1) by greater than or equal to 12% with bronchodilator administration is consistent with reversibility suggestive of asthma. This may not be exhibited by all asthmatics at each assessment, however. Patients with suspected asthma and otherwise normal spirometry results are candidates for a methacholine bronchial challenge. A 20% decrease in the FEV_1 is considered a positive result.

Some challenges may occur with patients with cough-variant asthma, because they may not have wheezing at all, but demonstrate airway responsiveness on methacholine challenge. In exercise-induced bronchoconstriction, physical activity may be the only trigger. Occupational asthma related to workplace exposures should be considered, particularly when symptoms are clearly made worse when at work, and improve when away, especially when a temporal association can be made with symptoms being absent before starting employment.

Patients may present with an acute asthma exacerbation, and it becomes important to assess the degree of severity of the episode because of the decisions that need to be made regarding triage (see Table 30-4).

Table 30-4. Asthma Exacerbation Severity

	Mild	Moderate	Severe	Imminent Respiratory Arrest
Breathless when …	Walking	Talking	At rest	
Able to talk in …	Sentences	Phrases	Words	
Respirations	Increased	Increased	>30/min	
Sensorium	May be agitated	Usually agitated	Usually agitated	May be drowsy or confused
Accessory muscle use	Usually not	Usually	Usually	Paradoxical thoracoabdominal movements
Wheeze	Moderate	Load	Usually load	May be absent
Pulse	<100	100–120	>120	Bradycardic
Pulsus paradoxus	<10 mm Hg	10–25 mm Hg	>25 mm Hg	Absence suggests fatigue
PEFR after bronchodilator	>80% predicted	60%–80% predicted	<60% predicted	
SaO_2 (%)	>95	91–95	<90	
Pao_2	Not usually tested	>60 mm Hg	<60 mm Hg	
Pco_2	<45 mm Hg	<45 mm Hg	>45 mm Hg	

Presence of several factors indicates severity.

Data from *Global Strategy for Asthma Management and Prevention,* Global Initiative for Asthma (GINA). <http://www.ginasthma.org/>; 2010 (update).

Treatment of Asthma

When the diagnosis of asthma is clearly established, it is important to determine the level of asthma control based on well-defined clinical characteristics (see Table 30-1).

Based on the level of control, an attempt should be made to adjust medications appropriately. The most common reason for uncontrolled asthma is nonadherence to medications, particularly ICSs; therefore, this should be assessed. Five treatment steps have been described that can guide the revision of the patient's

Table 30-5. Treatment Steps to Asthma Control

Controller therapy				
Step 1:	Step 2:	Step 3:	Step 4:	Step 5:
None	Select one:	Select one:	Step 3 + one or more:	Step 4 + one:
	Low-dose ICS	Low-dose ICS + LABA	Medium-/high-dose ICS + LABA	Oral glucocorticoid (lowest dose needed)
	Leukotriene modifier	Medium-/high-dose ICS	Leukotriene modifier	Anti-IgE therapy
		Low-dose ICS + leukotriene modifier	Sustained-release theophylline	
		Low-dose ICS + sustained-release theophylline		
Rapid therapy				
As needed SABA	As needed SABA	As needed SABA	As needed SABA	As needed SABA

Data from *Global Strategy for Asthma Management and Prevention*, Global Initiative for Asthma (GINA). <http://www.ginasthma.org/>; 2010 (update).

medication regimen (see Table 30-5). Basic therapy consists of inhaled SABAs (such as albuterol) as a reliever medication at all levels for rapid relief of symptoms. Additionally between steps 2 and 5, as symptoms become uncontrolled, the need to utilize controller medications, starting first with a low-dose ICS, is important. If uncontrolled symptoms continue to persist despite inhaled low-dose ICS, long-acting beta-2 agonists (LABAs) may be considered, as well as the use of medium- to high-dose ICS. Although less effective than LABAs, leukotriene modifiers and sustained-release theophylline can also be added in combination with low-dose ICS. If the patient is classified as difficult-to-treat or refractory, and nonadherence to the medical regimen has been excluded, the most aggressive step for obtaining asthma control is the use of both oral glucocorticoids and monoclonal antibody therapy with anti-IgE treatment, with omalizumab.

In acute severe asthma exacerbations, high-flow O_2 should be given to maintain O_2 saturation >90%. High doses of inhaled SABA should be given.

Intravenous beta-2 agonist therapy may be considered. An attempt should also be made to exclude concurrent illness, such as pneumonia, particularly if the history or physical examination is suggestive. Magnesium sulfate intravenously may be used adjunctively. In impending respiratory failure, wheezing may decrease, and Pao_2 may be deceptively normal or increased. In these instances, invasive mechanical ventilation may be necessary.

The Global Initiative for Chronic Obstructive Lung Disease (GOLD) has identified COPD as the sixth most common cause of death worldwide, and it is projected to become the third most common by 2020. It affects over 16 million people in the United States, and is the fourth leading cause of disease in this country. A causal relationship between cigarette smoking and the development of COPD has been proven. Although pack-years of cigarette smoking is the most significant predictor of FEV_1, this accounts for only 15% of the variability, suggesting that there are additional environmental and genetic factors that contribute.

While asthma is viewed as a primarily allergic phenomenon, COPD typically results from smoking-related inflammation and damage. A tendency for increased airway responsiveness is also present in COPD. The British hypothesis (which states that asthma and COPD are distinct entities) and the Dutch hypothesis (which states that they are intrinsically related disorders) are 2 models for understanding these diseases. Other possible contributing risk factors to COPD include respiratory infections, occupational exposures, ambient air pollution, and secondhand smoke exposure. Alpha 1-antitrypsin deficiency is a proven genetic risk factor for COPD. Individuals with 2 Z alleles or 1 Z and 1 null allele are referred to as PiZ, which is the most common form of severe alpha 1-antitrypsin deficiency.

As a result of accumulated damage, the effect on pulmonary function includes persistent reduction in the forced expiratory flow rate, which is not fully reversible, and ultimately an increased residual volume, which results in ventilation–perfusion mismatching. Airflow obstruction or limitation is characteristic, and this is measured as a decrease in the FEV_1 and FEV_1/FVC ratio to <70%. This chronic obstruction also causes "air trapping" or hyperinflation, which compensates for the obstruction, but also results in increased total lung capacity (TLC), flattened diaphragms, and an impediment to normal inspiration. The Pao_2 usually remains normal until FEV_1 is decreased to 50% predicted, and an elevated Pco_2 is not expected until the FEV_1 is <25% predicted.

Diagnosis of COPD

Cough, sputum production, and exertional dyspnea are the most common symptoms of COPD. These symptoms develop gradually, and may be punctuated by intermittent exacerbations of the disease. Some expected findings on physical examination may include the odor of smoke and nicotine stains on fingernails and teeth in cigarette smokers. A prolonged respiratory phase with expiratory wheezing may be present with advanced disease. Hyperinflation may be manifested by a barrel-chested appearance. Most people with COPD have a combination of bronchitis and emphysema, and therefore a clear distinction between "pink puffers" (thin and noncyanotic) and "blue bloaters" (heavy and cyanotic) is not always made. Severe disease may be accompanied by wasting and a paradoxical inward movement of the rib cage with inspiration (Hoover sign). Clubbing is not a typical sign of COPD, and its presence should alert you to other causes.

The classification of COPD is based on spirometric findings (see Table 30-2).

Treatment of COPD

Only 3 interventions have been demonstrated to influence the natural history of COPD. These include smoking cessation, oxygen therapy in chronic hypoxemia, and lung volume reduction in selected patients with emphysema. Similar to the asthma classification system, knowing the stage of COPD can be helpful in guiding therapy; however, spirometry stage alone has been shown to be a poor descriptor of disease status, and this must be combined with a knowledge of the patient's symptoms and future risk of exacerbations (see Tables 30-6 and 30-7).

An evidence-based method of approaching COPD management is stratifying the COPD population based on spirometric stage of disease, their frequency of exacerbations, and presence of symptoms. First choice therapy for GOLD Group A patients would be a SABA, such as albuterol, or short-acting anticholinergic (SAAC), such as ipratropium. While SABAs will still be important for rescue therapy in the other groups, Group B patients would benefit from using a long-acting anticholinergic (LAAC), such as tiotropium, or a LABA such as salmeterol or formoterol.

First choice therapy for Group C and D patients includes an ICS with LABA therapy or LAAC monotherapy. ICS, however, is associated with complications such as oropharyngeal candidiasis and decreased bone mass. Chronic oral glucocorticoid therapy is not recommended. Second-line therapy for both groups includes combined LABA and LAAC therapy. The newer PDE_4 inhibitor

Table 30-6. GOLD COPD Risk Stratification

	Group			
	A	**B**	**C**	**D**
GOLD stage	1–2	1–2	3–4	3–4
Exacerbations per year	≤1	≤1	≥2	≥2
Symptoms	Less	More	Less	More

Data from Global Initiative for Chronic Obstructive Lung Disease (GOLD). *Global Strategy for the Diagnosis, Management, and Prevention of Chronic Obstructive Pulmonary Disease.* Bethesda, MD: Global Initiative for Chronic Obstructive Lung Disease (GOLD); 2011 (update).

Table 30-7. COPD Treatment Strategy

| | Group | | | |
	A	B	C	D
First choice	SAAC or SABA	LAAC or LABA	ICS + LABA or LAAC	ICS + LABA or LAAC
Second choice	LAAC or LABA or SABA + SAAC	LAAC + LABA	LAAC + LABA	ICS + LAAC or LABA + LAAC ± ICS or ICS + LABA + PDE$_4$ inhibitor or LAAC + PDE$_4$ inhibitor
Alternative (may be used in combination with above)	Theophylline	SABA ± SAAC or theophylline	PDE$_4$ inhibitor or SABA ± SAAC or theophylline	Carbocysteine or SABA ± SAAC or theophylline
Non-pharmacologic	Smoking cessation, vaccination, physical activity	As for A + pulmonary rehabilitation	As for A + pulmonary rehabilitation	As for A + pulmonary rehabilitation

SAAC, short-acting anticholinergic; SABA, short-acting beta-2 agonist; LAAC, long-acting anticholinergic; LABA, long-acting beta-2 agonist.
Data from Global Initiative for Chronic Obstructive Lung Disease (GOLD). *Global Strategy for the Diagnosis, Management, and Prevention of Chronic Obstructive Pulmonary Disease.* Bethesda, MD: Global Initiative for Chronic Obstructive Lung Disease (GOLD); 2011 (update).

roflumilast may be considered as a second choice agent for Group D patients, and as an alternative agent for Group C patients. Theophylline can be used, but has a narrow therapeutic range, and is considered alternative therapy across all groups.

Supplemental O_2 is the only pharmacologic therapy that decreases mortality, and is indicated for patients with resting hypoxemia (O_2 saturations of <88% or <90% with signs of pulmonary hypertension or right heart failure). Other aspects of care for all groups include smoking cessation, influenza and polyvalent pneumococcal vaccination, and encouraging physical activity. For patients in Groups B to D, including those with lower GOLD stage 1 to 2 disease but with significant symptoms and those with more advanced GOLD stage 3 to 4 disease and more frequent exacerbations, pulmonary rehabilitation can improve health-related quality of life, dyspnea, and exercise capacity. Patients with upper lobe–predominant emphysema and a low postrehabilitation exercise capacity are most likely to benefit from lung volume reduction surgery.

COPD exacerbations are typical in the natural history of the disease. Bacterial infections and viral infections play a role in most COPD exacerbations. Because COPD patients are commonly colonized with potential pathogens, most are treated with antibiotics even without specific microbiologic data. *Mycoplasma pneumonia* and *Chlamydia pneumonia* are found in 5% to 10% of exacerbations. Other organisms include *Haemophilus influenza*, *Moraxella catarrhalis*, and *Streptococcus pneumoniae*. Choice of antibiotic should be based on local antibiotic susceptibility of the above organisms. A careful assessment of the distress of the patient should be undertaken. Concurrent pneumonia and/or congestive heart failure exacerbation should be excluded. Glucocorticoids reduce hospital length of stay, speed recovery, and reduce exacerbations for up to 6 months. The GOLD guidelines recommend 30 to 40 mg of oral prednisolone or equivalent for 10 to 14 days. Hyperglycemia should be monitored and treated, particularly in patients who are known diabetics. Supplemental O_2 should be used to maintain arterial saturation greater than 90%, and although a common concern, hypoxic respiratory drive only plays a small role, and does not justify withholding O_2 therapy. Arterial blood gas analysis is an important part of assessment of moderate-to-severe exacerbations. A Pco_2 >45 mm Hg warrants the use of noninvasive positive pressure ventilation (NIPPV). NIPPV reduces mortality and need for invasive ventilation, and decreases hospital length of stay and complications. It should be avoided in patients with cardiovascular/hemodynamic instability due to effects on systemic venous return. It should also be avoided in those with mental status impairment, inability to cooperate, severe burns, craniofacial trauma, extreme obesity, and copious secretions. Inability to respond to NIPPV, persistent severe respiratory distress, life-threatening hypoxemia, hypercapnia, acidosis, severely impaired mental status, hemodynamic instability, and respiratory arrest all warrant the use of invasive mechanical ventilation.

TIPS TO REMEMBER

- COPD is characterized by airflow limitation that is not fully reversible.
- Chronic bronchitis without airflow limitation is not COPD.
- Asthma is characterized by airflow limitation that is considered fully reversible (in its early stages).
- COPD and asthma can coexist.
- A diagnosis of asthma can be suspected using the patient's symptoms and medical history, and is suggested by a positive spirometric bronchodilator response (>12% increase in FEV_1). It can be confirmed with spirometry (methacholine challenge >20% decrease in FEV_1), and is classified by symptoms.

- The lowest dose of oral glucocorticoids should be used for the least amount of time, when necessary in the management of asthma.

- For COPD, spirometry stage alone has been shown to be a poor descriptor of disease status. This must be combined with a knowledge of the patient's symptoms and future risk of exacerbations.

- The 3 interventions that have been demonstrated to decrease mortality in COPD are smoking cessation, lung volume reduction surgery in selected patients, and O_2 supplementation when patients develop resting hypoxemia (O_2 saturation <88% or <90%) with signs of pulmonary hypertension or right heart failure.

COMPREHENSION QUESTIONS

1. A 55-year-old man presents to the clinic with worsening shortness of breath. He is a smoker and notes that he just visited his daughter in California last week. He had a scheduled pulmonary function test done and the results are available:

   FEV_1—55% predicted
   FEV_1/FVC—0.60
   Bronchodilator response—10% increase
   DLCO—normal

What is the most likely diagnosis?

2. A 25-year-old female with known asthma presents to the clinic and reports frequent use of her bronchodilator. She notes that she uses it about 4 times per week due to intermittent wheezing.

How would you classify her disease?

   A. Controlled
   B. Partially controlled
   C. Uncontrolled
   D. Need more information

3. What pharmacologic measure has been demonstrated to reduce mortality in COPD?

4. What is the most common reason for poor control of asthma?

Answers

1. The answer is COPD. The normal DLCO is not consistent with pulmonary embolism. The patient's age, bronchodilator response, and lack of intermittent symptoms by history do not suggest asthma. Based on his spirometric data, an FEV_1 at 55% is consistent with stage 1 COPD.

2. **D.** We need more information. Although use of the bronchodilator >2 times per week is among the "partially controlled" criteria, having knowledge of other symptoms, such as daytime symptoms more than 2 times per week, nocturnal awakening (any), limitation of activities (any), and PEFR <80% predicted, would help further classify her disease. More than 2 of the partially controlled criteria would place her disease in the uncontrolled category.

3. The answer is supplemental O_2. Supplemental O_2 is the only pharmacologic therapy that decreases mortality, and is indicated for patients with resting hypoxemia (O_2 saturation <88% or <90%) with signs of pulmonary hypertension or right heart failure. Nonpharmacologic therapies that have been shown to decrease mortality include smoking cessation and lung volume reduction surgery in selected patients.

4. The answer is nonadherence. Nonadherence to medication, particularly to ICSs, is noted to be the most common reason for poor asthma control.

SUGGESTED READING

Reilly JG Jr, Silverman EK, Shapiro SD. Chronic obstructive pulmonary disease. In: Fauci A, Braunwald E, Kasper D, et al, eds. *Harrison's Principles of Internal Medicine.* 17th ed. New York: McGraw Hill; 2008:1635–1643 [chapter 254].

Cancer Screening

Omar A. Vargas, MD, FACP

A 50-year-old Woman Requesting Cancer Screening

A 50-year-old Hispanic woman comes to your office for an annual examination. She has a medical history of hypertension for many years. She has no complaints and is interested in having all the cancer screening tests suggested for someone of her age. She still has menstrual periods. Her last Pap smear was normal 2 years ago. She has never had an abnormal Pap. She has never had a mammogram or a breast biopsy. She is the mother of 2 healthy young adults. Her menarche was at the age of 16. Family history is positive for colon cancer in her older sister diagnosed at age 45. The review of systems and physical examination is unremarkable.

1. Which cancers should you screen for?
2. Which tests will you use to screen?

Answers

1. At this time she should be screened for colon and breast cancer. Given her history of a first-degree relative diagnosed with colon cancer, she is considered a high-risk patient and should have started screening for colorectal cancer at the age of 40. She is an average-risk patient for breast cancer and she should start having biennial mammograms. Cervical cancer screening is still indicated but her next Pap smear should be done in 1 year (3 years after the last normal one).

2. To screen for colon cancer she should have a colonoscopy as she is considered a high-risk patient. For breast cancer film mammography is the test of choice.

A 55-year-old Man Interested in Cancer Screening

A 55-year-old Caucasian man comes to your clinic for an annual examination. He has no pertinent medical history and feels well. His family history is positive for dyslipidemia in his father. His review of systems and physical examination is unremarkable. He is interested in having all the recommended cancer screening tests suggested for someone of his age.

1. Which cancers should you screen for?

2. What tests will you use to screen?

Answers

1. He should be screened for colorectal cancer. He is at an average risk for colorectal cancer given his age (≥50) and the absence of other risk factors. He has no risk factors or symptoms of prostate cancer and there is no indication to perform a PSA. He has no risk factors for lung cancer.

2. To screen for colorectal cancer on this average-risk patient, there are 3 options: serial fecal occult blood testing (FOBT), flexible sigmoidoscopy, and optical colonoscopy. Given the similar performance, lower cost, minimal preparation, and minimal potential harm, FOBT is preferable. You advise the patient to collect 2 samples from 3 consecutive stools at home. If positive for blood, he will need to have an optical colonoscopy.

CANCER SCREENING

Breast Cancer

Breast cancer is the second leading cause of cancer-related death among women in the United States. Risk factors include older age, family history of breast cancer, early menarche, older age at the time of first childbirth, and a history of breast biopsy. A family history might suggest the presence of BRCA1 or BRCA2 mutations. Women with possible BRCA mutations should be referred for counseling.

Screening mammography reduces breast cancer mortality in women 50 to 70 years of age. There is ongoing debate about the benefit for women of ages 40 to 49.

The American College of Physicians (ACP) released guidelines on screening women in 2007 and they can be summarized as follows: clinicians should perform individualized assessment of risk factors for breast cancer periodically (1–2 years) to help guide the decision about screening. Women should be informed about potential benefits and harms related to screening mammography. Benefits and harms of screening, a woman's preferences, and breast cancer risk profile should guide the decision to screen.

The U.S. Preventive Service Task Force (USPSTF) also recommends an individualized decision based on a patient's values and the benefits and harms of screening in women younger than 50. The USPSTF recommends biennial screening mammography for women 50 to 74 years old. They state there is insufficient evidence to assess the benefits and harms of screening women ≥75 years old. The USPSTF recommends against the teaching of breast self-examination (BSE), and notes that there is insufficient evidence to assess the benefits or harms using digital mammography or breast MRI instead of film mammography.

Colorectal Cancer

Colorectal cancer is the third leading cause of cancer-related deaths among both men and women in the United States. Screening for colorectal cancer has led to a decrease in its incidence and mortality because early detection of premalignant polyps or cancer can prevent cancer-related deaths. Despite this evidence of a decrease in mortality, only 60% of adults older than 50 years of age get screened in the United States. Screening methods fall under 3 categories: stool-based tests, radiologic (imaging) tests, and endoscopic tests. Stool-based tests include guaiac-based fecal occult blood tests (gFOBT), immunochemical-based fecal occult blood tests (iFOBT), and stool DNA tests (sDNA). Radiologic tests include double-contrast barium enema (DCBE) and CT colonography (virtual colonoscopy). Endoscopic tests include flexible sigmoidoscopy and optical colonoscopy. Only flexible sigmoidoscopy and gFOBT have been evaluated in randomized controlled clinical trials and have shown a decrease in colorectal cancer mortality.

In 2012, after careful review of all available guidelines, the ACP published guidance statements to help internists and other providers make decisions about colorectal cancer screening. Following are the ACP guidance statements:

Clinicians should perform an individualized assessment of risk for colorectal cancer in all adults. High-risk patients include African Americans (who have the highest incidence of colorectal cancer compared with other races), a first-degree relative with colorectal cancer (especially before the age of 50), and a family history of less common conditions including hereditary nonpolyposis coli and familial adenomatous polyposis.

Screening in average-risk adults should start at the age of 50 years and in high-risk adults at the age of 40 years or 10 years younger than the age at which the youngest affected relative was diagnosed with cancer.

For average-risk adults screening can be done with a stool-based test, flexible sigmoidoscopy, or optical colonoscopy. For high-risk patients ACP recommends using optical colonoscopy. Benefits, harms, availability, and patient preferences should be considered.

ACP recommends stopping screening for colorectal cancer in adults older than 75 or in adults with a life expectancy of less than 10 years.

Proper gFOBT includes 2 samples for 3 consecutive stools at home. FOBT should be done yearly. An abnormal FOBT should be followed with optical colonoscopy. Flexible sigmoidoscopy requires bowel preparation, should be done every 5 years, and abnormal results followed by colonoscopy. Colonoscopy requires bowel preparation, and risks include perforation and bleeding. The screening interval is every 10 years.

Cervical Cancer

An estimated 12,200 new cases of cervical cancer and 4210 deaths occurred in the United States in 2010. Cervical cancer deaths have dramatically decreased since the implementation of widespread cervical cancer screening. HPV infection is associated with nearly all cases. HPV vaccination in young women is expected to decrease the incidence further. Other risk factors for cervical cancer include HIV, immunosuppression, in utero exposure to diethylstilbestrol, and previous treatment of a high-grade precancerous lesion or cervical cancer. Methods of screening include cytology and HPV testing. Evidence suggests there are no important differences between conventional and liquid-based cytology.

The USPSTF issued recommendations for screening in 2012. These recommendations apply to women who have a cervix regardless of sexual history. They do not apply to women at increased risk for cervical cancer including those with HIV or immunosuppression, in utero exposure to DES, or women who received a diagnosis of a high-grade precancerous cervical lesion or cervical cancer. These screening recommendations are summarized as follows:

Cytology (Pap) every 3 years for women 21 to 65 years of age.

Combination cytology *and* HPV testing every 5 years for women aged 30 to 65 who want to lengthen the screening interval.

Screening is not recommended in women <21 years old.

Screening is not recommended in women >65 years old who have had adequate prior screening and are not otherwise at increased risk for cervical cancer.

Screening is not recommended in women who have had a hysterectomy with removal of the cervix and who do not have a history of a high-grade precancerous lesion or cervical cancer.

HPV testing, alone or in combination with cytology, is not recommended for women younger than 30 years.

Adequate prior screening is defined as 3 consecutive negative cytology results or 2 consecutive negative HPV tests within 10 years before cessation of screening, with the most recent in the last 5 years. According to the American Cancer

Society, routine screening should continue for at least 20 years after either spontaneous resolution or adequate management of a high-grade precancerous lesion even if this extends beyond the age of 65. Women older than 65 should not resume screening on the basis of a new sexual partner. Individual risk assessment is advised for women older than 65 who have never had screening or in whom prior screening cannot be accurately accessed or documented.

Prostate Cancer

Prostate cancer is the number 1 cause of cancer in men in the United States (excluding skin cancer) with an incidence of 145 cases per 100,000 men. The death rate is approximately 23 deaths per 100,000. The incidence and death rates for African American patients are much higher at 218 and 50 per 100,000, respectively. Most deaths occur after the age of 75. Screening methods available include the PSA test and digital rectal examination. There is ongoing debate and disagreement about the benefits and harms associated with screening. The American Urological Association recommends that PSA and digital rectal examination be offered to asymptomatic men older than 40 if their life expectancy is greater than 10 years.

The American Cancer Society recommends that asymptomatic men with a life expectancy greater than 10 years be counseled about the potential benefits, harms, and uncertainties of screening so they can make an informed decision whether to be screened or not. This conversation should start at the age of 50 for average-risk men and at the age of 45 for African Americans or patients with a first-degree relative with prostate cancer diagnosed before the age of 65. In May 2012, the USPSTF published a recommendation statement against PSA-based screening for prostate cancer. The USPSTF based its recommendation on careful review of the evidence available from randomized controlled trials and concluded that the harms of screening outweigh the potential benefits.

Lung Cancer

Lung cancer is the third leading cause of cancer among men and women in the United States, but it is by far the deadliest of cancers with a death rate of approximately 50 per 100,000 people. Smoking is clearly the most important risk factor. Randomized controlled trials have failed to show a mortality benefit from screening with chest x-ray with or without sputum cytology. In August 2011, the National Cancer Institute published the results of the National Lung Screening Trial (NLST) that randomized heavy active or former smokers (>30 pack-year history) between 55 and 74 years of age to undergo either low-dose CT or PA chest x-ray. Screening with low-dose CT resulted in decreased lung cancer mortality. As a result of this trial, the American Lung Association (ALA) and the American Academy of Thoracic Surgery (AATS) have issued guidelines for screening patients for lung cancer. The ALA recommends screening with low-dose CT for patients meeting the following 4 criteria:

1. Current or former smokers
2. Ages 55 to 74
3. Smoking history of at least 30 pack years
4. No history of lung cancer

Other major organizations including the ACP and the USPSTF have not issued recommendations yet based on this new study. There is a concern that screening with low-dose CT will result in a significant number of repeated scans, procedures, and possible harm.

TIPS TO REMEMBER

- Film mammogram in women 50 to 74 years of age decreases breast cancer mortality and should be done every 2 years.
- In average-risk patients for colorectal cancer, a gFOBT annually is at least as good as colonoscopy and flexible sigmoidoscopy, with less side effects and potential complications.
- Prostate cancer screening recommendations are an ongoing debate. The USPSTF recommends against PSA-based screening.
- Heavy current or former smokers between 55 and 74 years of age are potential candidates for screening for lung cancer with low-dose CT.

COMPREHENSION QUESTIONS

1. A 60-year-old woman comes for her routine 6-month follow-up. She has a history of hypertension and dyslipidemia. She had a total hysterectomy 10 years ago due to abnormal bleeding. Her last mammogram 2 years ago was normal. Her gFOBT was negative for occult blood 1 year ago. Which of the following statements regarding cancer screening is true in this patient?

    A. She is due for breast cancer and colon cancer screening. Orders for a mammogram and a serial FOBT should be given.

    B. She is due for a mammogram, and given her age she should have an optical colonoscopy for colon cancer screening.

    C. She is due for breast cancer and colon cancer screening. A FOBT should be done during this visit and an order for a mammogram given.

    D. She is due for cervical cancer screening as her hysterectomy was performed less than 20 years ago. She is also due for a mammogram and a serial FOBT.

2. A 20-year-old woman comes to establish care with you. She is sexually active and reports inconsistent use of condoms or other methods of contraception. She has had 3 sexual partners in the last year. Regarding cervical cancer screening, which of the following statements is true?

  A. Given her age of greater than 18, a Pap smear is recommended.
  B. Given her risky sexual behavior, a Pap smear is recommended.
  C. Given her age of less than 21, a Pap smear is not recommended.
  D. Her sexual history does not put her at greater risk for cervical cancer; therefore, a Pap smear is not indicated.

Answers

1. **A.** This patient had her last mammogram 2 years ago. The current recommendation from the USPSTF is to screen women biennially after the age of 50, so a mammogram is indicated at this time. She is also due for a FOBT, which should be done yearly in average-risk patients. FOBT should *not* be done in the office as serial 2 samples from 3 different stools done at home increase the sensitivity of the test. Colonoscopy is not the best choice for screening in average-risk patients.

2. **C.** The current recommendation is to start screening at the age of 21 years regardless of sexual history, so a Pap is not indicated at this time.

SUGGESTED READINGS

American Lung Association. *Providing Guidance on Lung Cancer Screening to Patients and Physicians.* Report on Lung Cancer screening. Washington, DC: American Lung Association; April 2012.

Moyer VA, U.S. Preventive Services Task Force. Screening for cervical cancer: U.S. Preventive Services Task Force recommendation statement. *Ann Intern Med.* 2012;156(12):880–891.

Moyer VA, U.S. Preventive Services Task Force. Screening for prostate cancer: U.S. Preventive Services Task Force recommendation statement. *Ann Intern Med.* 2012;157:120–134.

Qaseem A, Denberg TD, Hopkins RH Jr, et al. Screening for colorectal cancer: a guidance statement from the American College of Physicians. *Ann Intern Med.* 2012;156(5):378–386.

The National Lung Screening Trial Research Team. Reduced lung-cancer mortality with low-dose computed tomographic screening. *N Engl J Med.* 2011;365:395–409.

U.S. Preventive Services Task Force. Screening for breast cancer: U.S. Preventive Services Task Force recommendation statement. *Ann Intern Med.* 2009;151(10):716–726.

Wolf AM, Wender RC, Etzioni RB, et al; American Cancer Society Prostate Cancer Advisory Committee. American Cancer Society guideline for the early detection of prostate cancer: update 2010. *CA Cancer J Clin.* 2010;60:70–98.

A 65-year-old Man With a GFR of 55

Omar A. Vargas, MD, FACP

65-year-old man with a history of diabetes mellitus type 2, hypertension, and obesity comes to your clinic for a 3-month follow-up visit. He was diagnosed with DM 15 years ago and HTN 20 years ago. He has no complaints and no episodes of hypoglycemia. He is eating better and has lost 10 lb in the last 1 year. On physical examination his BMI is 32, and BP 130/75. He has a normal heart examination. His foot examination demonstrates peripheral neuropathy with abnormal monofilament testing. His blood sugars have been better controlled in the last 6 months and his last HbA1C is 7.0%, which is an improvement from a previous 9.2%. Other test results include CBC with hemoglobin 11.0, normal WBC and platelets, creatinine 1.2, and glomerular filtration rate (GFR) 55. He has normal sodium, potassium, and calcium. Urine dipstick shows negative protein and urine microalbumin with 60 mg/g creatinine that has persisted for 6 months despite blood pressure control with a thiazide diuretic. His LDL is at goal. His last dilated eye examination showed nonproliferative retinopathy.

1. What complications is this patient at risk for given his chronic kidney disease (CKD)?

2. What are the common risk factors for CKD?

3. How do you screen for and decrease risk for complication of CKD?

Answers

1. Patient has CKD stage 3 given his GFR of 55. He is at risk for certain complications including anemia, metabolic acidosis, vitamin D deficiency, hyperparathyroidism, and metabolic bone disease.

2. Age is probably the most common risk factor for CKD as the GFR peaks at age 30 and slowly declines at a rate of 1 mL/min per year. However, diabetes and HTN, the 2 most common reasons for patients to develop atherosclerotic coronary heart disease, also account for most of the cases of CKD and the need for dialysis in the United States. Other risk factors include African ancestry, autoimmune diseases, autosomal dominant polycystic kidney disease (APKD), a history of acute renal failure, and chronic urinary tract infections, among many others.

3. Patient has multiple risk factors for the development of CKD including his age, diabetes, and hypertension. Moreover, he has evidence of microvascular complications from diabetes including neuropathy and retinopathy that makes the presence of nephropathy very likely. He has been screened appropriately with urine microalbumin measurements that have been confirmed on more than 1 occasion. In addition to treating his diabetes and HTN, the patient should be

started on an ACE inhibitor or an angiotensin receptor blocker (ARB) that will help delay the progression of his kidney disease.

CASE REVIEW

Patient's increased blood sugars and high blood pressures have injured and destroyed nephrons over time. For many years, his "healthy" nephrons likely maintained a normal GFR by hyperfiltration and hypertrophy. However, these maladaptive responses are not enough anymore as evidenced by his declining GFR of 55 mL/min.

Patient has reached CKD stage 3. He already has anemia that could be related to decreased erythropoietin (EPO) production unless another reason is found during his evaluation. He does not need a transfusion or EPO injection at this point. He should be screened for metabolic bone disease including 25-OH vitamin D, phosphorus, calcium, and PTH levels. His bicarbonate and anion gap should be measured to look for metabolic acidosis and he should receive bicarbonate supplementation if appropriate. As in any stage of CKD, his CV risk factors should be assessed and treated including blood pressure, blood sugar, and lipid control. To avoid or delay further progression, he should be started on an ACE inhibitor or an ARB (if unable to use an ACE inhibitor) with periodic monitoring of his microalbumin excretion.

Patient has no indications for dialysis at this point. It is also early to discuss renal replacement options and he can still be managed by his primary care physician. He should be referred to a nephrologist once he reaches CKD stage 4 or sooner if complications regarding his management arise.

Patient has CKD stage 3 as a result of diabetes and hypertension for many years. He should be screened for complications related to his CKD and his CV risk factors modified including strict control of blood sugar, blood pressure, and lipids. He should be started on an ACE inhibitor to help delay the progression of his kidney damage. Periodic monitoring of his GFR and urine albumin excretion should help you guide his proper treatment and timing for referral to a kidney specialist.

CHRONIC KIDNEY DISEASE

Diagnosis

The National Kidney Foundation has defined CKD as the persistence for more than 3 months of an abnormal GFR less than 60 mL/min or the persistence of abnormalities in the composition of blood and urine including proteinuria, hematuria, or an abnormal sediment, or the persistence of abnormalities of the kidneys on imaging tests.

Table 32-1. Staging of CKD

Stage	Severity	Glomerular Filtration Rate (GFR)
1	Mild	>90
2	Mild	60–89
3	Moderate	30–59
4	Severe	15–29
5	Renal failure	<15 or requiring dialysis

Your patient meets criteria for CKD given his abnormal GFR and his persistent microalbuminuria for more than 3 months.

Staging is based on the GFR that is derived from the Modification of Diet in Renal Disease (MDRD) study equation (Table 32-1). Using the GFR is useful as it correlates well with the onset of complications related to the decline in kidney function. For example, a patient with CKD stage 3 (GFR 30–59) could be expected to develop anemia, metabolic acidosis, and derangements in vitamin D, and calcium and phosphorus metabolism. Patients with CKD stage 4 (GFR 15–29) are at risk for the development of more serious complications including difficult-to-treat volume overload and hyperkalemia and should be prepared for renal replacement therapies. Staging according to GFR helps highlight that during stage 1 CKD (where the GFR is normal or increased), the kidney may be undergoing increased glomerular pressures with subsequent hyperfiltration that are the initial steps leading to irreversible nephron damage. This is also the time when the identification of risk factors for CKD and proper screening could stop the pathophysiologic process of nephron loss. Staging also helps primary care physicians identify patients who should be referred to a nephrologist, usually when they reach a GFR below 30 (CKD stage 4).

Staging of CKD does not take into account the etiology. The serum creatinine is not used for diagnosis or staging, since it is a poor predictor of kidney function and varies greatly depending on gender, muscle mass, protein intake, and catabolism, among other factors.

Currently there is much debate about modifying the classification and staging of CKD and a new equation for the estimation of GFR has emerged—the CKD-EPI. This equation might have better performance than the MDRD for accurate estimation of GFR especially at higher GFR levels. However, there is no consensus yet, and its role and application has not been well defined.

The identification of risk factors should alert the primary care physician to screen for nephropathy. There are different ways to screen including urinalysis, urine dipstick, 24-hour urine protein collection, measurement of GFR, and more. However, urine microalbumin measurement on a spot sample has emerged as the most popular test as it is easy to perform and it detects early glomerular damage. The presence of microalbuminuria also represents a marker of microvascular damage and is considered a cardiovascular risk factor. Microalbuminuria is present if the albumin/creatinine ratio is between 30 and 300 mg/g. Fever, exercise, and acute illness can all cause *transient* microalbuminuria without underlying kidney damage. Regardless of the cause (in most cases), ACE inhibitors and ARBs seem to delay the progression of kidney disease and the need for dialysis in patients with microalbuminuria.

The basic pathophysiology of CKD starts with nephron damage or loss related to 1 of the risk factors mentioned above. Irrespective of etiology, the maladaptive responses of the remaining nephrons are ultimately responsible for the progression of the disease. When nephron damage or loss occurs, different inflammatory cytokines, growth factors, and the renin–angiotensin–aldosterone system stimulate the healthy nephrons to undergo hypertrophy and hyperfiltration. This increase in pressure and flow promotes nephrosclerosis and eventual failure of remaining nephrons.

Treatment

The complications related to declining kidney function can be predicted based on the GFR. Patients with stage 1 and 2 CKD (GFR at or above 60 mL/min) are usually asymptomatic and free of complications but will exhibit symptoms related to the underlying etiology. For example, patients with nephrotic syndrome will have edema, APKD patients might have hypertension, etc. This is the time at which risk factor modification has a big impact. Risk factor modification includes treating the underlying etiology and the assessment of CV risk factors as most patients with CKD will die from cardiovascular complications.

Patients with stage 3 CKD (GFR 30–59 mL/min) are at risk for anemia, metabolic acidosis, vitamin D deficiency, calcium and phosphorus abnormalities, as well as secondary hyperparathyroidism with subsequent development of metabolic bone disease.

Anemia occurs secondary to decreased production of EPO by the kidney. It should be evaluated the same way as it is in the general population including reticulocyte count, iron studies, B_{12}, and folate levels. If no explanation for the anemia is found, then CKD is declared to be the cause. EPO level should not be measured as the test is expensive and optimal or normal levels have not been standardized. Patients should receive EPO-stimulating agents (ESAs) only if the hemoglobin level falls below 10 mg/dL to a target of 11 to 12 mg/dL. Higher hemoglobin values achieved with ESA have been associated with increased mortality in these patients.

Vitamin D deficiency occurs secondary to decreased production of 1,25-OH vitamin D (the active form) as the kidney is responsible for the 1-hydroxylation process. However, only 25-OH vitamin D levels should be measured as they represent the storage form and the 1,25-OH form has a very short half-life that makes testing difficult to interpret. Normalization of 25-OH vitamin D levels should occur before phosphorus, calcium, and PTH level abnormalities are addressed. A level of 25-OH vitamin D above 30 mg/mL is considered normal.

A non-anion gap metabolic acidosis occurs secondary to decreased bicarbonate reabsorption and generation by the kidneys. Treatment is easy with bicarbonate supplementation, usually in the form of sodium citrate tablets. Treatment should be started once bicarbonate falls below 18 mg/dL with a target level of 22 mg/dL.

Bone disease is secondary to abnormalities in the complex interaction between vitamin D, phosphorus, calcium, and PTH that result in either an excessive bone resorption (osteitis fibrosa cystica) or a state of bone quiescence (adynamic bone disease). Both result in a fragile bone matrix that increases the risk for fractures.

Patients with CKD stage 4 (GFR 15–29 mL/min) have more difficult-to-control hypertension and edema that requires large doses of loop diuretics. They also start having trouble maintaining normal potassium levels and can exhibit symptoms of uremia. They should be referred to nephrology and be ready to discuss renal replacement therapy options.

Patients with CKD stage 5 (GFR less than 15 mL/min) will need renal replacement or discussion regarding end-of-life measures. Their life expectancy once on dialysis is short with more than half of patients dying within 5 years. Most patients with CKD–ESRD die from complications of cardiovascular disease including MIs and strokes.

Renal replacement therapy, including dialysis and kidney transplantation, is usually not required until the GFR falls below 10 mL/min. There is much debate about the appropriate timing for dialysis as recent studies have shown that early initiation of dialysis might be related to poorer outcomes. However, it is also true that patients should be given ample time to discuss treatment options and prepare for replacement therapy. As mentioned before, this discussion should start once patients reach stage 4 CKD. There are multiple forms of renal replacement therapies, and their review is beyond the scope of this chapter.

The following is a list of some of the indications for dialysis:

1. Uremia including pericardial effusion and anion gap metabolic acidosis
2. Intractable hyperkalemia
3. Intractable volume overload

TIPS TO REMEMBER

- The diagnosis of CKD should be done after at least 3 months of abnormalities of the urine or an abnormal GFR.
- Urine microalbuminuria is probably the earliest marker of nephropathy.

● Patients with CKD should be started on an ACE inhibitor or an ARB to help delay the progression of kidney damage.

● The most common cause of death for CKD patients is ischemic heart disease, suggesting that CV risk factor assessment and modification should be done routinely.

● GFR and *not* creatinine is the best indicator of kidney function used in clinical practice.

COMPREHENSION QUESTIONS

1. A 70-year-old man with a long-standing history of hypertension and coronary artery disease is found to have abnormal laboratory test results including an elevated creatinine and a GFR of 45 mL/min. His electrolytes are normal. Urinalysis is negative for protein and blood. His hypertension is well controlled. His GFR 6 months ago was 55 mL/min. Which statement best describes his kidney function?

    A. He has acute kidney failure given the rapid deterioration of his GFR.
    B. He has a normal kidney function as evidenced by his normal urinalysis but he is at risk to develop CKD given his declining GFR.
    C. He has CKD stage 4 and should be referred to a nephrologist for further evaluation.
    D. He has CKD given his abnormal GFR that has persisted for longer than 3 months.

2. Your patient is a 55-year-old woman recently diagnosed with diabetes mellitus type 2. You would like to screen for microvascular complications related to her DM. What test is most appropriate to screen for diabetic nephropathy?

    A. Urine microalbumin excretion measurement
    B. Urine dipstick
    C. Serum creatinine
    D. Kidney ultrasound

3. A 65-year-old man with hypertension, diabetes, and recently diagnosed CKD stage 3 comes to your office asking about medications that could delay the progression of his kidney disease. Which of the following medications would you recommend?

    A. Loop diuretics
    B. Thiazide diuretics
    C. Calcium channel blockers
    D. ACE inhibitors
    E. Aldosterone antagonists

Answers

1. **D.** CKD is diagnosed after persistence for longer than 3 months of an abnormal GFR or abnormalities of the composition of the urine. This patient has a normal urinalysis but has had an abnormal GFR for 6 months indicating chronic kidney damage.

2. **A.** Urine microalbumin excretion measurement on a spot, random sample is a sensitive and easy way to screen for nephropathy. The presence of microalbuminuria (30–300 mg/g of albumin) is the earliest marker of nephropathy and an independent cardiovascular risk factor. Urine dipstick, serum creatinine, and kidney ultrasound are not sensitive enough to detect early kidney damage.

3. **D.** Regardless of the etiology, ACE inhibitors and angiotensin receptor blockers (ARBs) have been shown to delay the progression of kidney disease in most patients. All other medications are important in treating some of the complications related to declining GFR including hypertension and edema but are not superior to ACE inhibitors for kidney protection.

SUGGESTED READINGS

Bakris GL. Slowing nephropathy progression: focus on proteinuria reduction. *Clin J Am Soc Nephrol.* 2008;3:S3–S10.

Longo D, Fauci A, Kasper D, Hauser S, Jameson J, Loscalzo J. *Harrison's Principles of Internal Medicine.* 18th ed. New York: The McGraw-Hill Companies; 2012.

National Kidney Foundation. KDOQI clinical practice guidelines for chronic kidney disease: evaluation, classification, and stratification. *Am J Kidney Dis.* 2002;39:S1–S266.

UK Prospective Diabetes Study Group. Efficacy of atenolol and captopril in reducing the risk of macrovascular complications in type 2 diabetes (UKPDS 39). *BMJ.* 1998;317:713–720.

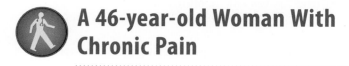

A 46-year-old Woman With Chronic Pain

Stacy Sattovia, MD, FACP

Ms Q is a 46-year-old female with a past medical history significant for depression, gastroesophageal reflux, and a motor vehicle accident 7 years ago. Over the last 3 years she has developed worsening low back pain that she feels is limiting her ability to carry out her activities of daily living. She works as a heavy equipment operator at a local factory. She denies fevers, chills, weight loss, and bladder or bowel habit changes. She denies radicular pain and numbness or weakness in her legs. Her vital signs include a blood pressure of 128/65, heart rate of 72 bpm, respiratory rate of 16/min, and temperature of 37.2°C. She is seeing you for the first time for pain control and is requesting opioid medication.

1. What is your differential diagnosis?

2. What are the key elements of the history and physical examination?

3. What diagnostic evaluation should be done for this patient?

4. What are the best treatment strategies for her pain?

Answers

Summary: This is a 46-year-old female with a history of depression, motor vehicle accident, and an occupation that involves heavy machine operation presenting with nonspecific low back pain that appears to be chronic in nature.

1. Subacute, nonspecific low back pain is the most likely diagnosis. Less likely etiologies include neoplasm, infection, and fracture.

2. Obtaining information to rule out neoplasm, infection, and fracture is key. A history of bacteremia or other disseminated infection as well as immunosuppression may heighten your suspicion for infection. Inquiring about fevers and chills is thus important. In addition, a history of unexplained weight loss or known malignancy may increase your concern for a neoplasm or complication of a malignancy. A recent history of trauma as well as risk factors for osteoporosis would increase your concern for fracture.

3. Physical examination should focus on location of tenderness on examination—percuss over each spinous process. True tenderness over the spine itself raises concern for neoplasm, infection, or fracture. Muscle tenderness is most likely seen in nonspecific back pain as well as fibromyalgia, myositis, and chronic muscle strain. A straight leg raise, performed with the patient supine, with

the knee in full extension is considered positive for nerve root compression if contralateral radiation of pain is elicited.

Numerous guidelines provide recommendations about diagnostic evaluation. The focus is primarily on identification of patients who are at high risk for pathology such as tumor, infection, and fracture. None of the guidelines advocate routine use of imaging, especially at the initial evaluation. Imaging is recommended primarily for those patients who exhibit red flags, such as fever, weight loss, or bowel or bladder incontinence. If red flags do exist, a plain film can be diagnostic of fracture, but for evaluation of infection and malignancy, MRI is typically advocated.

4. Because there are no red flags present on this patient's history or physical examination, she is most likely experiencing chronic, nonspecific back pain. Back pain is a common reason for seeking primary care services and a leading chronic pain condition in the United States. The approach to chronic pain will thus be discussed in detail.

CHRONIC PAIN IN AN AMBULATORY SETTING

The World Health Organization estimates that 20% of the world's population has some type of chronic pain. Chronic pain is defined as "pain lasting longer than 3 months or beyond the expected period of healing of tissue pathology." Characteristically, the nature and severity of the pain is not necessarily correlated with the degree of tissue injury. Specifically low back pain accounts for a majority of musculoskeletal and chronic pain visits to primary care.

Chronic pain typically affects all areas of a patient's life and can lead to significant loss of function, both physically and emotionally. In addition, there is a large burden to society due to this loss of function and productivity with studies indicating that the "total cost of chronic pain exceeds $210 billion annually in the United States."

Pathophysiology

Research done in osteoarthritis suggests that the OA is similar to other chronic pain states associated with "peripheral tissue injury and repair." As injury and remodeling occurs, "physiological mechanisms of pain operate at the local joint level, the dorsal root ganglion level and higher brain processing centers." The release of inflammatory mediators leads to sensitization of the nociceptive system creating "heightened sensitivity to noxious stimuli and to pain in response to non-noxious stimuli." This sensitization can occur at any of these 3 levels with the understanding that the nervous system demonstrates plasticity—and, in response to tissue injury and repair, can (among other mechanisms) upregulate or downregulate receptor expression, alter neuronal firing thresholds, and lead to "subsequent abnormal sensation of pain, unrelated to inflammation."

In addition, it is accepted that chronic pain is a complex interplay of "individuals' unique previous histories, any physiological abnormalities, their cognitive perceptions of nociception, emotional factors, coping styles and social and financial resources."

Treatment Strategies for Chronic Pain

Chronic pain is a condition that is typically multifactorial in etiology. Our understanding of triggers and mechanisms has improved in many aspects, but our therapeutic approach, specifically pharmacological approach, has changed very little. "Currently available treatments provide modest improvements in pain and minimum improvements in physical and emotional functioning." Unfortunately, the majority of evidence for pain control focuses on the acute setting with poor quality of evidence existing for chronic, noncancer pain control.

Pharmacological Treatments

Overall, the use of medications to treat pain has increased 188% between 1996 and 2005, with the majority of this increase related to increased use of opioid medications. A meta-analysis of randomized controlled trials addressing these agents in numerous noncancer chronic pain states revealed that opioids result in mild improvements in pain severity and function but are less effective than other analgesic agents. Therefore, opioids are considered second- or third-line agents in osteoarthritis, neuropathy, and low back pain. Studies have proven that tramadol, a combination of a mu-opioid agonist and serotonin and norepinephrine reuptake inhibitor (a distinct mechanism of action compared with other opioids), has been more effective than placebo in osteoarthritis and fibromyalgia.

Nonsteroidal anti-inflammatory drugs (NSAIDs) are generally considered first-line agents in osteoarthritis and low back pain and are thus highly recommended. Antidepressant drugs including tricyclic antidepressants and selective serotonin reuptake inhibitors have been proven to be more effective than placebo, particularly in neuropathic pain but also in fibromyalgia, back pain, and headaches. Anticonvulsant agents, specifically gabapentin, pregabalin, and carbamazepine, have good evidence for use in chronic neuropathic pain and fibromyalgia. They are also useful in low back pain with radiculopathy but appear to be less effective in nonspecific back pain. Skeletal muscle relaxants are frequently prescribed but with little evidence of effectiveness beyond adjuvant therapy with NSAIDs for acute pain relief. Topical drugs such as capsaicin and salicylate have proven more effective than placebo in chronic noncancer pain.

Complications of pharmacological therapies
The adverse effects of several of these medications can limit their effectiveness. Opioid therapy side effects produce significant attrition in clinical trials. Common

side effects include nausea, constipation, and somnolence. Rarely, patients maintained on opioid therapy chronically can begin to experience opioid-induced hyperalgesia. This "occurs when patients taking opioids become hypersensitive to nociceptive stimuli … postulated to result from changes in the peripheral and central nervous system that lead to facilitation of nociceptive pathways." If providers are unaware of this phenomenon, they can continue to escalate doses in the setting of little relief and actually increase pain symptomatology.

In addition, opioids carry a risk of misuse and abuse. According to the Office of National Drug Control Policy, "prescription drug abuse is the nation's fastest growing drug problem." This has led to increased emergency room visits, hospitalizations in addition to accidental overdose, and a mortality rate that exceeds that of heroin and cocaine. Therefore, caution in prescribing and monitoring for both side effects and misuse is critically important.

NSAIDs, which are considered first-line therapy, have several limiting side effects including NSAID gastropathy and exacerbation of renal failure and congestive heart failure. Antidepressant agents, specifically TCAs, carry the risk of arrhythmias, hypertension, and postural hypotension—with concern for falls in elderly patients. SSRIs have a more preferable side effect profile, but attention must be paid to doses and interactions with other medications that can increase serotonin levels and lead to a serotonin syndrome. Anticonvulsant drugs can commonly cause somnolence, weight gain, fatigue, and dizziness. Muscle relaxants, like many of the other agents used, can cause significant somnolence.

Thus, each class of medications imparts risk of adverse effects for patients, some of which can be particularly problematic in a patient who may be experiencing depressive symptoms secondary to a chronic pain state. A thorough discussion of risks and benefits, with setting of expectations, may enhance tolerability of pharmacological approaches to pain control.

Multidisciplinary Care

Of all the treatment modalities mentioned, the best evidence averages roughly ~30% relief in about half of all treated patients. To complicate the results, placebo response rates average 10% and use of an active placebo in trials yields a 21% improvement in symptoms. This effect underlies the complex nature of chronic pain—none of the most commonly prescribed treatments regimens are, by themselves, sufficient to eliminate pain and to have a major effect on physical and emotional function in most patients with chronic pain.

Interdisciplinary plan rehabilitation programs, which frequently include physician evaluation, physical therapy, exercise therapy, behavioral therapy with an emphasis on self-management and efficacy, and vocational rehabilitation (where necessary), actually provide results similar to traditional pharmacological treatments.

TIPS TO REMEMBER

- Chronic pain is difficult to manage, and therapy must be tailored to each individual patient.

- Currently available treatments provide modest improvements in pain and minimum improvements in physical and emotional functioning, so expectation setting is an important component of each treatment plan.

- A multidisciplinary approach to treatment is as successful as pharmacological treatments. This approach should be considered as many pharmacological treatments have unwanted side effects and complications.

COMPREHENSION QUESTIONS

1. A 52-year-old man with a history of hypertension presents to your acute care clinic with a 3-day history of severe low back pain. He has been unable to perform his occupation as a mail carrier during these 3 days and is seeking relief of his symptoms. He is interested in opioid therapy as this "happens a few times every year" and he believes "pain pills" will help prevent his symptoms from recurring. He has no fever, chills, weakness, numbness, or change in bladder or bowel habits. On examination, he is an obese gentleman with no spinal tenderness, but significant bilateral muscle tenderness. What is your first line of therapy?
    A. Oral opioid
    B. NSAID
    C. Muscle relaxant
    D. Intravenous opioid

2. A 35-year-old woman with a history of chronic abdominal pain is referred to your clinic from a local emergency room for continued opioid therapy and monitoring. She has not had a single primary care provider in adulthood. She is status postcholecystectomy and 2 exploratory laparotomies for severe abdominal pain with little change in her symptoms. On examination, she has vital signs within the normal range and diffuse tenderness to abdominal palpation. There is no rebound or guarding. What is the next best step?
    A. Refill opioid medications.
    B. Obtain a thorough social history.
    C. Abdominal CT scan.
    D. Abdominal ultrasound.

Answers

1. **B.** This 52-year-old gentleman most likely has acute, nonspecific low back pain, with intermittently recurrent symptoms. He has no elements on history or

physical examination that would suggest infection, malignancy, or trauma. The best first line of therapy is NSAIDs. Patient education regarding the most effective treatment for low back pain (NSAIDs vs opioid therapy) and counseling about weight loss and exercise may benefit this patient as well.

2. **B.** This 35-year-old female illustrates very well the complexity of chronic pain. Obtaining further information about contributing social and personal factors may be helpful to determine the next best therapeutic plan for her. She may benefit from social services to help address social stressors or counseling and therapy for a contributing and possibly undiagnosed psychiatric condition. Her care will most likely require repeat, frequent visits to establish rapport and explore contributors to her chronic pain.

SUGGESTED READINGS

LeBlond RF, Brown DD, DeGowin RL. *DeGowin's Diagnostic Evaluation.* 9th ed. New York: McGraw-Hill; 2009.

Lee M, Silverman S, Hansen H, Patel V, Manchikanti L. A comprehensive review of opioid-induced hyperalgesia. *Pain Physician.* 2011;14:145–161.

Noble M, Treadwell JR, Tregear SJ, et al. Long-term opioid management for chronic non-cancer pain [review]. *Cochrane Database Syst Rev.* 2010;(1):CD006605.

Office of National Drug Control Policy. Epidemic: responding to America's prescription drug abuse crisis. 2011 prescription drug abuse prescription plan. <www.whitehouse.gov/ondcp/prescription-drug-abuse>.

Sofat N, Ejindu V, Kiely P. What makes osteoarthritis painful? The evidence for local and central pain processing. *Rheumatology.* 2011;50:2157–2165.

Turk DC, Wilson HD, Cahana A. Treatment of chronic non-cancer pain. *Lancet.* 2011;377:2226–2235.

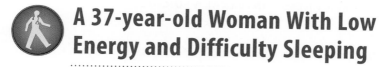

A 37-year-old Woman With Low Energy and Difficulty Sleeping

Tiffany Leung, MD, MPH

A 37-year-old woman presents to establish care with you in the office today. She complains of low energy levels and difficulty sleeping for the past 4 years. She has gained 30 lb over the past 2 years. She reports a family history of alcoholism in her mother and her older brother, and completed suicide in her father. She thinks her mother was hospitalized for a suicide attempt many years ago, but she does not know any more details. When you ask about her social history, she hesitates in giving her answer, and then becomes tearful as she tells you with great difficulty that she was in a physically and sexually abusive marriage for 10 years. The marriage finally ended over 1 year ago, but the patient still expresses guilt about its end and says she feels worthless every day. She admits that she had suicidal thoughts on and off in the past but has none currently. She has never had a suicide attempt. She drinks 3 beers nightly. Her vital signs and complete physical examination are normal except for a labile affect.

1. **What is the most likely diagnosis?**

2. **What is the next appropriate step in evaluation?**

3. **What therapeutic options can you offer to this patient?**

Answers

1. This patient presents with classic symptoms of major depressive disorder (MDD), and meets diagnostic criteria for MDD, according to the fourth edition of the *Diagnostic and Statistical Manual of Mental Disorders, Revised* (DSM-IV-R). She has depressed mood, insomnia, loss of energy, feelings of worthlessness, weight gain, and recurrent suicidal ideation without a specific plan. These symptoms have been present for 4 years, which is longer than the 2-week period required to meet DSM-IV-R criteria for MDD. She has multiple risk factors for MDD, most notably a family history of mood disorders and stressful life events, including a difficult marriage and history as a victim of intimate partner violence. She also drinks more than the recommended upper limit of alcohol daily for females, suggesting possible substance dependency or even abuse that needs further evaluation and directed management.

2. The next appropriate step is to evaluate her depressive symptoms in an objective manner to guide diagnosis, evaluate severity, and establish a baseline of severity that can later be compared with treatment response to pharmacologic and behavioral therapies. Multiple rating scales and scores exist to assist with quantifying the severity of depression symptoms and their level of functional impairment, which will be explored further in this chapter.

3. Therapeutic options for an episode of major depression include a wide variety of pharmacologic and behavioral therapies. Among pharmacologic therapies, selective serotonin reuptake inhibitors (SSRIs) are considered first-line agents in the treatment of an episode of major depression. The choice of SSRI depends in part on the side effect profiles for each medication in this class, as common side effects for each medication can be targeted to some of the specific symptoms that the patient is experiencing. It is important to recognize that all SSRIs are not immediately effective and must be titrated to a dose that will have maximum therapeutic effect over several weeks. Close follow-up is important to ensure that patients are deriving maximum benefit possible from adequate doses of medication, and if ineffective, then the medication is switched to an alternative agent. Eight weeks on a prescribed pharmacologic therapy is considered an adequate trial of a SSRI medication. SSRIs as a class carry a black box warning of initially increasing suicidal ideations, particularly in adolescents, and also have a high potential to interact with other medicines due to their effects on the cytochrome P450 systems of liver metabolism. Additional pharmacologic agents exist, and are alternatives for treatment of MDD as well.

The most common and well known of behavioral therapies is cognitive behavioral therapy (CBT), which is a form of therapy where awareness of dysfunctional thoughts as sources of depressed mood and appropriate coping techniques for these thoughts are fostered. Typically, a combination of pharmacologic therapy and CBT is the most effective treatment for MDD. Practically, affordable mental health services for the most vulnerable patients can often be challenging to access, and maintaining a supportive role as patient advocate can be vital to maintaining a therapeutic physician–patient relationship.

CASE REVIEW

This case clearly describes a patient with symptoms of untreated depression and with multiple risk factors for depression, including a family history of mood disorders and a personal history of excessive alcohol use and intimate partner violence. She clearly meets diagnostic criteria for a major depressive episode, as defined in DSM-IV (Table 34-1). Additionally, a family history of completed and attempted suicide increases her risk of suicide, even if she has never had a suicide attempt prior to her visit. Of her risk factors, the most modifiable is to abstain or at least limit alcohol consumption. It is important to recognize that substance abuse is a common comorbid condition in patients with mental health disorders, and intoxication or withdrawal from recreational or illicit substances can exacerbate the symptoms of a mood disorder, especially depression. Many subtypes of depression exist, including depression with melancholic, atypical, or psychotic features, dysthymia, and adjustment disorders. They are beyond the

Table 34-1. Criteria for Major Depressive Episode (*Diagnostic and Statistical Manual of Mental Disorders, Revised*)

Five or more of the following symptoms (1 of which is depressed mood or loss of interest or pleasure) have occurred together for a 2-week period and represent a change in previous functioning:

1. Depressed mood most of the day, nearly every day as self-reported or observed by others
2. Diminished self-interest or pleasure in all or almost all activities most of the day, nearly every day
3. Significant weight loss when not dieting, or weight gain; or decrease or increase in appetite nearly every day
4. Insomnia or hypersomnia nearly every day
5. Psychomotor agitation or retardation nearly every day
6. Fatigue or loss of energy nearly every day
7. Feelings of worthlessness or excessive or inappropriate guilt nearly every day
8. Diminished ability to concentrate or think every day
9. Recurrent thoughts of death, recurrent suicidal ideation without a specific plan

The symptoms cause clinically significant distress or impairment in social, occupational, or other areas of functioning

The symptoms are not due to the direct physiologic effects of a substance (drug or medication) or a general medical condition

The symptoms are not better accounted for by bereavement, or the symptoms persist for more than 2 months or are characterized by marked functional impairment, morbid preoccupation with worthlessness, suicidal ideation, psychotic symptoms, or psychomotor retardation

scope of this text, which will focus primarily on the management of MDD in a primary care setting.

MAJOR DEPRESSION

Diagnosis

Definitions
See Table 34-1.

Pathophysiology and Epidemiology

The neurobiological pathways affected in depression are complex and incompletely elucidated. Neuroendocrine abnormalities resulting from alterations in these pathways can explain some symptoms of depression. Genetic predisposition for developing depression can account for 40% to 50% of the risk for developing depression, but no specific gene for depression has been identified. Physical and emotional stress, as well as drugs and other ingested substances, also influences the pathways involved in depression. First-line therapeutic agents target pathways involved in serotonin and norepinephrine reuptake and, with time, neurobiological pathways of the brain adapt to the changes produced by antidepressant medications and ideally result clinically in mood elevation. More detailed neurobiological pathways are beyond the scope of this text.

The prevalence of major depression is approximately 5%, with about 15% of the population experiencing depression at least once during their lifetime. Milder forms of depression can have up to a 15% to 20% prevalence, and this excludes other mixed mood disorders that include symptoms that overlap with depression, such as bipolar disorder. Depression affects up to 10% of patients at any given time. Women are twice as likely as men to have depression. Depression is commonly underdiagnosed and undertreated. In the United States, an estimated $55.1 billion in lost productivity per year is attributed to all mood disorders, including depressive disorders, bipolar disorders, and depression associated with medical illness or substance abuse. About 10% to 15% of cases of depression can be explained by general medical illness or substance use. Depressive disorders manifest in about 20% to 30% of patients with cardiac disease; 25% to 50% of patients with cancer, with certain cancers being associated with a much higher prevalence; 8% to 27% of patients with diabetes mellitus; 22% to 45% of patients with HIV infection; and roughly 20% of patients with left-hemispheric stroke.

Rarely, a patient will present with a chief complaint of depressed mood. More commonly, an associated complaint is the first symptom identified, and more detailed history including a thorough review of symptoms is necessary to reveal symptoms of depression. Common symptoms include low energy levels and low motivation, poor sleep, lack of interest in previously enjoyable activities, and poor concentration. However, it is important to recognize that symptoms of depression are rarely the same between individual patients. Depression screening and diagnostic tools, which will be discussed further in this chapter, can be helpful to assess for symptoms of depression in a systematic, objective manner. A detailed medical history is important to identify potentially treatable etiologies of secondary depression or comorbid illness that, if better controlled, can improve symptoms of depression.

A careful review of medications and use of other substances is important to identify iatrogenic etiologies for depressive symptoms (Table 34-2). It is also important to ask the patient in a nonjudgmental manner about important

Table 34-2. Secondary Causes of Depression

Medications	Other substances
Antihypertensive drugs (eg, beta-blockers)	Psychostimulants, such as cocaine and amphetamines
Anticholesterolemic agents	
Antiarrhythmic agents (eg, digoxin)	Heroin and other opiates
Glucocorticoids	Ethanol
Antimicrobials (eg, mefloquine)	Marijuana, and related synthetic cannabinoids
Systemic analgesics (eg, opioid analgesics)	
Antiparkinsonian medications (eg, levodopa)	Phencyclidine
Anticonvulsants	Hypothyroidism
Contraceptive medications	Hypogonadism

components of the social and family history that may increase risk for and contribute to depression (Table 34-3). The family history should include mental health disorders, suicide attempts or completions, and substance abuse including alcoholism. The social history should address the patient's personal history of substance dependence or abuse, significant life events, as well as screening for intimate partner violence, which can include physical, verbal, or sexual abuse. Substance abuse history is essential, as intoxication or withdrawal from a substance also can cause depressive symptoms.

Multiple depression screening tools exist for use at the point of care. The shortest is the Primary Care Evaluation of Mental Disorders (PRIME-MD), which is a 2-item screening tool that asks the following 2 questions:

1. Over the past 2 weeks have you felt down, depressed, or hopeless?

2. Over the past 2 weeks have you felt little interest or pleasure in doing things?

A positive response, which is an answer of yes to any of the items, has a sensitivity of 96% and a specificity of 57%. More lengthy screening tools and depression scales exist that can be used in specific clinical situations. For example, the Geriatric Depression Scale (GDS) is intended for patients over 65 years of age, and the Edinburgh Postnatal Depression Scale is intended for use in postpartum women. The benefit of using a depression scale that assesses a more detailed inventory of symptoms is that the same scale may then be used to follow treatment responses. Common tools used to screen for depression and follow treatment response include the Patient Health Questionnaire (PHQ-9) and Beck Depression Inventory (BDI). The PHQ-9 and its score interpretation are included here (Tables 34-4 and 34-5). The 2-item screening tool is more efficient and can perform as

Table 34-3. Risk Factors for Depression

Older age (including associated neurologic conditions, such as Alzheimer disease and parkinsonism)

Recent childbirth

Neurologic conditions (multiple sclerosis, traumatic brain injury)

Stressful life events

Personal or family history of depression

Comorbid medical conditions (diabetes, coronary artery disease, stroke, obesity, HIV infection, cancer, hepatitis C)

Comorbid mental health conditions (eating disorders, anxiety disorders, somatoform disorders, psychotic disorders, personality disorders)

Chronic fatigue syndrome or fibromyalgia

Alarm symptoms[a]

- Past history of suicide attempts
- Profound hopelessness
- Substance abuse
- Social isolation

[a]Immediate mental health evaluation may be indicated if these significant risk factors are identified.

well as the longer instruments, but does not provide the level of detail needed to follow treatment response.

It is important to screen for risk of self-harm or harm to others through direct, nonjudgmental inquiry. Some depression scales, such as PHQ-9 and BDI, include questions about suicidal or homicidal ideation or intent, which, if marked affirmatively, should prompt more detailed questioning of the patient's imminent risk for harmful behaviors in order to guide triage and emergent psychiatric management.

Examine the patient for signs of a medical condition, substance use, or withdrawal that may be the cause of depressive symptoms. A social history indicating substance use can guide the physical examination, with attention to signs of withdrawal from or intoxication with the suspected substance(s). Attention to signs of intimate partner violence are also essential, including, for example, a detailed examination of injuries at varying stages of healing for which the patient is unable to adequately account.

Laboratory studies should be ordered judiciously based on the clinical suspicion for secondary causes of depression (Tables 34-2 and 34-3). Because a patient frequently presents with varied symptoms of depression, symptoms should guide indicated laboratory analyses. Common tests that are performed in a primary care

Table 34-4. Patient Health Questionnaire

Over the *last 2 weeks*, how often have you been bothered by any of the following problems?

	Not At All	Several Days	More Than Half the Days	Nearly Every Day
1. Little interest or pleasure in doing things	0	1	2	3
2. Feeling down, depressed, or hopeless	0	1	2	3
3. Trouble falling or staying asleep, or sleeping too much	0	1	2	3
4. Feeling tired or having little energy	0	1	2	3
5. Poor appetite or overeating	0	1	2	3
6. Feeling bad about yourself—or that you are a failure or have let yourself or your family down	0	1	2	3
7. Trouble concentrating on things, such as reading the newspaper or watching television	0	1	2	3
8. Moving or speaking so slowly that other people could have noticed? Or the opposite—being so fidgety or restless that you have been moving around a lot more than usual	0	1	2	3
9. Thoughts that you would be better off dead or of hurting yourself in some way	0	1	2	3
If you checked off *any* problems, how *difficult* have these problems made it for you to do your work, take care of things at home, or get along with other people?	Not difficult at all	Somewhat difficult	Very difficult	Extremely difficult

Table 34-5. PHQ-9 and Proposed Treatment Actions

PHQ-9 Score	Depression Severity	Proposed Treatment Actions
1–4	None	None
5–9	Mild	Watchful waiting; repeat PHQ-9 at follow-up
10–14	Moderate	Treatment plan, considering counseling, follow-up, and/or pharmacotherapy
15–19	Moderately severe	Immediate initiation of pharmacotherapy and/or psychotherapy
20–27	Severe	Immediate initiation of pharmacotherapy and, if severe impairment or poor response to therapy, expedited referral to a mental health specialist for psychotherapy and/or collaborative management

setting include thyroid-stimulating hormone, comprehensive metabolic panel, complete blood count, and free and total testosterone levels, although this list is by no means inclusive.

Treatment

Of primary importance is the recognition when a patient may need referral to a psychiatric specialist, or urgent psychiatric evaluation including possible hospitalization. These situations include suicidal or homicidal ideation, with or without intent and a plan. If initial depression screening indicates the presence of a depressive episode, pharmacologic and behavioral therapies may be recommended. Initial treatment choices should be selected based on the clinical context of the patient's depressive disorder (Table 34-6). First-line therapy is often an adequate trial of a SSRI. Combination therapy with pharmacologic therapy and psychotherapy, specifically CBT, can be a more effective method of treating depression. In CBT, patients learn and practice techniques, including role playing, imagery, problem-solving skills, and guided discovery, with the goal of identifying and modifying dysfunctional beliefs.

Close follow-up after initiation of medical therapy is essential. Initial follow-up within 2 weeks can be helpful to evaluate acceptance of the medication, reinforce educational messages, reassess suicidality, and address adverse events. Evidence of response to antidepressant medication is a 50% reduction in PHQ-9

Table 34-6. Medications for Treatment of Depression

Drug Class	Benefits	Side Effects	Notes
Selective serotonin reuptake inhibitor (SSRI) (citalopram, escitalopram, fluoxetine, fluvoxamine, paroxetine, sertraline)	Effective, well tolerated	Nausea, diarrhea, decreased appetite, anxiety, nervousness, insomnia, somnolence, sweating, impaired sexual function	Contraindicated with MAOIs Use with caution when also taking hepatically metabolized drugs If mental status changes occur while on SSRI, check electrolytes to rule out syndrome of inappropriate antidiuretic hormone (SIADH)
Serotonin and selective norepinephrine reuptake inhibitor (SNRI) (venlafaxine, duloxetine, mirtazapine)	Venlafaxine: effective, well tolerated Mirtazapine may be effective when other agents have not been	Venlafaxine: nausea, dry mouth, anorexia, constipation, dizziness, somnolence, insomnia, nervousness, sweating, abnormalities of sexual function, cardiovascular effects Mirtazapine: weight gain, somnolence, dizziness, increased cholesterol, elevated liver transaminases, orthostatic hypotension, agranulocytosis	Venlafaxine: contraindicated with MAOIs Monitor blood pressure Taper slowly due to potential for withdrawal syndrome Duloxetine: may be hepatotoxic with alcohol Mirtazapine: use caution with renal impairment; contraindicated with MAOIs; avoid benzodiazepines. Check fasting glucose and lipids

(continued)

Table 34-6. Medications for Treatment of Depression (*Continued*)

Drug Class	Benefits	Side Effects	Notes
Dopamine reuptake inhibitor (buproprion)	Less weight gain, fewer adverse effects on sexual functioning, approved for smoking cessation	Lowers seizure threshold, may exacerbate eating disorders, anorexia, rash, sweating, tinnitus, tremor, abdominal pain, agitation, anxiety, dizziness, insomnia, myalgia, nausea, palpitations, pharyngitis, urinary frequency	Contraindicated when there is a personal or family history of seizures, or with MAOIs, or with a history of bulimia or anorexia Use with caution with other drugs that may lower seizure threshold and in patients with impaired hepatic function
5-HT$_2$ receptor antagonist (trazodone)	May be used for insomnia Fewer adverse effect on sexual functioning; lower incidence of postural hypotension than TCAs, but higher than SSRIs	Somnolence, dry mouth, nausea, dizziness, constipation, asthenia, light-headedness, blurred vision, confusion, abnormal vision, priapism	Contraindicated with certain medications (carbamazepine, trazolam, alprazolam) Use with caution in cardiovascular, cerebrovascular, and seizure disorders Related medication nefazodone was removed from the market due to severe hepatotoxicity

(*continued*)

Medication		Side effects	Comments
Tricyclic antidepressant (TCA) (nortriptyline, amitriptyline, doxepin, desipramine, imipramine, clomipramine)	Desipramine least sedating. Amitriptyline and doxepin may be taken at bedtime to aid with sleep. Desipramine may be stimulating	Dry mouth, dizziness, nervousness, constipation, nausea, sedation, anticholinergic and orthostatic hypotension, may cause tardive dyskinesia and the neuroleptic malignant syndrome	Contraindicated with MAOIs, or in patients with prolonged QT interval or on drugs that may prolong QT interval. Use with caution in patients with cardiovascular disease and arrhythmia, patients prone to urinary retention and on thyroid medications. May precipitate attacks in narrow-angle glaucoma. Monitor EKG and orthostatic blood pressure changes
Monoamine oxidase inhibitor (MAOI) (phenelzine, isocarboxazid, tranylcypromine)	May be effective when other agents have not been. May be more effective in patients with atypical depression (hypersomnolence, hyperphagia, and rejection sensitivity)	Dizziness, headache, drowsiness, insomnia, hypersomnia, fatigue, weakness, tremors, twitching, myoclonic movements, hyperreflexia, constipation, dry mouth, gastrointestinal disturbances, elevated liver transaminases, weight gain, postural hypotension, edema, sexual disturbances	Infrequently used in primary care. Contraindicated when there is a history of cerebrovascular and cardiovascular disease, pheochromocytoma, liver disease; many drug interactions. Increases risk for hypertensive crisis and serotonin syndrome (hypertension, hyperthermia, tachycardia, death). Extensive patient education is required

(continued)

Table 34-6. Medications for Treatment of Depression (*Continued*)

Drug Class	Benefits	Side Effects	Notes
5HT$_{A1}$ receptor partial antagonist (buspirone)	May be used in second- and third-line treatment to augment antidepressant therapy in treatment-resistant depression	Insomnia, dizziness, headache, light-headedness, nausea, gastrointestinal side effects	Use with caution when also taking hepatically metabolized drugs
Atypical antipsychotics (olanzapine, aripiprazole, quetiapine)	May be used in third-line treatment to augment antidepressant therapy in treatment-resistant depression. Specialty referral is likely needed	Olanzapine is most likely to have side effects of weight gain, insulin resistance, elevated cholesterol, sedation	Check fasting glucose and lipids at baseline and annually. Check EKG in patients >40 years old or with cardiac risk factors

score by 6 weeks. Continued follow-up for a minimum of 6 to 9 months on drug therapy should be considered. Patient counseling regarding expectations of treatment response must be clear in order to optimize treatment adherence.

Treatment-resistant depression can occur in up to 40% of patients, but treatment resistance or nonresponse should be differentiated from inadequate treatment or pseudoresistance. First, adherence to the recommended treatment regimen should be assessed, as patients with depression are at risk for nonadherence to all medications, including antidepressants. Nonadherence to antidepressant medication occurs in approximately 28% of patients after 1 month and 44% after 3 months. Specific patient educational messages that promote adherence include the following 5 messages:

1. Take the medication daily.
2. Antidepressants must be taken for 2 to 4 weeks for a noticeable effect.
3. Continue taking the medicine even if feeling better.
4. Do not stop taking the antidepressant without checking with the physician.
5. Provide specific instructions regarding what to do to resolve questions regarding antidepressants.

Second, an adequate trial is considered: 8 weeks of treatment with an optimal dose of an antidepressant medication. Subsequent management may include switching to an alternative medication of the same class (eg, switch to a different SSRI) or to a different class of medication (eg, selective norepinephrine reuptake inhibitor [SNRI], or buproprion), combining with another medication (eg, buproprion), or augmenting with another class of medication (eg, buspirone or atypical antipsychotics) or with psychotherapy.

Complementary and alternative medicines have also been considered in the treatment of mild depression. Dietary supplements including omega-3 fatty acids, St. John's wort, and valerian are alternative treatments for depression. Complementary health practices that can be used in the treatment of depression include massage, yoga, and relaxation techniques. It is important to recognize that complementary medicines and practices are not regulated or well studied, and supplements can potentially interact with numerous prescription medicines. Careful discussion of the benefits and risks of each of these therapies is essential to guide an informed decision regarding their use.

TIPS TO REMEMBER

- Depression is common in the general population and incurs significant direct and indirect health care costs in the United States.
- Depression is frequently underdiagnosed and undertreated. Screening for depressive symptoms using evidence-based tools should be incorporated into routine clinical practice. Close follow-up and monitoring is necessary to ensure adherence to therapy and adequate treatment response.

COMPREHENSION QUESTIONS

1. A 55-year-old woman with diabetes, a history of depression, and a history of sexual abuse in childhood presents after being lost to follow-up when her primary care provider moved. She states that she has not taken any medications for over 1 year. What is the next best step in evaluation in the office?

    A. Check hemoglobin A1c to evaluate diabetes control.

    B. Start an antidiabetic medication.

    C. Start an antidepressant medication.

    D. Both B and C.

    E. Screen for depression to guide further management.

2. A 32-year-old man with a history of alcoholism and depression sees you for a 4-week follow-up after starting low-dose sertraline for symptoms meeting criteria for an episode of MDD, without suicidal thoughts or ideation. His PHQ-9 score was 21 at his initial office visit. His current PHQ-9 score is 8, and he reports that he is taking his antidepressant daily and that his energy levels have improved slightly. What is the next best step in management?

    A. No change in medication dose, and recommend follow-up in 4 weeks.

    B. Increase medication dose, and recommend follow-up in 4 weeks.

    C. Change medication because sertraline was ineffective, and recommend follow-up in 4 weeks.

    D. Refer to a psychiatrist because he has treatment-resistant depression.

3. A 25-year-old female presents to the emergency department via ambulance after she was found unconscious on her bedroom floor by her roommate. Paramedics report that when she was found, there were empty, unlabeled prescription bottles scattered on the bedroom floor. She was intubated for airway protection and treated in the ambulance with the usual medications in a suspected case of poisoning with an unknown substance, and intravenous fluids were started. She is hypotensive and tachycardic, and an EKG shows a QTc interval of 520 milliseconds. What is 1 of the likely substances that she overdosed on based on the limited information available so far?

    A. Benzodiazepine

    B. Beta-blocker

    C. Acetaminophen

    D. Tricyclic antidepressant

    E. SSRI

Answers

1. **E.** The next best step in evaluation is to use a depression screening questionnaire, such as PHQ-9 or BDI, to establish a baseline of severity of depressive

symptoms and their impact on overall function. Adequate treatment of depression will be essential to satisfactory management of diabetes, a common comorbid condition and risk factor for depression.

2. **B.** The next best step in management is to optimize the dose of sertraline for treatment response. He is demonstrating some improvement in symptoms based on self-reported symptoms and reassessment with the PHQ-9 scale; however, his response can be improved. Increasing sertraline and reevaluating with the PHQ-9 in 4 weeks is the most reasonable option. Not changing the dose is not appropriate because his treatment response is not optimal. Changing medication or referring for specialist evaluation and management of his depression suggests that he has treatment-resistant depression, which he does not have because he has not tried an adequate trial of first-line treatment as of this office visit.

3. **D.** In this case, it is unclear how many substances this patient may have overdosed upon, and a broad workup and management for suspected substances to guide therapeutic management and monitoring is necessary. Additionally, it is important to contact the local Poison Control Center (800-222-1222) for assistance in managing suspected poisonings. In this case, at a minimum, 1 of the suspected substances should include tricyclic antidepressants, and monitoring for cardiac arrhythmias should be instituted, because they may be preceded by a prolonged QTc.

SUGGESTED READINGS

American College of Physicians. ACP depression care guide: team-based practices for screening, diagnosis, and management in primary care settings. American College of Physicians. <http://depression.acponline.org/>; 2012. Accessed March 2012.

Fancher TL, Kravitz RL. In the clinic. Depression. *Ann Intern Med.* 2010;152:ITC51–ITC15 [quiz ITC5–ITC6].

Longo D, Fauci A, Kasper D, Hauser S, Jameson J, Loscalzo J. *Harrison's Principles of Internal Medicine.* 18th ed. New York: The McGraw-Hill Companies; 2012.

WEB SITES

Search for mental health centers supported by county public health departments and other local mental health resources:

National Association of State Mental Health Directors: http://www.nasmhpd.org/mental_health_resources.cfm#State.

National Suicide Hotlines USA: http://www.suicidepreventionlifeline.org (toll-free, available 24 hours a day, 7 days a week); 1-800-SUICIDE (784-2433); 1-800-273-TALK (8255); TTY: 1-800-799-4TTY (4889).

National Domestic Violence Hotline: http://www.thehotline.org; 1-800-799-SAFE (7233); TTY: 1–800–787–3224.

National Institutes of Mental Health: http://www.nimh.nih.gov/health/topics/depression/index.shtml.

A 55-year-old Woman is Diagnosed with Diabetes

Owaise M. Y. Mansuri, MD and Michael Jakoby, MD, MA

A 55-year-old African American female presents to clinic as a new patient. She has not seen a physician in many years and would like a general health checkup. The patient is not treated for any chronic health problems. However, her mother had type 2 diabetes, and she would like to be screened.

Physical examination is unremarkable except for weight of 180 lb (81.8 kg; height 165 cm, BMI 30.3 kg/m²). The patient has multiple risk factors for type 2 diabetes including age, ethnicity, and family history that justify screening. Since the patient is not fasting, hemoglobin A1c (HbA1c) is measured and found to be elevated at 6.8%. Morning fasting plasma glucose is 145 mg/dL.

The patient returns to the office to discuss management of her newly diagnosed type 2 diabetes. She is started on metformin and titrated to 1000 mg twice daily without side effects. She also modifies her diet and starts an exercise program. Three months later, capillary blood glucose measurements are consistently below 130 mg/dL, and HbA1c improves to 6.0%. Four years later, HbA1c increases steadily to 7.5% despite compliance with diet, exercise, and metformin. Dilated fundoscopy and foot examination are unremarkable, and urine albumin/Cr ratio remains below 30 mg/g.

Initially, HbA1c improves with the addition of glimepiride to metformin. Exenatide is then started 18 months later due to worsening glycemic control. Two years later, the patient returns to discuss treatment options. Despite taking maximal effective doses of metformin (1000 mg BID), glimepiride (8 mg QD), and exenatide (10 µg BID), HbA1c is 8.5%. Fasting glucose measurements fall mostly in the range of 140 to 180 mg/dL, and glucose measurements during the day increase steadily and are often more than 200 mg/dL.

1. **Who should be screened for type 2 diabetes mellitus?**

2. **How is type 2 diabetes initially managed?**

3. **What regular screening is necessary for type 2 diabetes patients?**

4. **What additional therapies can be added if metformin monotherapy is ineffective?**

5. **What is the next step in management for patients with progressively worsening glycemic control despite multiple oral medications or glucagon-like peptide-1 (GLP-1) analog therapy?**

Table 35-1. Risk Factors for Type 2 Diabetes Mellitus

Physical inactivity

First-degree relative with diabetes

High-risk ethnicity (African American, Latino, Native American, Asian American, Pacific Islander)

Women with history of gestational diabetes or baby weighing >9 lb

Hypertension (treated or screening blood pressure ≥140/90 mm Hg)

HDL <35 mg/dL or triglycerides >250 mg/dL

Polycystic ovary syndrome (PCOS)

Cardiovascular disease

Pre–diabetes mellitus

Conditions associated with insulin resistance (obesity, acanthosis nigricans)

Answers

1. All adults with BMI ≥25 kg/m^2 and 1 or more risk factors summarized in Table 35-1 should be screened annually. Individuals aged 45 years or older without risk factors should be screened every 3 years.

2. Therapeutic lifestyle change (TLC), which consists of diet and aerobic exercise, and metformin are the initial interventions for type 2 diabetes.

3. Complete physical examination including dilated fundoscopy and foot examination with monofilament evaluation should be performed at least annually. HbA1c should be checked at 3- to 6-month intervals depending on glycemic control. Fasting lipid panels and urine albumin/Cr ratio should also be checked at least yearly.

4. Sulfonylureas, thiazolidinediones (TZDs), dipeptidyl peptidase-IV (DPP-IV) inhibitors, GLP-1 analogs, and insulin are all potential add-on therapies to metformin (see Appendix 1).

5. Insulin therapy is required when combinations of alternative therapies fail to keep HbA1c <7%. Basal insulin or the combination of basal and mealtime insulin may be required.

CASE REVIEW AND DIAGNOSIS

Type 2 diabetes mellitus is caused by impaired insulin signaling in key organ systems such as skeletal muscle, liver, and adipose tissue and relative insulinopenia. Nearly 20 million Americans have been diagnosed with diabetes mellitus, with approximately 95% of patients qualifying for a diagnosis of type 2 diabetes. It is estimated that 7 million Americans have undiagnosed type 2 diabetes.

All adult patients with BMI ≥25 kg/m^2 and 1 or more risk factors (Table 35-1) should be screened for type 2 diabetes. Patients older than 45 years should be screened every 3 years regardless of risk.

The American Diabetes Association (ADA) recently accepted HbA1c ≥6.5% as diagnostic of type 2 diabetes. Other screening tests include fasting plasma glucose ≥126 mg/dL (minimum 8-hour fast), 2-hour plasma glucose ≥200 mg/dL during a 75 g oral glucose tolerance test, and random plasma glucose ≥200 mg/dL with symptoms of hyperglycemia such as polyuria and polydipsia. Unless there is unequivocal hyperglycemia, a positive test should be confirmed by repeat testing.

Before starting treatment, patients with newly diagnosed diabetes mellitus should undergo screening for potential complications of hyperglycemia. For example, some degree of retinopathy was present in over 10% of patients newly diagnosed with type 2 diabetes in the Diabetes Prevention Program.

Treatment

Diabetes management requires a team including physicians, nurse diabetes educators, and dietitians. Lifestyle modification (healthy diet, regular aerobic exercise) and metformin are recommended as initial therapy for most patients in guidelines published by the ADA and American College of Endocrinology and a recent update published by ADA and the European Association for the Study of Diabetes. However, patients with HbA1c >7.5% at diagnosis may require initial treatment with metformin and a second oral medication or even insulin, depending on the degree of hyperglycemia. Dietitians can help patients choose appropriate foods, particularly when they face multiple restrictions such as low-sodium diet for hypertension and low-fat diet for dyslipidemia. The Centers for Disease Control recommends 150 minutes of exercise per week, with a target heart rate of 70% of maximum for age.

Metformin is a biguanide class drug that lowers glucose primarily by decreasing hepatic glucose output. Key characteristics are summarized in Appendix 1. Metformin is highly potent at reducing plasma glucose but does not cause hypoglycemia or weight gain. Side effects are typically gastrointestinal and include abdominal discomfort, nausea, bloating and cramping, and diarrhea. Metformin is contraindicated in patients with renal impairment due to risk of lactic acidemia. The drug should not be prescribed if serum creatinine exceeds 1.4 mg/dL in women or 1.5 mg/dL in men. It is typically started at 500 mg twice daily and then advanced in 500 mg weekly increments to the maximally effective dose of 1000 mg twice daily. As monotherapy, metformin lowers HbA1c by 1% to 2%.

Patients with diabetes are at risk for both microvascular (retinopathy, nephropathy, and neuropathy) and macrovascular (coronary artery disease, cerebrovascular disease, and peripheral artery disease) complications. A complete physical examination and dilated fundoscopic evaluation should be performed at least once a year. A foot examination that includes monofilament testing and evaluation of vibratory sensation and proprioception should be performed at routine office visits. Blood pressure should be measured at each visit and treated to goal <130/80 mm Hg. Patients with diabetes and hypertension should be managed with a regimen that includes either an angiotensin-converting enzyme inhibitor (ACE inhibitor) or an angiotensin receptor blocker (ARB).

HbA1c is a marker of glycemic control over 2 to 3 months and strongly correlated with risk of microvascular complications. It should be checked every 3 months in patients starting or changing glucose-lowering therapy or who have not achieved HbA1c <7%. HbA1c may be checked twice yearly when stable glycemic control is achieved. Target HbA1c for most patients is ≤7.0%, although some patients may be able to achieve HbA1c ≤6.5% without significant risk of hypoglycemia. For patients with frequent hypoglycemia, hypoglycemia unawareness, or limited life expectancy, higher HbA1c (eg, ≤8.0%) is acceptable.

Fasting lipid profile (total cholesterol, HDL cholesterol, LDL cholesterol, and triglycerides) should be checked at least once yearly. Target LDL is <100 mg/dL for most patients, although patients with cardiovascular disease have a target of <70 mg/dL. Other lipid targets are HDL >40 mg/dL in men and >50 mg/dL in women, and triglycerides <150 mg/dL. HMG CoA reductase inhibitor ("statin") therapy is indicated in all diabetes patients with cardiovascular disease or who are over age 40 years and should be considered in patients under age 40 with baseline LDL cholesterol over 100 mg/dL.

Patients should be screened annually for proteinuria by measurement of urine albumin to creatinine ratio on a spot urine sample. A ratio of 30 to 300 mg/g is considered microalbuminuria, and ratio >300 mg/g indicates overt proteinuria. Several factors can lead to spurious elevation of the ratio such as vigorous exercise or urinary tract infection. An abnormal result should be confirmed on at least 2 additional urine samples obtained within 3 to 6 months of the initial abnormal test.

Type 2 diabetes is a slowly progressive disease, primarily due to a steady decline in beta-cell function but also an increase in insulin resistance. In the United Kingdom Prospective Diabetes Study (UKPDS), fewer than half of patients maintained HbA1c <7% in their original treatment arms 3 years after randomization. Patients should be educated regarding the natural history of type 2 diabetes and advised that changes in treatment are likely to be required to maintain appropriate glycemic control. Depending on the decrement in glycemic control, combinations of oral medications, oral medications and GLP-1 analogs, oral medications and insulin, or insulin monotherapy may be required to improve blood glucose control. Appendix 1 contains a complete list of glucose-lowering therapies, and specific insulin preparations are presented in Appendix 2.

Sulfonylureas are the oldest class of oral diabetes medications. They act by binding to the sulfonylurea receptor (SUR-1), inhibiting potassium efflux, and increasing transmembrane potential. Voltage-gated calcium channels are then activated, and insulin release is increased for any given plasma glucose level.

Glipizide, glimepiride, and glyburide are the most commonly prescribed sulfonyl-ureas. Anticipated improvement in HbA1c is 1% to 2%, particularly when sulfonylureas are used as initial therapy. Weight gain and hypoglycemia are the 2 most common side effects of treatment with sulfonylureas.

Nateglinide and repaglinide are collectively called "glinides" and bind to the sulfonylurea receptor at sites distinct from sulfonylurea class drugs. They are also insulin secretagogues but have a shorter duration of activity than sulfonylureas and are dosed before meals. Blood glucose-lowering potency is somewhat lower than the sulfonylureas. Weight gain and hypoglycemia are potential side effects.

DPP-IV inhibitors are a new class of insulin secretagogue. GLP-1 is an incretin class hormone that augments prandial insulin release, and these drugs increase GLP-1 levels by inhibiting DPP-IV, the enzyme that inactivates GLP-1. Sitagliptin, saxagliptin, and linagliptin are the currently available DPP-IV inhibitors. HbA1c improves by 0.5% to 1.0% when DPP-IV inhibitors are used as monotherapy. DPP-IV inhibitors are generally well tolerated, although long-term safety remains to be established. They do not cause weight gain or hypoglycemia. In a recent meta-analysis, there were modest increases in risk of nasopharyngitis, urinary tract infection, and headache associated with DDP-IV inhibitors.

TZDs are agonists of peroxisome proliferator–activated receptor gamma (PPAR-γ) that improve hyperglycemia primarily by improving the insulin sensitivity of skeletal muscle. Troglitazone has been withdrawn from the market due to hepatotoxicity, and rosiglitazone was withdrawn from retail pharmacies and restricted to a special access program due to increased risk of cardiovascular events such as myocardial infarction. Pioglitazone is the remaining TZD in widespread clinical use. Anticipated improvement in HbA1c is 0.5% to 1.5%, including when pioglitazone is used as a second-line agent. Weight gain and edema are the most common untoward effects of therapy, and TZDs are contraindicated when patients are predisposed to fluid retention (eg, heart failure, hepatic insufficiency).

Acarbose and miglitol are alpha-glucosidase inhibitors. Alpha-glucosidases are enzymes in the small intestines that break down complex polysaccharides into monosaccharides. These drugs delay glucose absorption to the distal small bowel and better match glucose absorption with prandial insulin release. Improvement in HbA1c is modest (approximately 0.5%), and the drugs are often poorly tolerated due to gastrointestinal side effects such as diarrhea, abdominal pain, and flatulence.

GLP-1 analogs, exenatide and liraglutide, are a relatively new class of antidiabetic therapy. GLP-1 is a hormone secreted by L-cells in the ileum in response to carbohydrate intake. Prandial insulin is consequently increased in a glucose-dependent manner. GLP-1 also delays gastric emptying, inhibits glucagon release, and acts on satiety centers in the hypothalamus to reduce food intake. It is quickly degraded by the enzyme DPP-IV, making it difficult to utilize as a diabetes therapy. However, GLP-1 analogs exenatide and liraglutide have been developed that are resistant to degradation by DPP-IV and have significantly longer half-lives. Both agents are administered subcutaneously. Exenatide branded as Byetta™ is dosed twice daily, and a new preparation of exenatide branded as Bydureon™ is administered once weekly. Liraglutide is dosed once daily. Both medications are approved as add-on therapies for patients failing to control hyperglycemia adequately with oral medications and lifestyle changes. Anticipated improvement in HbA1c is 1.0% to 1.5%. Weight loss is also common with both agents, particularly when added to treatment with metformin. Most patients experience mild nausea and abdominal discomfort at start of therapy that resolves spontaneously, although up to 10% of patients may not be able to tolerate therapy with a GLP-1 analog due to persistent gastrointestinal side effects. There is concern for risk of acute pancreatitis in GLP-1 analog–treated patients, although rates from postmarketing surveillance are similar to the background rate for all patients with diabetes. Liraglutide was associated with benign and malignant C-cell tumors in rodents, and it is contraindicated in patients with a personal or family history of medullary thyroid cancer or multiple endocrine neoplasia 2A or 2B.

Amylin is a peptide cosecreted with insulin. It appears to improve glucose control by slowing gastric emptying, decreasing postprandial glucagon, and reducing food intake. Pramlintide is a synthetic amylin analog and is subcutaneously dosed prior to meals. The drug is approved for patients with type 1 or type 2 diabetes who are taking mealtime insulin. Patients typically experience a 0.5% to 1% improvement in HbA1c and some degree of weight loss (1–2 kg). Nausea is the most common side effect. Patients may need to reduce mealtime insulin doses to avoid hypoglycemia when initiating treatment with pramlintide.

Insulin is the most effective therapy for controlling hyperglycemia and always an option for patients who are unable to achieve adequate glycemic control with lifestyle changes and oral medications. Odds of requiring insulin for successful management increase substantially with increasing duration of type 2 diabetes. American Association of Clinical Endocrinologists (AACE) guidelines recommend starting insulin for patients with HbA1c 7.6% to 9.0% 2 to 3 months after adding a second oral agent or GLP-1 analog if glucose control fails to improve and immediately for patients with HbA1c >9.0%. Appendix 2 contains a complete list of currently available insulins and their pharmacokinetics. Many patients may achieve good glycemic control by adding a basal insulin (NPH, glargine, detemir) to oral medications and adjusting the dose in a stepwise manner to achieve morning fasting glucose 80 to 110 mg/dL. Hypoglycemia and weight gain are the most common adverse effects of insulin therapy.

Declining insulin secretory reserve is an important part of the natural history of type 2 diabetes, and most patients will require therapy with insulin, often both prandial and basal preparations, to achieve and maintain desirable glycemic control. Unfortunately, insulin therapy may be delayed for several years due to patient or health care provider reluctance despite suboptimal glycemic control. In a retrospective study conducted in the United Kingdom, 25% of patients delayed initiating insulin for 18 months and 50% of patients delayed starting insulin for almost 5 years despite HbA1c ≥8% and treatment with multiple oral medications.

Patients should be prepared for the possibility that insulin will be required for optimal glycemic control early in the course of treatment. The patient in this vignette requires both prandial and basal insulin to restore good blood glucose control. The most common approaches are to use premix insulin with fixed ratios of NPH insulin and prandial insulin (eg, NovoLog 70/30 mix, Humalog 75/25) or basal/bolus insulin combining a rapid-acting insulin analog (lispro, aspart, glulisine) dosed before meals with a basal insulin analog (glargine or detemir) dosed once daily.

Insulin doses are adjusted to achieve premeal and bedtime blood glucose measurements generally in the range of 90 to 130 mg/dL. When prandial insulin is prescribed, insulin secretagogues such as glimepiride and GLP-1 analogs are typically stopped. Insulin may be combined with metformin or pioglitazone as these oral agents may reduce total daily insulin requirements. Because patients with type 2 diabetes are insulin resistant, total daily insulin doses of 1 U/kg or higher are not uncommon.

TIPS TO REMEMBER

- Type 2 diabetes mellitus is caused by relative insulinopenia in the setting of significant insulin resistance.

- Diagnostic criteria for type 2 diabetes include plasma glucose ≥126 mg/dL after an 8-hour fast, 2-hour glucose ≥200 mg/dL on a 75 g oral glucose tolerance test, random glucose ≥200 mg/dL with symptoms of hyperglycemia such as polyuria or polydipsia, and HbA1c ≥6.5%.

- Initial therapy for most patients includes lifestyle modification (diet and exercise) and metformin; multiple therapies may be required if HbA1c is >7.5% at initial presentation, and insulin is recommended if HbA1c is >9.0%.

- Type 2 diabetes is a progressive disease with loss of beta-cell function over time resulting in need for multiple oral medications, GLP-1 analog therapy, or insulin to maintain satisfactory glycemic control.

- The general goal of glycemic therapy is to maintain HbA1c <7%, although some patients can be managed more aggressively if hypoglycemia risk is low and other patients may be more safely managed to higher HbA1c targets in the setting of hypoglycemia unawareness or limited life expectancy.

Appendix 1. Glucose-Lowering Therapies

Therapy	Expected Decrease in HbA1c With Monotherapy (%)	Advantages	Disadvantages
Metformin	1.0–2.0	Weight neutral	GI side effects, contraindicated with renal insufficiency
Insulin	1.5–3.5	No dose limit, rapidly effective, improved lipid profile	One to 4 injections daily, monitoring, weight gain, hypoglycemia, analogs are expensive
Sulfonylureas	1.0–2.0	Rapidly effective	Weight gain, hypoglycemia
TZDs	0.5–1.4	Improved lipid profile	Fluid retention, CHF, weight gain, bone fractures, bladder cancer
GLP-1 agonist	0.5–1.0	Weight loss	Injections, GI side effects, long-term safety not established
α-Glucosidase inhibitor	0.5–0.8	Weight neutral	Frequent GI side effects, frequent dosing
Glinide	0.5–1.5	Rapidly effective	Weight gain, frequent dosing, hypoglycemia
Pramlintide	0.5–1.0	Weight loss	Three injections daily, frequent GI side effects, long-term safety not established
DPP-IV inhibitors	0.5–0.8	Weight neutral	Long-term safety not established

Modified from Nathan DM, Buse JB, Davidson MB, et al. Medical management of hyperglycemia in type 2 diabetes: a consensus algorithm for the initiation and adjustment of therapy: a consensus algorithm for the initiation and adjustment of therapy. *Diabetes Care.* 2008;31:1–11.

Appendix 2. Insulin Preparations and Pharmacokinetics

Insulin	Onset	Peak	Duration
Prandial			
Lispro (Humalog)	5–15 min	30–90 min	5 h
Aspart (NovoLog)	5–15 min	30–90 min	5 h
Glulisine (aspart)	5–15 min	30–90 min	5 h
Regular	30–60 min	2–3 h	5–8 h
Basal			
NPH	2–4 h	4–10 h	10–16 h
Glargine (Lantus)	2–4 h	None	20–24 h
Detemir (Levemir)	2–4 h	None	16–22 h[a]

[a]Dose dependent.

SUGGESTED READINGS

American Diabetes Association. Standards of medical care in diabetes—2012. *Diabetes Care*. 2012; 35(suppl 1):S11–S63.

Amori RE, Lau J, Pittas AG. Efficacy and safety of incretin therapy in type 2 diabetes: systematic review and meta-analysis. *JAMA*. 2007;298:194–206.

Bailey CJ, Turner RC. Metformin. *N Engl J Med*. 1996;334:574–583.

Centers for Disease Control and Prevention. *National Diabetes Fact Sheet: National Estimates and General Information on Diabetes and Prediabetes in the United States, 2011*. Atlanta, GA: U.S. Department of Health and Human Services, Centers for Disease Control and Prevention; 2011.

Groop L. Sulfonylureas in NIDDM. *Diabetes Care*. 1992;15:737–747.

Hirsch IB, Bergenstal RM, Parkin CG, et al. A real-world approach to insulin therapy in primary care practice. *Clin Diabetes*. 2005;23:78–86.

Hollander PA, Levy P, Fineman MS, et al. Pramlintide as an adjunct to insulin therapy improves long-term glycemic and weight control in patients with type 2 diabetes: a 1-year randomized controlled trial. *Diabetes Care*. 2003;26(3):784–790.

Inzucchi SE, Berganstal RM, Buse JB, et al; American Diabetes Association (ADA); European Association for the Study of Diabetes (EASD). Management of hyperglycemia in type 2 diabetes: a patient-centered approach: position statement of the American Diabetes Association (ADA) and the European Association for the Study of Diabetes (EASD). *Diabetes Care*. 2012;35:1364–1379.

Knowler WC, Barrett-Connor E, Fowler SE, et al; Diabetes Prevention Program Research Group. Reduction in the incidence of type 2 diabetes with lifestyle intervention or metformin. *N Engl J Med*. 2002;346:393–403.

Malaisse WJ. Pharmacology of the meglitinide analogs: new treatment options for type 2 diabetes mellitus. *Treat Endocrinol*. 2003;2:401–414.

Monnier L, Colette C. Contributions of fasting and postprandial glucose to hemoglobin A1c. *Endocr Pract*. 2006;12(suppl):42–46.

Nathan DM, Buse JB, Davidson MB, et al. Medical management of hyperglycemia in type 2 diabetes: a consensus algorithm for the initiation and adjustment of therapy: a consensus algorithm for the initiation and adjustment of therapy. *Diabetes Care*. 2008;31:1–11.

Richter B, Bandeira-Echtler E, Bergerhoff K, et al. Dipeptidyl peptidase-4 (DPP-4) inhibitors for type 2 diabetes mellitus. *Cochrane Database Syst Rev*. 2008;(2):CD006739.

Rodbard HW, Jellinger PS, Davidson JA, et al. Statement by an American Association of Clinical Endocrinologists/American College of Endocrinology consensus panel on type 2 diabetes mellitus: an algorithm for glycemic control. *Endocr Pract*. 2009;15:540–559.

Rubino A, McQuay LJ, Gough SC, Kvasz M, Tennis P. Delayed initiation of subcutaneous insulin therapy after failure of oral glucose-lowering agents in patients with type 2 diabetes: a population-based analysis in the UK. *Diabet Med*. 2007;24:1412–1418.

Shyangdan DS, Royle P, Clar C, Sharma P, Waugh N, Snaith A. Glucagon-like peptide analogues for type 2 diabetes mellitus. *Cochrane Database Syst Rev*. 2011;(10):CD006423.

The International Expert Committee. International Expert Committee report on the role of the A1C assay in the diagnosis of diabetes. *Diabetes Care*. 2009;32:1327–1334.

Turner RC, Cull CA, Frighi V, Holman RR. Glycemic control with diet, sulfonylurea, metformin, or insulin in patients with type 2 diabetes mellitus: progressive requirement for multiple therapies (UKPDS 49). UK Prospective Diabetes Study (UKPDS) Group. *JAMA*. 1999;281:2005–2012.

UKPDS Study Group (UKPDS 16). Overview of six years' therapy of type 2 diabetes—a progressive disease. *Diabetes*. 1995;44:1249–1258.

US Department of Health and Human Services. *2008 Physical Activity Guidelines for Americans*. Hyattsville, MD: US Department of Health and Human Services. www.health.gov/PAGuidelines/guidelines/default.aspx; 2008.

Van de Laar FA, Lucassen PL, Akkermans RP, et al. Alpha-glucosidase inhibitors for type 2 diabetes mellitus. *Cochrane Database Syst Rev*. 2005;(2):CD003639.

Weyer C, Bogardus C, Mott DM, Pratley RE. The natural history of insulin secretory dysfunction and insulin resistance in the pathogenesis of type 2 diabetes mellitus. *J Clin Invest*. 1999;104:787–794.

Yki-Jarvinen H. Drug therapy: thiazolidinediones. *N Engl J Med*. 2004;351:1106.

A 69-year-old Man Diagnosed With Metastatic Non-small Cell Lung Cancer

Vajeeha Tabassum, MD, FACP

John is a 69-year-old man married to Mary, 68, for 43 years. They have just moved to live close to their daughter and have always had active lifestyles. They invested their retirement funds in a condominium near a golf course. John was doing well at home until about 2 months ago when he noticed shortness of breath on exertion. Mary had suffered a fall around the same time with a fracture of her hip requiring hospitalization. John as well as his family considered John's shortness of breath to be due to ongoing stress and anxiety.

One week ago John fell on the left side of his chest, and since then his pain and shortness of breath have continued to increase and are persistent with rest. He went to the ER and was diagnosed with pulmonary emboli with a left upper lobe infiltrate with bilateral hilar and mediastinal lymphadenopathy. John was admitted for further evaluation. John, Mary, and their daughter are very optimistic about the workup and reassure themselves that everything will be fine. John was ultimately diagnosed with metastatic non-small cell lung cancer. He was very frightened and angry when he was told about the biopsy results. His family wanted to get all possible treatments done. They want to have a meeting with the oncologist to discuss the possible treatment options and plan for the future.

1. **Assuming that the chances of complete remission are very small, what is the most appropriate course of action?**

Answer

1. After establishing a trusting relationship, the physician should assess the patient's understanding of the illness and then gently share the information that will bring the patient's understanding closer to medical reality. Offering false reassurance is unkind and unethical. Additionally, symptom control, emotional support, and a caring presence are necessary and appropriate.

   If the patient is terminally ill but not yet psychologically ready to hear bad news, a palliative care consult will help to define the goals of care and services available.

PALLIATIVE CARE

The palliative model of care recognizes the importance of symptom control, relief of suffering, and support for the best quality of life for patients and their families, regardless of the stage of illness or need for other therapies. Table 36-1 compares the characteristics of curative and palliative care.

Table 36-1. Characteristics of Curative Versus Palliative Care Models

Curative Model	Palliative Model
The primary goal is cure	The primary goal is relief of suffering
The objective of analysis is the disease process	The objective of analysis is the patient and the family
Symptoms are treated primarily as clues to the diagnosis	Distressing symptoms are treated as entities in themselves
Primary value is placed on measurable date, for example, lab tests	Both measurable and subjective dates are valued
This model tends to devalue information that is subjective, immeasurable, or unverifiable	This model values the patient's experience of an illness
	Therapy is medically indicated if it controls symptoms and relieves suffering
Therapy is medically indicated if it eradicates or slows progression of disease	The patient is viewed as a complex being comprising physical, emotional, social, and spiritual dimensions
The patient's body is differentiated from the patient's mind	Enabling a patient to live fully and comfortably until he or she dies is a success
Death is the ultimate failure	

CASE REVIEW

John and Mary decide to think about the options discussed and schedule an office visit. During the office visit, in which the daughter accompanies John and Mary, John mentions that he is ready to fight the cancer and has decided to undergo chemotherapy. His decision is applauded by his family. John also mentions that he has an upcoming follow-up appointment with the oncologist in 3 days. The physician acknowledges the difficulty of their situation, and mentions that most people in John and Mary's case feel frightened and anxious about the best course of action. The physician asks about their main concerns and stops talking for a long enough time for them to consider the question.

John mentions he is most bothered by his lack of appetite and fatigue. He wants to seek treatment immediately and get back to his golfing. Mary mentions that the oncologist also discussed the hospice/palliative care options; however, John is interested in treatment. They mention that the oncologist gave them a hospice brochure to look at and scheduled a follow-up appointment in 2 weeks. Mary stated that John makes comments such as "I'm going to take any treatment; I am young and can fight this cancer." The physician notes tears in Mary's eyes and asks Mary, "I see tears in your eyes. Can you tell me something about what is going on in your mind?" Mary cries quietly for some time and states that she was with her father who also died of cancer and that he suffered terribly during the process. It was very hard to cope with it. Mary also mentions that she had some of her friends who have used hospice care and they have good things to say about it. She asks John to consider hospice for her sake. John becomes angry and states that he plans to live for a long time.

Two days later John develops fever and shortness of breath and is taken to the emergency room, where he is told that he has multiple blood clots in his lungs.

Treatment

1. What is the most appropriate course of action?

Answer

1. Meeting with John and Mary to discuss their concerns and talk about the change in John's condition will provide John with another opportunity to come to terms with his diagnosis and prognosis. Involving the palliative care team will provide John and his family with an ability to discuss specific concerns.

Palliative interventions are primarily designed to provide comfort, not cure disease or extend life. Because palliative interventions control distressing symptoms and provide psychological and spiritual support, they may prolong a patient's life and improve its quality.

The essential components of hospice and palliative care include:

- Alleviating the suffering of patients and families by focusing on all aspects of total pain: physical, emotional, spiritual, and social
- Improving the patient's quality of life
- Helping patients and families make the transition from health to illness to death to bereavement
- Participating in the patient's and family's search for meaning
- Helping patients achieve the developmental goals and dreams or aspirations of the dying according to their specific needs and wishes

Table 36-2 lists a set of core principles for end-of-life care that were published by the Milbank Report in December 1999, which are embraced by a substantial number of medical societies and the Joint Commission on the Accreditation of Healthcare Organizations.

The case of the 69-year-old man continues: John is started on a heparin drip, and after 3 days he feels slightly better and wishes to talk with his oncologist. The oncologist informs John that chemotherapy is not the best choice in his case now. He suggests that John meet with the hospice team to discuss services that could help him remain at home and provide assistance for Mary. The oncologist

Table 36-2. Core Principles of End-of-life Care

Respect the dignity of both the patient and caregivers
Be sensitive to and respectful of the patient's and family's wishes
Use the most appropriate measures that are consistent with patient choices
Encompass alleviation of pain and other physical symptoms
Assess and manage psychological, social, and spiritual or religious problems
Offer continuity (eg, the patient should be able to receive continued care by primary care provider or specialist providers, if so desired)
Provide access to any therapy that may realistically be expected to improve the patient's quality of life, including alternative or nontraditional treatments
Provide access to palliative and hospice care
Respect the right to refuse treatment
Respect the physician's professional responsibility to discontinue some treatments when appropriate, with consideration for both patient and family preferences
Promote clinical and evidence-based research on providing care at the end of life

promises that he will be available to discuss any concerns, however recommends that John follow up with his primary care and hospice program. John then asks about the charges for hospice care.

The physician reassures John that, in his case, hospice services are covered in full by Medicare and discusses the core principles of end-of-life care with John and his family. John agrees to talk with the hospice representative. The physician calls the hospice office and arranges for a referral. Mary cries quietly, however thanks the physician for supporting them.

The hospice representative arrives, asks about John and Mary's situation, describes the hospice services that are offered, and tailors it to their needs. She emphasizes the program focuses on keeping patients at home and as independent as possible, controlling pain and other symptom management so patients can remain as active as possible. She also discusses available help for spouses. John mentions that he wants his primary care doctor to act as the attending physician.

John is discharged from the hospital to hospice home care. He begins to acknowledge his situation gradually and begins completing a number of tasks, including financial planning and saying goodbye to his family and friends. John remains comfortable and alert for the next 3 weeks and dies peacefully at home amidst family and friends. Mary is very grateful to the physicians involved and the hospice program.

In hospice and palliative care settings, treatment decisions are linked to the primary task of the physician, which is helping patients choose the best interventions for specific situations and then providing the best possible care.

Table 36-3 describes some of the roles that physicians who practice hospice and palliative care play.

Table 36-3. Role of Physicians Practicing Hospice and Palliative Medicine

Care for patients

Provide guidance and support as patients make the transition from curative to palliative care

Provide competent assessments and diagnosis

Provide information about diagnosis, prognosis, and treatment options

Provide guidance during the process of making treatment decisions

Respect the patient's beliefs, values, and goals

Provide skilled, effective interventions that meet the patient's needs

Collaborate with the patient's attending physician and with members of the interdisciplinary team to achieve outcomes that meet the patient's needs

Offer caring presence

Support the patient's search for a renewed sense of meaning, purpose, and hope

Serve as an advocate to help patients receive needed services

Participate in teaching and research activities to improve the standards of patient care

Care for family members

Provide guidance and support as families make transition from curative to palliative goals for continued care

Provide information about diagnosis, prognosis, and treatment options

Provide guidance during the process of making treatment decisions so that the patient's wishes are honored

Adjust therapies to meet the capabilities of family members, and teach patient care techniques

Provide ongoing emotional support and reassurance

Care for self

Attain professional competence

Seek peer support

Learn stress management techniques and practice self-care activities, including taking time for exercise, interactions with family members, and vacations

Table 36-4. Development Tasks of People Who Are Dying

Develop a renewed sense of personhood and meaning
Find meaning of life through life review and personal narrative
Develop a sense of worthiness, both in the past and in the current situation
L'earn to accept love and caring from other people
Bring closure to personal and community relationships
Say goodbye to family members and friends with expressions of regret, gratitude, appreciation, and affection
Ask for and grant forgiveness to estranged friends and family members so that reconciliation can occur
Say goodbye to community relationships
Bring closure to worldly affairs
Arrange for the transfer of fiscal, legal, and social responsibilities

Everyone involved in this process—patient, family members, and health care professionals—struggles with the challenging task of envisioning meaningful roles for a person who is dying but who may continue to live for many months. Researchers have identified some activities described as developmental tasks of dying patients. These tasks may help support a sense of meaning for persons during the final stages of their lives. However, caution should be taken as to not place burdens by insisting that dying patients engage in these activities. Listed in Table 36-4 are some of the activities described as developmental tasks.

The case of the 69-year-old man—follow-up: Over the next several months, hospice bereavement program volunteers contact Mary at regular intervals and invite her to bereavement support groups.

Mary also has regular follow-up visits scheduled with her primary care doctor. She misses John deeply, however is more involved with life after 3 months and is extremely thankful for the team effort.

TIPS TO REMEMBER

- Anyone with a serious illness, regardless of life expectancy, can receive palliative care.
- Anyone with an illness—with a life expectancy measured in months, not years—qualifies for hospice care.
- In almost all states, Medicare pays all charges related to hospice care.
- Respect the patient's beliefs, values, and goals.
- Offering false reassurance is unkind and unethical.

COMPREHENSION QUESTIONS

1. Which term refers to a medical specialty that focuses on patients experiencing a debilitating chronic or life-threatening illness, condition, or injury?
>   A. Hospice care
>   B. Oncology
>   C. Hospice and palliative medicine
>   D. End of life care

2. When a terminally ill patient is losing weight because of difficulties in swallowing, which of the following is the most appropriate first step?
>   A. Surgical resection of the obstructing lesion
>   B. Assess for the presence of oral candidiasis
>   C. Placement of an esophageal stent
>   D. Radiation therapy

3. Which answer best describes the Core Principles of End-of-life Care?
>   A. Respect the right to refuse
>   B. Respect the dignity of both the patients and caregivers
>   C. Respect the physicians' professional responsibility to discontinue some treatments when appropriate, with consideration for both patient and family preferences
>   D. All of the above

Answers

1. **C.** Hospice and palliative medicine refers to a medical specialty that focuses on patients experiencing a debilitating chronic or life-threatening illness, condition, or injury. Physicians in this subspecialty have advanced knowledge and skills to prevent and relieve the suffering experienced by patients with life-limiting, life-threatening, and terminal illnesses. This specialist has expertise in the assessment of patients with advanced disease and catastrophic injury, the relief of distressing symptoms, the coordination of interdisciplinary patient and family-centered care in diverse settings, the use of specialized care systems including hospice, the management of the imminently dying patient; and legal and ethical decision making in end-of-life care.

2. **B.** Impaired oral intake could be a consequence of dry mouth, altered taste or small, stomatitis, odynophagia, dysphagia, severe constipation, bowel obstruction, nausea, vomiting or uncontrolled pain, or dyspnea. Clinicians should focus on the identifiable treatable causes of difficulty swallowing.

3. **D.** The core principles of end-of-life care are designed to provide comfort and alleviate the sufferings of patients and families by focusing on all the aspects of pain, improving the quality of life, and helping the patients and families search for meaning in life.

SUGGESTED READINGS

American Academy of Hospice and Palliative Medicine. <www.aahpm.org>.

Center to Advance Palliative Care. <http://www.capc.org>.

Education in Palliative and End of Life Care (EPEC). <http://www.epec.net>.

End of Life—Palliative Education Resource Center. <http://www.eperc.mcw.edu>.

National Hospice and Palliative Care Organization (including state-specific advance directives). <http://www.nhpco.org>.

NCCN. *The National Comprehensive Cancer Network Palliative Care Guidelines.* <http://www.nccn. org>.

Maxwell TL, Martinez JM, Knight CF. The hospice and palliative medicine approach to life-limiting illness. In: Storey P, Levine, J, Shega J. /Unipac Series/. Glenview IL: Mary Ann Liebert, Inc; 2008:1-71.

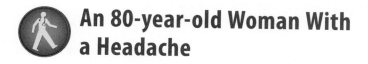

An 80-year-old Woman With a Headache

Siegfried W. B. Yu, MD, FACP

An 80-year-old female presents to the outpatient clinic complaining of headache in the bilateral frontal and temporal regions. She says the headache has been present for at least a couple of years, but has recently become worse over the past few months. It is described as squeezing in character with muscle tightness, graded around 8/10 in severity. She notes occasional nausea without vomiting. No sensitivity to light or sound is noted. She denies having any problems with vision, eye tearing, swallowing, or speech, or neck pain. No bladder or bowel movement problems are noted. No complaints of new numbness or weakness are noted. The headache occurs throughout most of the day, every day, and it can happen any time. She has a background of hip arthritis, with prior hip replacement, and has been on chronic oral narcotic therapy. Due to the increase in headache severity, she has been taking more of her pain medication, without much benefit.

On examination, she is anxious and in mild distress due to the headache. She is afebrile, with a heart rate of 78 bpm and a blood pressure of 130/85 mm Hg. She is alert and oriented, and speech and expression are intact. Palpation of her temporal regions bilaterally does not elicit tenderness. Her face appears symmetric. Fundoscopy does not reveal papilledema. Cardiac examination and lung examination are normal. Normal sensory function is noted with light touch. Muscle strength is graded as 5/5 throughout with deep tendon reflexes 1+ throughout. There is pain with internal and external rotation of her right hip. Gait and stance including tiptoe and heel walking is normal, but unsteady on tandem walk. Romberg sign is negative. Finger-to-nose testing does not reveal ataxia.

1. **In light of her reported symptoms by history, what is the patient's most likely primary diagnosis?**

2. **What may be the precipitating factor in this case?**

3. **What management decision would you need to make at this time?**

Answers

1. The patient's baseline chronic headache seems to have worsened with her increased narcotic pain medication use, which she originally started for her arthritic pain. In light of her reported symptoms by history, and lack of other striking features on her history and examination, the patient's most likely primary diagnosis is a medication-overuse headache, with a likely underlying preceding tension-type headache (TTH).

2. Narcotic pain medications are the likely precipitating factor.

3. It would be reasonable to attempt a taper off of her narcotic pain medications and reassess her symptoms. Due to her age, it would be also appropriate to exclude secondary causes of her headache.

CASE REVIEW

Although the character of the patient's headache does not appear to suggest a very specific cause, her presentation forces one to think about the various potential causes of headache. Because of her advanced age, it is important that we start by excluding specific secondary causes of headache, such as temporal arteritis, and vascular dissection. Migraine-type symptoms, such as aura, laterality, nausea, and vomiting, are not present, but likewise, because of her age at onset, these symptoms would still prompt a search for a secondary cause of the headache. Likewise, a thorough physical examination, with careful attention to neurologic function, is important for assessing the cause of the headache. Ultimately, the most prominent feature of her headache was the increased use of narcotic pain medication, which is the most likely cause. In order to fully exclude other causes of headache, however, it would be appropriate to assess inflammatory markers, such as the erythrocyte sedimentation rate (ESR), and an advanced imaging study, such as CT or MRI, because of her advanced age.

HEADACHES

Pathophysiology

Headache may originate from 1 of the following 2 mechanisms of pain perception: (1) pain that is the result of a normal physiologic response from a healthy nervous system or (2) pain that results when pain-producing pathways are damaged or activated inappropriately. Pain, in general, usually occurs when peripheral nociceptors are stimulated in response to tissue injury, visceral distention, or other factors. In regard to headache, the scalp, middle meningeal artery, dural sinuses, falx cerebri, and proximal segments of the large pial arteries are the pain-producing structures. The primary structures involved in primary headache include the large intracranial vessels and dura mater, the peripheral terminals of the trigeminal nerve that innervate these structures, the caudal portion of the trigeminal nucleus (the trigeminocervical complex), and the pain modulatory systems in the brain that receive input from the trigeminal nociceptors. The trigeminovascular system is composed of the trigeminal innervation of the large intracranial vessels and respective dura mater (see Figure 37-1). It is not surprising that lacrimation and nasal congestion are prominent in the trigeminal autonomic cephalgias (TACs), such as cluster headache and paroxysmal hemicranias, as well as some migraine headaches.

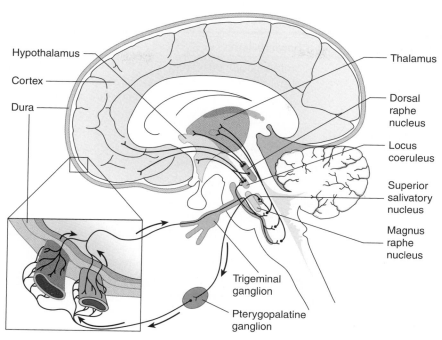

Figure 37-1. Brainstem pathways that modulate sensory input. (Reproduced with permission from Fauci AS, Braunwald E, Kasper DL, et al, eds. *Harrison's Principles of Internal Medicine.* 17th ed. New York: McGraw-Hill; 2008:97 [Figure 15-1].)

Diagnosis

A thorough history is the most important way to differentiate among the different causes of headache, which are many (Table 37-1). A classification dividing the headache types into primary headache (those in which headache and its associated features are the primary disorder) and secondary headache (those in which the headaches are secondary to another distinct disorder) has been developed by the International Headache Society (IHS). See Table 37-2 for common causes of headache.

Primary headache disorders often result in significant disability and decreased quality of life. Among them, the most common are TTH, migraine headache, and idiopathic stabbing headache. TTH describes a chronic headache syndrome characterized by bilateral tight, band-like discomfort, with pain that builds slowly, fluctuates in severity, and may persist continuously for many days. It can be episodic or chronic (>15 days in a month). An approach to TTH may clearly delineate them based on the absence of nausea, vomiting, photophobia, phonophobia, osmophobia, throbbing, and aggravation with movement. This simplifies TTH in

Table 37-1. Differential Diagnosis of Headache

Disease	Characteristics
Tension-type headache	Common; duration 30 min–7 days; typically bilateral, nonpulsating pressing quality; mild to moderate in intensity without prohibiting activity; no nausea or vomiting (anorexia may occur)
Cluster headache	Uncommon; sudden onset; duration, minutes to hours; repeats over a course of weeks, and then disappears for months or years; often unilateral tearing and nasal congestion; pain is severe, unilateral, and periorbital; more common in men
Frontal sinusitis	Usually worse when lying down; associated with nasal congestion; tenderness over affected sinus
Cervical spondylosis	Worse with neck movement; posterior distribution; pain is neuralgic and sometimes referred to vertex or forehead; more common in elderly patients
Greater occipital neuralgia	Occipital location; tenderness at base of skull; pain is neuralgic in character and sometimes referred to vertex or forehead; more common in elderly patients
Postconcussion syndrome	History of antecedent head trauma; vertigo (often positional), light-headedness, or giddiness; poor concentration and memory; lack of energy; irritability and anxiety
Trigeminal neuralgia	Brief episodes of sharp, stabbing pain with trigeminal nerve distribution
TMJ dysfunction	Pain generally involves the TMJ and temporal areas and is associated with symptoms when chewing
Medication-induced headache	Chronic headache with a few features of migraine; tends to occur daily; HRT and hormonal contraceptives are frequent culprits
Subarachnoid hemorrhage	Explosive onset of severe headache; 10% preceded by "sentinel" headaches
Acute or chronic subdural	History of antecedent trauma; may have subacute onset; altered level of consciousness or neurologic deficit, hematoma may be present
Meningitis	Fever; meningeal signs
Encephalitis	Associated with neurologic abnormalities, confusion, altered mental state, or change in level of consciousness

(continued)

Table 37-1. Differential Diagnosis of Headache (*Continued*)

Disease	Characteristics
Intracranial neoplasms	Worse on awakening; generally progressive; aggravated by coughing, straining, or changing position
Benign intracranial hypertension (pseudotumor cerebri)	Often abrupt onset; associated with nausea, vomiting, dizziness, blurred vision, and papilledema; may have CN VI palsy; headache aggravated by coughing, straining, or changing position
Temporal arteritis	Occurs almost exclusively in patients aged over 50; associated with tenderness of scalp or temporal artery, and jaw claudication; visual changes
Acute severe hypertension	Marked BP elevation (systolic ≥ 210 mm Hg; diastolic ≥ 120 mm Hg); may have symptoms of encephalopathy (eg, confusion, irritability)
CO poisoning	May be insidious or associated with dyspnea; occurs more commonly in the colder months
Acute glaucoma	Associated with blurred vision, nausea, vomiting, and seeing halos around lights; ophthalmologic emergency
Carotid dissection	Cause of stroke; can be spontaneous or following minor trauma or sudden neck movement; unilateral headache or face pain; ipsilateral Horner syndrome; ophthalmologic emergency

BP, blood pressure; CN VI, cranial nerve VI; CO, carbon monoxide; HRT, hormone replacement therapy; TMJ, temporomandibular joint.
Data from Wilson JF. In the clinic. Migraine. *Ann Intern Med.* 2007;147(9):ITC11-1–ITC11-6.

Table 37-2. Common Causes of Headache

Primary Headache		Secondary Headache	
Type	%	Type	%
Migraine	16	Systemic infection	63
Tension-type	69	Head injury	4
Cluster	0.1	Vascular disorders	1
Idiopathic stabbing	2	Subarachnoid hemorrhage	<1
Exertional	1	Brain tumor	0.1

Source: Data from Olesen J, Goadsby PJ, Ramadan N, et al. *The Headaches.* Philadelphia: Lippincott Williams & Wilkins; 2005.

contrast to migraine headache; however, the IHS definition does allow for degrees of nausea, photophobia, and phonophobia. TTH may represent a primary disorder of central nervous system pain modulation.

Migraine headache is the second most common cause of headache and is usually associated with triggers. It is episodic and has features such as light, sound, and movement sensitivity, as well as nausea and vomiting. It affects 15% of women and 6% of men. It is a syndrome of recurring headache, which is generally benign, and associated with other symptoms of neurologic dysfunction. A useful mnemonic for the symptoms of migraine headache is POUND. P indicates a pulsatile quality of headache. O indicates 1-day duration (<4 hours suggests TTH). U indicates unilateral location. N indicates the presence of nausea or vomiting. D indicates a disabling intensity. The presence or absence of these features can be used to formulate the probability that the headache is a migraine headache versus a TTH (see Table 37-3).

Idiopathic stabbing headaches are the third most common primary headache and represent TACs that include a number of subtypes, including cluster headache, paroxysmal hemicranias, and short-lasting unilateral neuralgiform

Table 37-3. Elements of Patient History for Clinical Diagnosis of Migraine Versus Tension-type Headache

Clinical Feature	Sensitivity (%)	Specificity (%)	Positive Likelihood Ratio	Negative Likelihood Ratio
Nausea or vomiting	42–60	81–93	6	0.62
Duration 4–72 h	74	53	1.6	0.49
Pounding or throbbing character	64–87	22–83	3.8	0.43
Unilateral head pain	65–75	60–85	4.3	0.41
Disabling for usual activities	59–87	52–76	2.5	0.54
Presence of ≥4 of the above symptoms	29	100	23	0.71
Presence of ≥3 of the above symptoms	80	94	13	0.21
Presence of ≥2 of the following 3 symptoms: nausea, photophobia, and headache-related disability (any day in the previous 3 months)	81	75	3.25	0.25

headache attacks with conjunctival injection and tearing (SUNCT). These are characterized by relatively short-lasting attacks of head pain with associated lacrimation, conjunctival injection, or nasal congestion (see Table 37-4).

Table 37-4. Clinical Features of the Trigeminal Autonomic Cephalalgias

	Cluster Headache	**Paroxysmal Hemicrania**	**SUNCT**
Gender	M > F	F = M	F ~ M
Pain type	Stabbing, boring	Throbbing, boring, stabbing	Burning, stabbing, sharp
Severity	Excruciating	Excruciating	Severe to excruciating
Site	Orbit, temple	Orbit, temple	Periorbital
Attack frequency	1/alternate day to 8/day	1–40/day (>5/day for more than half the time)	3–200/day
Duration of attack	15–180 min	2–30 min	5–240 s
Autonomic features	Yes	Yes	Yes (prominent conjunctival injection and lacrimation)[a]
Migrainous features[b]	Yes	Yes	Yes
Alcohol trigger	Yes	No	No
Cutaneous triggers	No	No	Yes
Indomethacin effect	—	Yes[c]	—
Abortive treatment	Sumatriptan injection or nasal spray, oxygen	No effective treatment	Lidocaine (IV)
Prophylactic treatment	Verapamil, methysergide, lithium	Indomethacin	Lamotrigine, topiramate, gabapentin

Note: SUNCT, short-lasting unilateral neuralgiform headache attacks with conjunctival injection and tearing.

[a]If conjunctival injection and tearing not present, consider SUNA.

[b]Nausea, photophobia, or phonophobia; photophobia and phonophobia are typically unilateral on the side of the pain.

[c]Indicates complete response to indomethacin.

Other variants of headache include medication-overuse headache, which typically occurs in the context of overuse of narcotic or barbiturate-containing analgesics, which results in a daily or near-daily headache that is refractory. This headache should be strongly considered in patients who may be overusing these types of medications. This is not likely a separate headache entity, but a consequence of overuse of this type of medication. Likewise, another broad diagnosis is chronic daily headache (CDH) that is present when a patient experiences headache more than 15 days per month, and while it may also encapsulate medication-overuse headache, it may also be caused by secondary causes of headache, such as trauma, infection, inflammation, low cerebrospinal fluid (CSF) volume headache, and raised CSF pressure headache.

Secondary causes of headache are many, and it is paramount that these are appropriately excluded before assuming a headache is due to a primary cause. Much of this can be determined by a thorough history and physical examination. Some major causes to take note of include meningitis, intracranial hemorrhage, brain tumor, temporal arteritis, and glaucoma. It is important to assess for alarm features that suggest headache due to a secondary, nonbenign cause (see Table 37-5).

The physical examination should be directed to evaluate features suggestive of a secondary headache. This includes evaluation of blood pressure, the presence of fever, meningeal signs or other signs of infection, neurologic deficits, visual

Table 37-5. "Red Flag" or Alarm Features That Suggest Headache is Due to Nonbenign, Secondary Causes

Daily headache

Blurred vision

Dizziness, syncope, discoordination, or focal neurologic abnormality

Sudden, explosive onset

Pain worse with coughing or movement

Change in personality or mental status

Headache awakens person from sleep

Onset after 50 years of age

Fever

Meningeal signs

Diastolic blood pressure >120 mm Hg

Diminished pulse or tenderness of temporal artery

Papilledema

Necrotic or tender scalp lesions

Increased intraocular pressure

acuity changes, increased intraocular pressure, and mental status changes. As noted above, combined with thorough history taking, a thorough physical examination plays an essential role in diagnosis of headache syndromes.

Depending on the clinical impression, and what causes of headache are necessary to confirm and exclude, laboratory testing should proceed in an evidence-based manner. For example, for a patient with a new-onset headache after 50 years of age, it would be important to obtain an ESR to exclude secondary causes of headache such as temporal arteritis and other vasculitides. If elevated, this would lead to a temporal artery biopsy to confirm the diagnosis. On the other hand, if fever and neck rigidity were the prominent features, performing a lumbar puncture would be more important to establish the diagnosis. Laboratory testing may also need to be done if the patients' symptoms are severe enough to cause significant metabolic derangements that may require correction.

Advanced neuroimaging, such as MRI, should be performed particularly in patients with atypical headache features, substantial changes in headache pattern, or symptoms or signs of neurologic abnormalities. It is also important to note, however, that certain instances may occur in which serious causes of headache exist and neuroimaging may be normal (see Table 37-6).

Treatment

Once the diagnosis is clearly established, treatment may be pursued. Standard treatment for TTH can generally be managed with simple analgesics such as acetaminophen, NSAIDs, or aspirin. Relaxation can be effective. Triptans are only useful if the patient also has migraine headache. For chronic TTH, amitriptyline is the only proven treatment. Other pharmacologic treatments such as other tricyclics, selective serotonin reuptake inhibitors, and benzodiazepines have not been shown to be effective.

Table 37-6. Serious Causes of Headache in Which Neuroimaging Findings May Be Normal

Giant cell or temporal arteritis
Glaucoma
Trigeminal or glossopharyngeal neuralgia
Lesions around sella turcica
Warning leak of aneurysm (sentinel bleed)
Inflammation, infection, or neoplastic invasion of leptomeninges
Cervical spondylosis
Pseudotumor cerebri
Low intracranial pressure syndromes (cerebrospinal fluid leaks)

For mild-to-moderate migraine headaches not associated with vomiting, over-the-counter analgesics such as acetaminophen, aspirin, or NSAIDs (alone or in combination) may be sufficient. Standard treatment for severe acute migraine headache, however, typically includes the use of triptan medications (see Table 37-7),

Table 37-7. Short-term Drug Treatment for Migraine and Migraine-specific Medications

Agent (Route)	Mechanism of Action	Dosage	Notes
Sumatriptan (subcutaneous)	Selective serotonin (5-HT1B/1D) agonist	6 mg at onset (may repeat after 1 h; maximum 12 mg/day)	Rapid onset of action; little sedation; treatment of choice for moderate-severe attacks; not effective if given during aura; contraindicated in patients with CAD, uncontrolled hypertension, or strictly basilar or hemiplegic migraine; pregnancy category C
Sumatriptan (oral)	Selective serotonin (5-HT1B/1D) agonist	25–100 mg at onset (may repeat after 2 h; maximum 200 mg/day)	Well tolerated; little sedation; less rapid onset; may be used again for recurrent headache; no evidence of teratogenicity
Sumatriptan (nasal)	Selective serotonin (5-HT1B/1D) agonist	20 mg at onset (may repeat after 2 h; maximum 40 mg/day)	Well tolerated; little sedation; speed of action and effectiveness similar to oral sumatriptan; useful when nonoral route of administration needed; no evidence of teratogenicity
Almotriptan (oral)	Selective serotonin (5-HT1B/1D) agonist	6.25–12.5 mg at onset (maximum 25 mg/day)	Similar efficacy to oral sumatriptan
Eletriptan (oral)	Selective serotonin (5-HT1B/1D) agonist	20–40 mg at onset (may repeat after 2 h; maximum 80 mg/day)	Highly effective oral triptan; rapid onset of action; slightly higher efficacy compared with oral sumatriptan

(continued)

Table 37-7. Short-term Drug Treatment for Migraine and Migraine-specific Medications (*Continued*)

Agent (Route)	Mechanism of Action	Dosage	Notes
Frovatriptan (oral)	Selective serotonin (5-HT1B/1D) agonist	2.5 mg at onset (may repeat after 2 h; maximum 7.5 mg/day)	Well tolerated; little sedation; effective for prevention of menstrual migraine
Naratriptan (oral)	Selective serotonin (5-HT1B/1D) agonist	1.0–2.5 mg at onset (may repeat after 4 h; maximum 5 mg/day)	Possibly lower risk for headache recurrence than other oral triptans; relatively lower efficacy and incidence of side effects than other triptans
Rizatriptan (oral)	Selective serotonin (5-HT1B/1D) agonist	5–10 mg at onset (may repeat after 2 h; maximum 30 mg/day)	Available in a fast-melt preparation, which may be no faster in providing pain relief than the regular tablet; slightly higher efficacy compared with oral sumatriptan
Zolmitriptan (oral)	Selective serotonin (5-HT1B/1D) agonist	1.25–2.5 mg at onset (may repeat after 2 h; maximum 10 mg/day)	Similar efficacy to oral sumatriptan; also available in a rapidly dispersing tablet formulation
Dihydroergotamine (nasal)	Nonselective serotonin agonist	1 spray (0.5 mg) into each nostril (may repeat after 15 min; maximum 4 sprays/day, 8/week)	No sedation; should not be used with a 5-HT1B/1D; pregnancy category X
Dihydroergotamine (all other routes)		1 mg SC/IM/IV (may repeat after 1 h; maximum 2 mg/dose, 3 mg/attack, 6 mg/week)	Useful in status migrainosus; contraindicated in patients with CAD; pregnancy category X

although other classes of medications can also be used with good effectiveness (see Table 37-8). Less effective nonspecific short-term drug treatments for migraine include acetaminophen, chlorpromazine, prochlorperazine, topical lidocaine, isometheptene-containing preparations, and codeine combinations. Codeine, and other narcotics, has high potential for "rebound" headaches and opiate dependence and should generally be avoided. Conflicting evidence for migraine treatment exists for ergotamine/caffeine oral preparations, and dexamethasone or other corticosteroids.

Table 37-8. Short-term Drug Treatment for Migraine and Non-migraine-specific Medications

Agent (Route)	Mechanism of Action	Dosage	Notes
Naproxen and other NSAIDs (oral)	Inhibits cyclooxygenase, decreases prostaglandin synthesis	500 mg at onset (may repeat after 6–8 h)	Well tolerated; treatment of choice for mild-to-moderate attacks; may be given with antiemetic; avoid in pregnancy after 32-week gestation; pregnancy category B
Aspirin/ metoclopramide (oral)	Blocks dopamine receptors in CTZ; increases response to acetylcholine in upper GI tract	650/10 mg at onset (may repeat after 3–4 h)	Antinausea effect; elderly are more likely to develop dystonic reactions than younger adults; use lowest recommended doses initially; pregnancy category C (D in third trimester)
Butorphanol (nasal)	Opiate agonist–antagonist	1 spray in 1 nostril (may repeat after 1 h)	Well-tolerated rescue medication; risk for opiate dependence; pregnancy category C
Metoclopramide/ diphenhydramine (intravenous)	Blocks dopamine receptors in CTZ	20–25 mg over 20 min (may repeat after 1 h)	Antinausea effect; recent RCT showed equal effectiveness to sumatriptan; pregnancy category C

It is important to note that triptans do not have a class effect; therefore, lack of efficacy or intolerance of side effects to 1 triptan does not predict a patient's response to other triptans. Additionally, the dose may need to be repeated in order to be effective. Triptans are contraindicated in patients with coronary artery disease (CAD) or uncontrolled hypertension. Antiemetic agents can be used in conjunction with analgesics and migraine-specific medications to address migraine-associated nausea and vomiting. In particular, metoclopramide may address both pain and nausea symptoms.

Preventive migraine treatment should be considered in patients with frequent disabling migraine headaches (>2 per month), and may reduce frequency by one third to one half. Other appropriate candidates include those who have contraindications or intolerance to acute therapies, failure or overuse of acute therapies, or preference for preventive therapy (see Table 37-9). Other available options, which have lower efficacy and/or limited strength of evidence for prophylactic

Table 37-9. Preventive Drug Treatment for Migraine With Medium-to-high Efficacy

Agent	Mechanism of Action	Dosage	Notes
Amitriptyline	Inhibits norepinephrine	Amitriptyline, 30–150 mg PO qd	Anticholinergic effects, dry mouth, drowsiness; weight gain
Divalproex sodium, other anticonvulsants (eg, sodium valproate, gabapentin, topiramate)	Unknown	Divalproex sodium, 250–500 mg PO bid	Bone marrow suppression, liver inflammation, alopecia, tremors, weight loss with topiramate
Propranolol, other non-ISA beta-adrenergic antagonists (eg, timolol, atenolol, metoprolol, nadolol)	Beta-adrenergic antagonists	Propranolol, 120–240 mg PO qd in divided doses	Fatigue, bradycardia, hypotension (check blood pressure and heart rate before prescribing)
Methysergide	Selective serotonin agonist (5-HT2); constricts cranial and peripheral blood vessels	4–8 mg PO qd	Limited by side effect concerns. Retroperitoneal fibrosis, pulmonary fibrosis, nausea, vomiting; no longer available in the United States

migraine therapy, include fluoxetine, verapamil, naproxen, feverfew, riboflavin, magnesium, and ACE inhibitors/angiotensin II receptor blockers.

Treatment of the TAC primary headache category is reviewed in Table 37-4. Treatment of secondary headaches from a variety of causes should be targeted to the particular etiology at hand.

CDH that has evolved from medication-overuse headache is usually due to the overuse (>2 days per week) of ergotamine tartrate, triptans, analgesics (especially those combined with barbiturates), narcotics, and possibly benzodiazepines. Some physicians think that even simple analgesics taken more than 2 days a week can cause a daily headache syndrome. The overuse of triptan drugs (more than 3 days a week, for 2 or more weeks) is now becoming a common cause of this syndrome. In order to obtain control of these headaches, the medications have to be discontinued. Not only does the overuse of these medications cause the daily headache, but the daily use of these medications also prevents other medications from working effectively. Treatment may require hospitalization with supervised withdrawal, and treatment with IV dihydroergotamine combined with an antiemetic, such as metoclopramide. NSAIDs, beta-blockers, calcium channel blockers, and tricyclics do not cause a withdrawal syndrome.

TIPS TO REMEMBER

- A thorough history is the most important way to differentiate among the different causes of headache, which are many.
- A useful mnemonic for the symptoms of migraine headache is POUND. P indicates a pulsatile quality of headache. O indicates 1-day duration (<4 hours suggests TTH). U indicates unilateral location. N indicates the presence of nausea or vomiting. D indicates a disabling intensity.
- Medication-overuse headache should be strongly considered in patients who may be overusing narcotic or barbiturate-containing analgesics, which results in a refractory daily or near-daily headache.
- The overuse of triptan drugs (more than 3 days a week, for 2 or more weeks) is now becoming a common cause of medication-overuse headache.
- It is important to assess for alarm features that suggest headache due to a secondary, nonbenign cause.
- There are serious causes of headache that exist and for which neuroimaging may be normal.
- For migraine treatment, codeine, and other narcotics, has high potential for "rebound" headaches and opiate dependence and should generally be avoided.
- It is important to note that triptans do not have a class effect; therefore, lack of efficacy or intolerance of side effects to 1 triptan does not predict a patient's response to other triptans.

- Triptans are contraindicated in patients with CAD or uncontrolled hypertension.
- Preventive migraine treatment should be considered in patients with frequent disabling migraine headaches (>2 per month), and may reduce frequency by one third to one half.

COMPREHENSION QUESTIONS

1. A 25-year-old man presents to the clinic complaining of severe headaches near his frontal sinus region that have been more frequent over the past week. They occur multiple times a day, and he notes some associated tearing and nasal stuffiness. Between the short attacks he feels okay. The headaches are described as sharp in character. No fever noted. He has not responded to nasal spray given at his last visit. On examination you don't find any sign of sinus tenderness or nasal congestion.
    What is the diagnosis?
        A. Migraine headache
        B. Acute sinusitis
        C. Brain tumor
        D. Cluster headache

2. A 60-year-old woman presents to the clinic with 10 days of headache that is severe. It is pounding in character, primarily on the right side, and is associated with some difficulty chewing her food. She is trying to read you a list of medications she has brought with her; however, she is having difficulty seeing out of her right eye.
    What test would best confirm your diagnosis?
        A. ESR
        B. Temporal artery biopsy
        C. MRI
        D. Antineutrophilic cytoplasmic antibody (ANCA)

3. A 50-year-old man complains of sudden headache associated with tearing neck pain, dizziness, and vomiting. On your neurologic examination, you find leftward rapid eye movements, with drooping of his eyelid. He has lost sensation to his left face, and his right arm and leg. What is going on?
        A. Paroxysmal hemicrania
        B. Complicated migraine
        C. Vertebral artery dissection
        D. Normal pressure hydrocephalus

Answers

1. **D.** Based on the clinical features in this patient's history, the headache is not compatible with the typical migraine character of symptoms. Remember the mnemonic POUND. P indicates a pulsatile quality of headache. O indicates 1-day

duration (<4 hours suggests TTH). U indicates unilateral location. N indicates the presence of nausea or vomiting. D indicates a disabling intensity. Although there is some suggestion of nasal congestion, the patient's history of short, frequent headaches without fever and examination findings absent for sinus tenderness do not suggest the problem is acute sinusitis. Brain tumor, though not fully excluded, would be expected to produce identifiable neurologic deficits and/or signs and symptoms of increased intracranial pressure.

2. **B.** The patient has a number of "red flags" in her history including her age, associated vision impairment, and a constellation of findings suggestive of temporal arteritis. ESR would be useful supportive testing; however, it would not necessarily be the best test to confirm the diagnosis. The association between giant cell arteritis and ANCA remains obscure despite several published studies.

3. **C.** This patient also has a number of "red flags" in his history, including his age, explosive onset, and neurologic deficits. The tearing neck pain suggests dissection may be the etiology in light of the associated symptoms. Paroxysmal hemicrania is one of the TACs and is characterized by multiple short headaches affecting the orbit or temple, which are throbbing, boring, or stabbing in character. Complicated migraine would have a pain presentation of migraine character, which does not fit with this patient, and would have associated neurologic deficits. The patient's symptoms and findings do not fit with normal pressure hydrocephalus either, which is not in the differential diagnosis for headache. Furthermore, the headache is slow in onset, and associated with symptoms of walking difficulty, slowing of mental function, and urinary incontinence.

SUGGESTED READINGS

Brian A, Crum M, Benarroch EE, Brown Jr RD. Neurology. Part II: general principles from the level of the cerebral cortex through the neuraxis to muscle. In: Ghosh AK, ed. *Mayo Clinic Internal Medicine Board Review*. 9th ed. New York: Oxford University Press; 2010 [chapter 19].

Goadsby PJ, Ruskin NH. Headache. In: Fauci AS, Braunwald E, Kasper DL, et al, eds. *Harrison's Principles of Internal Medicine*. 17th ed. New York: McGraw Hill; 2008:95–106 [chapter 15].

Wilson JF. In the clinic. Migraine. *Ann Intern Med*. 2007;147(9):ITC11-1–ITC11-16.

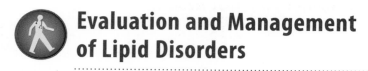

Evaluation and Management of Lipid Disorders

Chaitanya K. Mamillapalli, MD and
Michael Jakoby, MD, MA

A 31-year-old Male With Severe Hypercholesterolemia

A 31-year-old male is referred for lipid management. The patient recently was diagnosed with multivessel coronary artery disease (CAD) and underwent 3-vessel bypass surgery. The patient's father experienced an acute myocardial infarction at age 39 years and required bypass surgery for management. The patient has no history of hypertension, diabetes, or tobacco use. Examination revealed a generally fit-appearing young man with bilateral tendon xanthomas. Preoperative fasting lipid panel was notable for total cholesterol 331 mg/dL, high-density lipoprotein (HDL) cholesterol 44 mg/dL, low-density lipoprotein (LDL) cholesterol 266 mg/dL, and triglycerides 104 mg/dL.

1. What is the patient's primary lipid disorder?

2. What is the patient's cholesterol treatment target, and what are his therapeutic options?

Answers

1. Familial hypercholesterolemia (FH).

2. LDL cholesterol <100 mg/dL; best treatment option is a 3-hydroxy-3-methylglutaryl-coenzyme A (HMG-CoA) reductase inhibitor ("statin").

CASE REVIEW

Lipids are sparingly soluble molecules that include cholesterol, fatty acids, and their derivatives. They are transported in the circulation by lipoprotein particles composed of proteins called apolipoproteins and phospholipids. Human plasma lipoproteins are classified into 5 major classes based on density: chylomicrons (least dense), very-low-density lipoprotein (VLDL), intermediate-density lipoprotein (IDL), LDL, and HDL. A sixth class called lipoprotein(a) (Lp(a)) resembles LDL in lipid composition and has density that overlaps that of both LDL and HDL.

There are 3 major lipid metabolic pathways. In the exogenous pathway, dietary long-chain fatty acids and cholesterol are esterified and assembled into chylomicrons as triglycerides and cholesterol esters, respectively. The primary structural protein on chylomicrons is apolipoprotein B48 (apo-B48). Chylomicrons are secreted into the lymphatic circulation by small bowel enterocytes and enter the venous circulation from the thoracic duct. Triglycerides are hydrolyzed to nonesterified fatty acids by the activity of the enzyme lipoprotein lipase (LPL), with apo-CII on chylomicrons serving as an essential cofactor. Triglyceride-depleted chylomicrons are called chylomicron remnants and are cleared by the LDL receptor–like protein (LRP) in an interaction with apo-E.

Hepatic triglycerides and cholesterol esters are assembled into VLDL particles and secreted into the portal venous circulation in the endogenous lipid pathway. The main structural protein on VLDL particles is apo-B100, a high-affinity ligand for the LDL receptor. Triglycerides are hydrolyzed by LPL (with apo-CII as cofactor) to create triglyceride-depleted IDL. IDL can be cleared by binding to either LRP or LDL receptor or can undergo further delipidation by LPL to create cholesterol ester–enriched LDL particles. Apo-B100 is the only structural protein on LDL particles, and LDL is cleared by interaction of apo-B100 with LDL receptors expressed by liver and extrahepatic tissues.

HDL is the key lipoprotein in the reverse cholesterol pathway. Nascent HDL is secreted from the liver and small intestines as small apo-AI-containing discs. The discs acquire free cholesterol from peripheral tissues through activity of the cholesterol efflux regulatory protein ABC1. Cholesterol is then esterified by the enzyme lecithin:cholesterol acyltransferase (LCAT), with apo-AI serving as cofactor. At this time, the particles are termed HDL3. Larger HDL2 particles are formed by the acquisition of apolipoproteins and lipids released from delipidated chylomicrons and VLDL particles. HDL2 is converted back to HDL3 after removal of triglycerides by hepatic lipase or transfer of cholesterol esters to apo-B100-bearing lipoproteins (VLDL, IDL, or LDL particles) catalyzed by cholesterol ester transport protein (CETP), resulting in reverse cholesterol transport.

Lipid disorders are usually multifactorial in etiology and reflect the effects of uncharacterized genetic influences coupled with diet, inactivity, tobacco, alcohol, and comorbid conditions such as obesity and diabetes mellitus. However, some lipid abnormalities can be linked to specific causes, such as severe elevations of LDL cholesterol caused by inactivating LDL receptor mutations in FH or severe triglyceride elevations in LPL deficiency states. The differential diagnosis of major lipid disorders is presented in Table 38-1.

Table 38-1. Differential Diagnosis of Major Lipid Abnormalities

Lipid Abnormality	Primary Disorder	Secondary Disorder
Hypercholesterolemia	Polygenic, familial hypercholesterolemia, familial defective apo-B100	Hypothyroidism, nephrotic syndrome
Hypertriglyceridemia	Lipoprotein lipase deficiency, apo-CII deficiency, familial hypertriglyceridemia	Diabetes mellitus, obesity, metabolic syndrome, alcohol use, oral estrogens
Combined hyperlipidemia	Familial combined hyperlipidemia, Type 3 hyperlipoproteinemia	Diabetes mellitus, obesity, metabolic syndrome, hypothyroidism, nephrotic syndrome
Low HDL	Familial hypoalphalipopro-teinemia, Tangier disease, familial HDL deficiency, LCAT deficiency	Diabetes mellitus, metabolic syndrome, tobacco, anabolic steroids, hypertriglyceridemia

Diagnosis

LDL cholesterol over 200 mg/dL strongly suggests a genetic disorder of choles-terol metabolism. The patient's age, history of premature CAD, family history of early CAD, tendon xanthomas, and significant elevations of total and LDL cho-lesterol are consistent with a diagnosis of heterozygous FH. FH is an autosomal dominant disorder with gene frequency approximately 1:500. Plasma total cho-lesterol is usually greater than 300 mg/dL, and LDL cholesterol usually exceeds 250 mg/dL. Premature heart disease is common with onset before age 45 years in men and 55 years in women. Most affected patients have tendon xanthomas, and other findings on examination include xanthelasmas and premature corneal arcus. Homozygous FH is rare (approximately 1 per 1,000,000 population) and leads to severe hypercholesterolemia (total cholesterol >600 mg/dL, LDL choles-terol >500 mg/dL) and very early CAD. Homozygous FH patients develop planar xanthomas at areas of skin trauma, such as elbows and knees.

Familial defective apolipoprotein B-100 (FDB) is caused by mutations in the apo-B100 gene that reduce the affinity of apo-B100 for the LDL receptor.

Prevalence is slightly less than FH at 1:700 to 1:1000. LDL levels range from 160 to 300 mg/dL, and premature CAD is common. Polygenic hypercholesterolemia is the most common etiology of significant hypercholesterolemia, with prevalence 1:10 to 1:20. LDL levels are greater than 160 mg/dL, and there is a 3- to 4-fold increase in prevalence of CAD. Cholesterol levels are less elevated than in heterozygous FH, and tendon xanthomas are not observed.

Treatment

Animal models, epidemiological studies, and genetic causes of hypercholesterolemia establish a strong causal relationship between increasing total and LDL cholesterol levels and risk of CAD. LDL cholesterol–lowering therapy, particularly with HMG-CoA reductase inhibitors, lowers the risk of CAD-related death, morbidity, and revascularization procedures in hypercholesterolemia patients with (secondary prevention) or without (primary prevention) CAD (see Appendix). Adult Treatment Panel III (ATP III) classification of patients by coronary risk is presented in Table 38-2. ATP III can be reviewed online at http://www.nhlbi.nih.gov/guidelines/cholesterol. The Framingham Risk Score calculator takes into account multiple factors including age, gender, total cholesterol, HDL cholesterol, blood pressure, treatment with antihypertensive agents, and tobacco use. An online calculator is available at http://www.nhlbihin.net/atpiii/calculator.asp.

Table 38-2. ATP III Categories of CAD Risk and LDL Cholesterol Treatment Target

Secondary prevention	**Very-high-risk category:** CAD and other high-risk factors such as diabetes mellitus, hypertension, tobacco use, or low HDL cholesterol (<40 mg/dL)	<70 mg/dL
	High risk: Isolated CAD or CAD risk equivalent such as diabetes mellitus, stroke, abdominal aortic aneurysm, or 20% risk of CAD in 10 years by Framingham Risk Score	<100 mg/dL
Primary prevention	**Moderately high risk:** >2 risk factors and 10-year CAD risk 10%–20%	<130 mg/dL (<100 mg/dL optional)
	Moderate risk: Patients with 2 or more risk factors and 10-year risk less than 10%	<130 mg/dL
	Low risk: 0–1 risk factors	<160 mg/dL

Since this patient has isolated CAD, his LDL cholesterol treatment target is <100 mg/dL. Therapeutic lifestyle changes (TLC), including saturated fat-restricted diet, regular aerobic exercise, and weight loss, are initial interventions that reduce LDL cholesterol by 10% to 15%. However, most patients need TLC combined with cholesterol-lowering medications to achieve their LDL cholesterol treatment targets.

HMG-CoA reductase inhibitors ("statins") are the most potent class of cholesterol-lowering drugs and have the most evidence of clinical cardiovascular benefit. They reduce endogenous cholesterol synthesis by competitively inhibiting HMG-CoA reductase and increasing expression of hepatic LDL receptors. Lipid-lowering effects are measurable within the first week of therapy and are stable after approximately 4 weeks. Doubling the dose of a statin lowers LDL cholesterol by an additional 5% to 10%, and maximum reduction in LDL cholesterol from baseline is 24% to 60% depending on the potency of the drug prescribed. Currently available statins and their lipid-lowering effects are presented in Table 38-3.

Response to therapy is assessed after 6 weeks, and statin dose is advanced if LDL cholesterol is not at treatment target. ATP III recommends monitoring LDL cholesterol at 6-week intervals until treatment target is achieved and then every 6 to 12 months when patients are at goal. Failure to achieve target LDL cholesterol after 12 weeks of therapy may require a second lipid-lowering agent or referral to a specialist. Markers of liver function should be checked before starting treatment, although the Food and Drug Administration (FDA) has revised statin drug labels to advise subsequent monitoring of liver function only if there are clinical indications. Statin-induced elevations of liver enzymes are dose dependent and reversible. Statin dose should be reduced or an alternative drug started if alanine aminotransferase (ALT) is persistently more than 3-fold elevated or 3-fold above baseline before starting treatment.

Muscle toxicity is a concern during statin treatment, with complications ranging from myalgias to rhabdomyolysis. Myalgias may occur without elevation of creatinine kinase (CK) levels. Routine CK monitoring is not recommended, although a baseline measurement before starting therapy can be useful. Care should be taken when interpreting CK levels because factors unrelated to statin therapy, such as hypothyroidism or vigorous activity, can raise CK levels. Approximately 2% to 10% of patients will experience muscle-related side effects during statin therapy, and renal failure, obstructive liver disease, and hypothyroidism increase the risk of side effects.

Patients with chronic renal or liver impairment require special consideration if cholesterol-lowering therapy is required to mitigate CAD risk. Atorvastatin and fluvastatin do not require dose adjustments in the setting of severe renal impairment (creatinine clearance <30 mL/min). Patients with well-compensated noncholestatic liver disease and baseline elevations of liver enzymes have been demonstrated to tolerate pravastatin without exacerbation

Table 38-3. HMG-CoA Reductase Inhibitors

Name	Atorvastatin (Lipitor)	Fluvastatin (Lescol)	Lovastatin (Mevacor)	Pitavastatin (Livalo)	Pravastatin (Pravachol)	Rosuvastatin (Crestor)	Simvastatin (Zocor)
Dose (mg)	10–80	20–80	10–80	1–4	10–80	5–40	10–80
LDL effect (%)	38–54	17–36	29–48	32–43	19–34	41–65	28–46
TG effect (%)	13–32	5–35	2–13	15–19	3–15	10–35	12–36
HDL effect (%)	4.8–5.5	0.9–12	4.6–8	5–8	3–9.9	10–14	5.2–10

of underlying liver disease. However, significant elevations of transaminase levels were common in a small study of atorvastatin in patients with primary biliary cirrhosis.

Other drugs that lower LDL cholesterol include bile acid sequestrant resins ("resins"), ezetemibe, and niacin. Cholestyramine, colestipol, and colesevelam are the currently available resins. Resins interrupt the enterohepatic recirculation of bile salts and reduce LDL cholesterol by 15% to 30%. They are not absorbed and do not cause systemic side effects, although they may cause abdominal discomfort, bloating, flatulence, and constipation. Resins are usually titrated slowly to desired therapeutic effect to minimize the risk of side effects. Many drugs bind to resins, limiting their oral bioavailability. Care must be taken when timing the administration of other drugs during resin treatment. Resins may worsen hypertriglyceridemia and should not be used as monotherapy when triglycerides exceed 250 mg/dL.

Ezetemibe is a drug that inhibits dietary cholesterol absorption. It reduces LDL cholesterol approximately 15% to 20% when prescribed as monotherapy, and an additional 25% reduction in LDL cholesterol is achieved when ezetemibe is combined with a statin. Incidence of side effects is low, with no increased risk of muscle symptoms or liver function abnormalities when the drug is used as monotherapy. Liver enzymes should be monitored when used in conjunction with a statin, however, as there appears to be a slightly increased incidence of enzyme elevations with combined therapy. There are no dosing adjustments for renal failure, mild hepatic impairment, or elderly patients. Ezetemibe is not recommended for use in the setting of moderate-to-severe hepatic impairment.

Nicotinic acid (niacin) inhibits production of VLDL and its metabolite LDL. Niacin is most useful in treatment of hypertriglyceridemia and low HDL cholesterol, although at high doses (eg, 1.5 g 3 times daily) it lowers LDL cholesterol by approximately 20%. Use of niacin is often limited by poor tolerability. The majority of patients who take immediate-release crystalline niacin experience flushing, although this can be mitigated by taking aspirin or ibuprofen prior to dosing. Other untoward effects include hepatocellular injury, ranging from asymptomatic elevations of liver enzymes to symptomatic hepatitis, hyperglycemia, hyperuricemia, and worsening of gout, and hypotension in patients treated with vasodilators. Immediate-release crystalline niacin is started at 100 mg 3 times daily and slowly titrated to therapeutic effect (maximum dose 1.5 g TID). Sustained-release niacin (Niaspan®) has reduced incidence of flushing. Starting dose is 500 mg at bedtime, and the maximum dose is 2000 mg. Addition of niacin to statin therapy in patients with CAD or a CAD risk equivalent reduced carotid intima-media thickness and a composite cardiovascular end point compared with ezetemibe in the ARBITER 6-HALTS trial, but addition of sustained-release niacin to statin therapy did not reduce cardiovascular event rates in the AIM-HIGH trial.

A Middle-aged Woman With Combined Hyperlipidemia

A 48-year-old woman seeks health care after her older sister (age 52 years) was diagnosed with CAD. The patient reports that her sister was told she has "high cholesterol." The patient is not taking any medications and is a nonsmoker. Blood pressure is 155/90 mm Hg, but the rest of physical examination is unremarkable. The patient agrees to screening laboratories including a fasting lipid panel. Total cholesterol is 270 mg/dL, HDL cholesterol 34 mg/dL, LDL cholesterol 178 mg/dL, and triglycerides 292 mg/dL. Fasting plasma glucose, serum creatinine, and markers of liver function are unremarkable. The patient agrees to take atorvastatin 10 mg daily. Six weeks later, a repeat fasting lipid panel shows total cholesterol 209 mg/dL, HDL cholesterol 36 mg/dL, LDL cholesterol 124 mg/dL, and triglycerides 248 mg/dL.

1. Who should be screened for lipid disorders?
2. What is the patient's lipid abnormality?
3. How should the patient's dyslipidemia be managed?
4. What can be done to improve hypertriglyceridemia?

Answers

1. All adults 20 years or older should be screened at least every 5 years. Individuals with cardiovascular risk factors (eg, tobacco use, family history, hypertension, diabetes mellitus), established cardiovascular disease, and under treatment for dyslipidemia should be checked more frequently.

2. History and lipid panel suggest familial combined hyperlipidemia (FCHL).

3. Since triglycerides are <500 mg/dL, an HMG-CoA reductase inhibitor ("statin") is the initial treatment of choice.

4. Diet restricted in saturated fat, regular aerobic exercise, and adding a fibric acid derivative, niacin, or pharmacological doses of omega-3 fatty acids (fish oil supplements) are all interventions that are likely to improve hypertriglyceridemia.

CASE REVIEW

Screening for dyslipidemias should begin in all adults aged 20 years or older. Screening is usually performed with a standard lipid profile (total cholesterol, HDL cholesterol, and triglycerides) obtained after a 12-hour fast. LDL cholesterol is then calculated from the Friedewald equation, although LDL cholesterol cannot be calculated when triglyceride levels exceed 400 mg/dL. Assays to directly measure LDL cholesterol are now available.

If a fasting lipid panel cannot be obtained, total and HDL cholesterol should be measured. A fasting lipid panel is indicated if the total cholesterol exceeds

200 mg/dL or HDL cholesterol is less than 40 mg/dL. If lipid levels are unremarkable and the patient has no major risk factors for cardiovascular disease, subsequent screening can be performed at 5-year intervals. Patients with multiple cardiovascular risk factors (eg, hypertension, tobacco use, family history) should be screened more frequently. Patients hospitalized for an acute coronary syndrome or coronary revascularization should have a lipid panel obtained within 24 hours of admission if lipid levels are unknown.

Diagnosis

The patient has a newly diagnosed Fredrickson Type IIb combined hyperlipidemia. The Fredrickson classification of hyperlipidemias and corresponding lipoprotein abnormalities is presented in Table 38-4. The differential diagnosis of lipid disorders was presented previously in Table 38-1.

Although there is insufficient information to make a definitive diagnosis, the patient's pattern of lipid abnormalities and history of a sibling with dyslipidemia and premature CAD raises concern for FCHL. FCHL is an autosomal dominant disorder that occurs in 1% to 2% of the general population and is a potent risk factor for CAD. In a genetic analysis of 157 hyperlipidemic myocardial infarction survivors, 30% were found to have FCHL.

FCHL shows phenotypic heterogeneity, with affected family members and patients also potentially manifesting Fredrickson Type IIa and IV hyperlipidemias over time. It is caused by overproduction of apo-B100; phenotypic variability appears to be a consequence of LDL particle subtype and possible coexisting deficiency of LPL activity. Variability in the type of dyslipidemia is a clue to diagnosis. Historically, diagnosis has been made through demonstration of the phenotype in an affected subject and family members and exclusion of other disorders that may cause combined hyperlipidemia (eg, diabetes mellitus). A nomogram to diagnose FCHL based on measurements of triglycerides, total cholesterol, and apo-B100 has been published.

Table 38-4. Fredrickson Classification of Dyslipidemias

Phenotype	Lipoprotein Abnormality	Lipid Abnormality
I	Chylomicrons	Hypertriglyceridemia
IIa	LDL	Hypercholesterolemia
IIb	VLDL and LDL	Combined hyperlipidemia
III	Chylomicron remnants and IDL	Combined hyperlipidemia
IV	VLDL	Hypertriglyceridemia
V	Chylomicrons and VLDL	Hypertriglyceridemia

Treatment

Since the patient has no symptoms, findings, or history of cardiovascular disease, she falls into one of the ATP III primary prevention risk categories (see Table 38-2). The first step in treatment is to determine the patient's non-LDL CAD risk factors (age, family history, hypertension, tobacco use, HDL cholesterol <40 mg/dL). She has 3—family history of premature CAD, hypertension, and low HDL cholesterol—placing her in either the moderate or moderately high-risk categories. For patients with 2 or more risk factors, a Framingham Risk Score is calculated (http://www.nhlbihin.net/atpiii/calculator.asp). The patient's Framingham Risk Score is 16 and predicts a 4% risk of CAD in the next 10 years. Consequently, the patient falls in the moderate-risk category. In patients with combined hyperlipidemia and triglycerides <500 mg/dL, LDL cholesterol is the primary treatment target. The patient's LDL cholesterol treatment target is <130 mg/dL, and an HMG-CoA reductase inhibitor is the best initial choice for cholesterol reduction.

Non–HDL cholesterol (total cholesterol–HDL cholesterol) is a measure of cholesterol in partially delipidated VLDL and is a secondary treatment target in patients with elevated triglycerides but levels <500 mg/dL. Non–HDL cholesterol treatment targets are 30 mg/dL higher than the corresponding LDL cholesterol treatment target for a given level of cardiovascular risk. The relationship between LDL cholesterol and non–HDL cholesterol treatment targets is shown in Table 38-5.

TLC is emphasized as the initial intervention to lower triglycerides. Non-pharmacological treatments are important in the therapy of hypertriglyceridemia and include low-fat diet, aerobic exercise, weight loss, decreasing or eliminating alcohol intake, changing oral estrogen to transdermal preparations, and good glycemic control in patients with diabetes mellitus.

Fibric acid derivatives (fibrates) are most potent at lowering triglyceride levels and include fenofibrate, gemfibrozil, bezafibrate, and ciprofibrate (bezafibrate and ciprofibrate are not available in the United States). Triglyceride reductions are

Table 38-5. LDL Cholesterol and Non–HDL Cholesterol Targets by CAD Risk Category

Category	LDL-C Target (mg/dL)	Non-HDL-C Target (mg/dL)
Very high risk	<70	<100
High risk	<100	<130
Moderately high risk	<130	<160
Moderate risk	<130	<160
Low risk	<160	<190

dose dependent and range 20% to 50% from baseline. Fibrates are agonists for peroxisome proliferator–activated receptors (PPARs) that reduce VLDL secretion and enhance LPL activity by downregulating apo-CIII expression. They increase HDL cholesterol levels 5% to 20% in part by inducing expression of the major HDL structural proteins apo-AI and apo-AII, although the largest improvements in HDL cholesterol are observed in patients with triglycerides over 500 mg/dL. Muscle toxicity is a potential complication of fibrate therapy, particularly when gemfibrozil is prescribed in combination with statins cleared through the CYP3A4 pathway. Pravastatin and fluvastatin are preferred in combination with gemfibrozil because they are not extensively metabolized by CYP3A4. In the Fenofibrate Intervention and Event Lowering in Diabetes (FIELD) study, there was no increased risk of side effects when fenofibrate was combined with statins, making it the preferred fibrate in treatment regimens that include a CoA reductase inhibitor.

The effects of fibrate therapy on CAD risk in randomized controlled trials are mixed. In the Bezafibrate Infarction Prevention (BIP) trial, Helsinki Heart Study (HHS), and VA High-density Lipoprotein Cholesterol Intervention Trial (VA-HIT), patients with hypertriglyceridemia experienced significant reductions in primary end points. However, in FIELD and the Action to Control Cardiovascular Risk in Diabetes (ACCORD) lipid studies, there was no significant reduction in cardiovascular events among patients with diabetes taking fenofibrate as monotherapy (FIELD) or in addition to simvastatin (ACCORD lipid study).

Niacin is also potent at lowering triglyceride levels, with reductions of 30% to 40% from baseline at doses of 1.5 to 2.0 g daily. Mechanisms of action, untoward effects of therapy, and results of clinical trials have been presented in discussion of the hypercholesterolemia case. HMG-CoA reductase inhibitors may also reduce triglyceride levels by 30%, particularly at high doses (Table 38-3).

Concentrated fish oil supplements contain omega-3 fatty acids (eicosapentaenoic acid [EPA] and docosahexaenoic acid [DHA]) and reduce triglyceride levels 30% to 50% from baseline at high doses (6 g daily or more) by decreasing synthesis of apo-B100 and hepatic triglycerides, with no significant impact on other lipid fractions. Fish oil supplements can be combined with fibrates or niacin to reduce triglyceride levels by an additional 30%. In addition to preparations available over the counter, the FDA has approved a prescription fish oil preparation called Lovaza˙. The most common side effects are gastrointestinal and include nausea and "fishy taste" after eructation (burping). A recent meta-analysis of placebo-controlled trials found no significant impact of omega-3 fatty acid supplements on cardiovascular events among patients with preexisting cardiovascular disease. An earlier meta-analysis of prospective cohort studies and randomized trials found that relatively modest consumption of fish high in omega-3 fatty acids was associated with significant reductions in risk of both coronary and total mortality.

Severe hypertriglyceridemia (triglyceride level >1000 mg/dL) is a risk factor for acute pancreatitis. Hypertriglyceridemia is the third leading cause of acute pancreatitis after alcohol and gallstones. Fredrickson Type I, IV, and V hyperlipidemias may lead to severe hypertriglyceridemia and predisposition to acute pancreatitis. On acute presentation, patients should be managed with total fat restriction until triglyceride level is below 1000 mg/dL. After recovery from acute pancreatitis, patients require management with a fat-restricted diet (<10% cal from fat) and a potent triglyceride-lowering medication such as a fibrate or niacin. Secondary factors such as diabetes mellitus, obesity, or alcohol consumption also need to be addressed.

A 56-year-old Male With Low HDL Cholesterol

A 56-year-old male is referred for lipid management after undergoing 3-vessel bypass grafting. Fasting lipid panel on atorvastatin (Lipitor) 10 mg daily revealed total cholesterol 137 mg/dL, HDL cholesterol 25 mg/dL, LDL cholesterol 92 mg/dL, and triglycerides 98 mg/dL. The patient reports his HDL has historically been <30 mg/dL. The patient's brother also has been diagnosed with CAD and low HDL cholesterol. Medical history is notable for hypertension. The patient is a nonsmoker.

1. What is the patient's most likely lipid disorder?
2. What is the next appropriate step in lipid management?

Answers

1. Familial hypoalphalipoproteinemia.
2. Adjust atorvastatin or add an additional cholesterol-lowering agent to achieve LDL cholesterol <70 mg/dL.

CASE REVIEW AND DIAGNOSIS

Obesity, metabolic syndrome, physical inactivity, tobacco, diabetes mellitus, hypertriglyceridemia, and certain medications (eg, androgens, progestins, beta-blockers, and benzodiazepines) are potential causes of low HDL cholesterol. However, genetic factors also play an important role for some patients. Isolated low HDL cholesterol is defined as HDL cholesterol levels <40 mg/dL in the absence of hypertriglyceridemia, and a genetic disorder of HDL metabolism should be considered.

Familial hypoalphalipoproteinemia is an autosomal dominant disorder characterized by HDL cholesterol less than the 10th percentile for men (<30 mg/dL) and 15th percentile for women (<40 mg/dL) and increased risk of premature cardiovascular disease. It is an autosomal dominant disorder with gene frequency approximately 1:400. The underlying metabolic defect leading to low HDL cholesterol remains unknown, although approximately half of cases can be linked to the apo-AI/CIII/AIV/AV gene locus on chromosome 11. The diagnosis is suggested in this patient's case by persistently low HDL cholesterol and early CAD and first-degree relative with both cardiovascular disease and low HDL. Other hereditary causes of low HDL cholesterol are presented in Table 38-6.

Treatment

Prospective studies in several countries provide convincing evidence for an inverse association between HDL cholesterol level and cardiovascular risk. An important change in ATP III is redefining low HDL cholesterol as <40 mg/dL. HDL cholesterol is important in CAD risk stratification. It is 1 of the 5 non–LDL cholesterol risk factors and an important component of the Framingham Risk Score. Low HDL cholesterol also moves patients with established CAD from the high-risk to very-high-risk category and reduces LDL cholesterol treatment target to <70 mg/dL.

The mechanisms by which low HDL cholesterol leads to atherosclerosis and cardiovascular disease are not fully understood. HDL promotes efflux of cholesterol from foam cells in atherosclerotic lesions, and diminished reverse cholesterol transport from arterial vasculature to liver may be a key factor. Low HDL levels also tend to occur with other atherogenic risks such as hypertriglyceridemia, elevated remnant lipoprotein levels, increased levels of small, dense LDL, and insulin resistance. Low HDL often occurs in the setting of hypertriglyceridemia and metabolic syndrome. Management of these conditions may result in a secondary improvement of HDL cholesterol levels.

There is no formal ATP III treatment target for low HDL level. Although clinical trial data suggest that raising HDL cholesterol will reduce cardiovascular risk, currently available evidence is not sufficient to specify a therapeutic target for HDL. ATP III guidelines emphasize lifestyle modifications including regular aerobic exercise, smoking cessation, moderate alcohol consumption, and higher intake of monounsaturated fatty acids as first-line therapy for low HDL-C. Medications generally have modest effects on HDL cholesterol levels. Statins raise HDL cholesterol 3% to 10%, with rosuvastatin showing highest efficacy. Fibrates raise HDL levels 5% to 20%, although best results are observed in patients with hypertriglyceridemia. Niacin is the most potent agent for raising HDL levels and may increase HDL cholesterol by as much as 35% from baseline.

Optimal treatment for low HDL cholesterol is determined in part by the presence or absence of other lipid abnormalities. In patients with elevated LDL cholesterol level, the primary therapeutic goal is treating to LDL target. Based on ATP III guidelines, the patient's constellation of coexisting CAD, low HDL cholesterol, and hypertension places him in the very-high-risk patient category. Although he is already treated with atorvastatin, LDL cholesterol remains above target (<70 mg/dL), and atorvastatin should be advanced, with addition of a second-line agent such as ezetimibe if necessary, until LDL cholesterol is at goal.

Table 38-6. Hereditary HDL Cholesterol Disorders

Disorder	Mutation	Inheritance	Frequency	HDL (mg/dL)	CVD	Corneal Opacifications
Familial hypoalphalipoproteinemia	Unknown	Dominant	1:400	20–30	+	—
Familial apo-AI deficiency	Apo-AI	Recessive	Rare	<5	+	+
Apo-AI Milano	Apo-AI	Dominant	Rare	~10	—	—
LCAT deficiency	LCAT	Recessive	Rare	<10	+	+
Fish eye disease	LCAT	Recessive	Rare	<10	—	+
Tangier disease	ABCA1	Recessive	Rare	<5	+	+
CETP deficiency	CETP	Recessive	Rare	>100	—	—

TIPS TO REMEMBER

- Lowering total and LDL cholesterol reduces the risk of coronary death, myocardial infarction, stroke, and need for coronary revascularization.
- All adults aged 20 years or older should be screened for hyperlipidemia and treated based on risk assessment. High-risk patients should be treated to LDL cholesterol <100 mg/dL, and very-high-risk patients should be treated to LDL cholesterol <70 mg/dL.
- All patients with elevated lipids should implement TLC including reduced fat diet and regular aerobic exercise.
- HMG-CoA reductase inhibitors ("statins") are treatment of choice for lowering LDL cholesterol. Other options for patients who cannot tolerate a statin include bile acid sequestrant resins, niacin, and ezetemibe.
- Fibrates, niacin, and high-dose fish oil supplements are effective in treating hypertriglyceridemia. Additional interventions including low saturated fat diet, exercise, reduction or cessation of alcohol, and control of hyperglycemia also significantly lower triglyceride levels.

Appendix. Selected Clinical Trials of HMG-CoA Reductase Inhibitors

	Drug	Key Outcome
Primary prevention		
WOSCOPS	Pravastatin	31% reduction in nonfatal MI or CAD death
AFCAPS/TexCAPS	Lovastatin	37% reduction in fatal/nonfatal MI, unstable angina, or sudden death
ASCOT-LLA	Atorvastatin	36% reduction in nonfatal MI or fatal CAD
JUPITER	Rosuvastatin	44% reduction in first major cardiovascular event
Secondary prevention		
4S	Simvastatin	30% reduction in mortality
LIPID	Pravastatin	22% reduction in mortality
CARE	Pravastatin	22% reduction in fatal coronary event or nonfatal MI
TNT[a]	Atorvastatin	22% reduction in major cardiovascular events

[a]Comparison of atorvastatin 80 mg daily with atorvastatin 10 mg daily.

SUGGESTED READINGS

ACCORD Study Group, Ginsberg HN, Elam MB, et al. Effects of combination lipid therapy in type 2 diabetes mellitus. *N Engl J Med.* 2010;362(17):1563–1574.

AIM-HIGH Investigators, Boden WE, Probstfield JL, et al. Niacin in patients with low HDL cholesterol levels receiving intensive statin therapy. *N Engl J Med.* 2011;365(24):2255–2267.

Downs JR, Clearfield M, Tyroler HA, et al. Air Force/Texas Coronary Atherosclerosis Prevention Study (AFCAPS/TEXCAPS): additional perspectives on tolerability of long-term treatment with lovastatin. *Am J Cardiol.* 2001;87(9):1074–1079.

Expert Panel on Detection, Evaluation, and Treatment of High Blood Cholesterol in Adults. Executive summary of the third report of the National Cholesterol Education Program (NCEP) Expert Panel on Detection, Evaluation, and Treatment of High Blood Cholesterol in Adults (Adult Treatment Panel III). *JAMA.* 2001;285(19):2486–2497.

Frick MH, Elo O, Haapa K, et al. Helsinki Heart Study: primary-prevention trial with gemfibrozil in middle-aged men with dyslipidemia. Safety of treatment, changes in risk factors, and incidence of coronary heart disease. *N Engl J Med.* 1987;317(20):1237–1245.

Goldenberg I, Boyko V, Tennenbaum A, Tanne D, Behar S, Guetta V. Long-term benefit of high-density lipoprotein cholesterol-raising therapy with bezafibrate: 16-year mortality follow-up of the Bezafibrate Infarction Prevention trial. *Arch Intern Med.* 2009;169(5):508–514.

Goldstein JL, Brown MS. Familial hypercholesterolemia. In: Scriver CR, Beaudet AL, Sly WS, Valle D, eds. *The Metabolic Basis of Inherited Disease.* New York: McGraw-Hill; 1995:1981–2030.

Goldstein JL, Schrott HG, Hazzard WR, Bierman EL, Motulsky AG. Hyperlipidemia in coronary heart disease. II. Genetic analysis of lipid levels in 176 families and delineation of a new inherited disorder, combined hyperlipidemia. *J Clin Invest.* 1973;52(7):1544–1568.

Grundy SM, Cleeman JI, Merz CN, et al. Implications of recent clinical trials for the National Cholesterol Education Program Adult Treatment Panel III guidelines. *Circulation.* 2004;110(2):227–239.

Jones PH, Davidson MH, Stein EA, et al. Comparison of the efficacy and safety of rosuvastatin versus atorvastatin, simvastatin, and pravastatin across doses (STELLAR* Trial). *Am J Cardiol.* 2003;92(2):152–160.

Knopp RH. Drug treatment of lipid disorders. *N Engl J Med.* 1999;341(7):498–511.

Kwak SM, Myung SK, Lee YJ, Seo HG; Korean Meta-analysis Study Group. Efficacy of omega-3 fatty acid supplements (eicosapentaenoic acid and docosahexaenoic acid) in the secondary prevention of cardiovascular disease: a meta-analysis of randomized, double-blind, placebo-controlled trials. *Arch Intern Med.* 2012;172:686–694. <http://www.ncbi.nlm.nih.gov/pubmed/22493407>.

LaRosa JC, Grundy SM, Waters DD, et al. Intensive lipid lowering with atorvastatin in patients with stable coronary disease. *N Engl J Med.* 2005;352(14):1425–1435.

National Cholesterol Education Program (NCEP) Expert Panel on Detection, Evaluation, and Treatment of High Blood Cholesterol in Adults (Adult Treatment Panel III). Third report of the National Cholesterol Education Program (NCEP) Expert Panel on Detection, Evaluation, and Treatment of High Blood Cholesterol in Adults (Adult Treatment Panel III) final report. *Circulation.* 2002;106(25):3143–3421.

Prevention of cardiovascular events and death with pravastatin in patients with coronary heart disease and a broad range of initial cholesterol levels. The Long-term Intervention with Pravastatin in Ischaemic Disease (LIPID) Study Group. *N Engl J Med.* 1998;339(19):1349–1357.

Randomised trial of cholesterol lowering in 4444 patients with coronary heart disease: the Scandinavian Simvastatin Survival Study (4S). *Lancet.* 1994;344(8934):1383–1389.

Ridker PM, Danielson E, Fonseca FA, et al. Rosuvastatin to prevent vascular events in men and women with elevated C-reactive protein. *N Engl J Med.* 2008;359(21):2195–2207.

Robins SJ, Collins D, Wittes JT, et al. Relation of gemfibrozil treatment and lipid levels with major coronary events: VA-HIT: a randomized controlled trial. *JAMA.* 2001;285(12):1585–1591.

Rosenson RS. Low HDL-C: a secondary target of dyslipidemia therapy. *Am J Med.* 2005;118(10):1067–1077.

Sacks FM, Pfeffer MA, Moye LA, et al. The effect of pravastatin on coronary events after myocardial infarction in patients with average cholesterol levels. Cholesterol and Recurrent Events Trial Investigators. *N Engl J Med.* 1996;335(14):1001–1009.

Schaefer EJ, Lamon-Fava S, Ordovas JM, et al. Factors associated with low and elevated plasma high density lipoprotein cholesterol and apolipoprotein A-I levels in the Framingham Offspring Study. *J Lipid Res.* 1994;35(5):871–882.

Scott R, Best J, Forder P, et al. Fenofibrate Intervention and Event Lowering in Diabetes (FIELD) study: baseline characteristics and short-term effects of fenofibrate [ISRCTN64783481]. *Cardiovasc Diabetol.* 2005;4:13.

Sever PS, Dahlöf B, Poulter NR, et al. Prevention of coronary and stroke events with atorvastatin in hypertensive patients who have average or lower-than-average cholesterol concentrations, in the Anglo-Scandinavian Cardiac Outcomes Trial–Lipid Lowering Arm (ASCOT-LLA): a multicentre randomised controlled trial. *Drugs.* 2004;64(suppl 2):43–60.

Shepherd J, Cobbe SM, Ford I, et al. Prevention of coronary heart disease with pravastatin in men with hypercholesterolemia. West of Scotland Coronary Prevention Study Group. *N Engl J Med.* 1995;333(20):1301–1307.

A 55-year-old Man With a History of Diabetes Mellitus Type 2 and Hypertension

Omar A. Vargas, MD, FACP

A 55-year-old man with a history of diabetes mellitus type 2 comes to your clinic for a 1-month follow-up visit. His blood pressures in the last 2 visits have been 145/90, 140/85, 140/90, and 135/90 mm Hg. Today his blood pressure shows similar numbers. You explain to the patient that he likely has hypertension and appropriate management is important to prevent complications.

Important considerations include blood pressure target lifestyle modifications, medical therapy and additional testing.

CASE REVIEW

Given his history of diabetes, his blood pressure target is <130/80 mm Hg. The BP goal for the general population is <140/90 mm Hg.

You should recommend dietary changes including decrease of sodium intake to less than 2400 mg per day and adoption of the DASH (Dietary Approaches to Stop Hypertension) diet, which is rich in fruits, vegetables, and potassium and low in saturated fats. Weight loss for those who are overweight and aerobic exercise most days of the week for 20 to 30 minutes are also recommended.

Patients with diabetes and hypertension should be treated with ACE inhibitors or angiotensin receptor blockers (ARBs) as they help delay the onset and progression of diabetic nephropathy.

All patients with a new diagnosis of HTN should be assessed for organ damage and the presence of other cardiovascular risk factors. Complete blood count (CBC), basic metabolic profile (BMP), urinalysis (for microalbuminuria), EKG, lipid profile, and fasting blood sugar (or HbA1C) should be obtained at the time of diagnosis.

The *Seventh Report of the JNC-7* defines hypertension as systolic pressure ≥140 mm Hg or diastolic pressure ≥90 mm Hg for the general population, and ≥130 or ≥80 mm Hg for certain groups including patients with diabetes and chronic kidney disease.

Epidemiology

Hypertension affects about 30% of the adult population in the United States and is one of the leading causes of cardiovascular disease including coronary artery disease, stroke, and congestive heart failure. Along with diabetes, it is also responsible for many cases of end-stage renal disease, retinopathy, and peripheral arterial disease (PAD). Approximately 30% of adults in the United States who have hypertension are unaware, and only about 50% of those diagnosed are adequately controlled. The prevalence continues to increase as our population ages and obesity worsens. Hypertension affects all races but African Americans in general have an earlier onset, are more difficult to control, and have a higher rate of complications than Caucasian Americans.

Classification

According to the JNC-7 report, blood pressure is classified as normal, prehypertension, stage 1 hypertension, and stage 2 hypertension. See Table 39-1.

This classification is important as it guides therapy including lifestyle modifications and the choice of medications, and correlates well with the risk of cardiovascular complications. Starting at 115/75 mm Hg, for every 20/10 mm Hg of systolic/diastolic blood pressure elevation, the risk of cardiovascular disease doubles. Patients with prehypertension should be counseled on lifestyle modifications to prevent progression to hypertension. Patients with stage 1 and 2 hypertension should be counseled on lifestyle modifications and started on pharmacologic treatment. In patients with systolic pressures ≥20 mm Hg or diastolic pressures ≥10 mm Hg above goal, initial treatment with 2 medications should be strongly considered.

Diagnosis

This includes proper measurement, confirmation on separate visits, and consideration of ambulatory blood pressure monitoring (ABM) for certain patients.

Proper measurement
Blood pressure should be taken after the patient has been seated quietly for at least 5 minutes, with feet on the floor and the arm supported at the level of the heart. The cuff should cover about 80% of the arm.

Confirmation
Abnormal blood pressure readings should be confirmed on separate visits, and the average of these measurements should be used before making a diagnosis of hypertension.

Ambulatory blood pressure monitoring
Through a portable device, ambulatory BP monitoring provides information on blood pressure during activities of daily living and sleep. There is increasing evidence that ABM might correlate better with end-organ damage and the risk for complications. Blood pressure during sleep should decrease about 10% compared with diurnal measurements. Patients without a nocturnal "dip" (nondippers) have an increased cardiovascular risk. Patients with discrepancies between office and home BP readings (eg, white-coat hypertension) and patients not

Table 39-1. Classification and Management of Blood Pressure for Adults Aged 18 Years or Older

BP Classification	Systolic BP (mm Hg[a]) And/ Or Diastolic BP (mm Hg[a])	Lifestyle Modification	Management[a]		
				Initial Drug Therapy	
			Without Compelling Indication	With Compelling Indication[b]	
Normal	<120 and <80	Encourage			
Prehypertension	120–139 or 80–89	Yes	No antihypertensive drug indicated	Drug(s) for the compelling indications[c]	
Stage 1 hypertension	140–159 or 90–99	Yes	Thiazide-type diuretics for most; may consider ACE inhibitor, ARB, β-blocker, COB, or combination	Drug(s) for the compelling indications Other antihypertensive drugs (diuretics, ACE inhibitor, ARB, β-blocker, CCB) as needed	
Stage 2 hypertension	≥160 or ≥100	Yes	2-Drug combination for most (usually thiazide-type diuretic and ACE inhibitor or ARB or β-blocker or CCB)[d]	Drug(s) for the compelling indications Other antihypertensive drugs (diuretics, ACE inhibitor, ARB, β-blocker, CCB) as needed	

Abbreviations: ACE, angiotensin-converting enzyme; ARB, angiotensin-receptor blocker; BP, blood pressure; CCB, calcium channel blocker.

[a]Treatment determined by highest BP category.

[b]See Table 6 in JNC-7 report in JAMA (below).

[c]Treat patients with chronic kidney disease or diabetes to BP goal of less than 130/80 mm Hg.

[d]Initial combined therapy should be used cautiously in those at risk for orthostatic hypotension.

Reproduced from Chobanian AV, Bakris GL, Black HR, et al. Joint National Committee on Prevention, Detection, Evaluation, and Treatment of High Blood Pressure. National Heart, Lung, and Blood Institute; National High Blood Pressure Education Program Coordinating Committee. The seventh report of the Joint National Committee on Prevention, Detection, Evaluation and Treatment of High Blood Pressure. *JAMA.* 2003;289:2560–2572.

adequately controlled on multiple medications (eg, resistant hypertension) should be considered for ABM. Availability, coverage by insurance, and cost continue to be limitations for widespread use of ABM. Home blood pressure measurement done by the patient (self-BP monitoring) is a reasonable alternative to ABM in those patients.

Approach to the Patient With a New Diagnosis of Hypertension

After making the diagnosis of hypertension, the initial evaluation of the patient should include 3 major goals:

1. Assessment of major cardiovascular risk factors: See Table 39-2.

   A successful reduction in cardiovascular morbidity and mortality depends not only on adequate blood pressure control but also, more importantly, on the modification of *all other* risk factors that together increase cardiovascular events. Patients should have a thorough history and physical examination that focus on the identification of smoking, physical inactivity, obesity, and a family history of premature cardiovascular disease. Laboratory tests for assessment of risk factors should include screening for diabetes, dyslipidemia, and proteinuria. Management of identified risk factors should be done according to established evidence-based guidelines.

Table 39-2. Cardiovascular Risk Factors (Major Risk Factors)

Hypertension[a]
Cigarette smoking
Obesity (BMI ≥30)[a]
Physical inactivity
Dyslipidemia[a]
Diabetes mellitus[a]
Microalbuminuria or estimated GFR <60 mL/min
Age (>55 years for men, >65 years for women)
Family history of premature cardiovascular disease (men <55 years or women <65 years)

[a]Major risk factor.

Reproduced from Chobanian AV, Bakris GL, Black HR, et al. Joint National Committee on Prevention, Detection, Evaluation, and Treatment of High Blood Pressure. National Heart, Lung, and Blood Institute; National High Blood Pressure Education Program Coordinating Committee. The seventh report of the Joint National Committee on Prevention, Detection, Evaluation and Treatment of High Blood Pressure. *JAMA.* 2003;289:2560–2572.

Table 39-3. Target Organ Damage

Heart
Left ventricular hypertrophy
Angina or prior myocardial infarction
Prior coronary revascularization
Heart failure
Stroke or transient ischemic attack
Chronic kidney disease
Peripheral arterial disease
Retinopathy

Reproduced from Chobanian AV, Bakris GL, Black HR, et al. Joint National Committee on Prevention, Detection, Evaluation, and Treatment of High Blood Pressure. National Heart, Lung, and Blood Institute; National High Blood Pressure Education Program Coordinating Committee. The seventh report of the Joint National Committee on Prevention, Detection, Evaluation and Treatment of High Blood Pressure. *JAMA.* 2003;289:2560–2572.

2. Assessment of target organ damage: See Table 39-3.

Heart: Left ventricular hypertrophy caused by long-standing high blood pressure is the initial pathologic change that predisposes to systolic and diastolic heart failure and increases cardiac oxygen demand. High blood pressure promotes atherosclerosis of all vascular beds including the coronary arteries decreasing myocardial oxygen supply and leading to ischemic heart disease. A 12-lead EKG is a useful test for identification of left ventricular hypertrophy and previous or current ischemia or infarction. An abnormal EKG and/or symptoms and signs suggestive of heart failure should be evaluated with an echocardiogram.

Brain: High blood pressure is the number 1 cause of ischemic and hemorrhagic strokes in this country. History should focus on previous symptoms suggestive of transient ischemic attacks or stroke. If present, evaluation of the cerebral circulation and brain parenchyma including carotid Doppler, head and neck magnetic resonance angiogram (MRA), and brain MRI should be considered.

Kidneys: Microalbuminuria (urinary albumin excretion of 30–300 mg/g Cr) is not only an established cardiovascular risk factor but also likely the earliest marker of nephropathy. Chronic hypertension increases glomerular pressure with the development of nephrosclerosis and continuous loss of nephrons. Hypertension is a major cause of end-stage renal disease. The JNC-7 report lists microalbuminuria as an optional test but the European

Society of Hypertension and other organizations recommend it routinely as part of the initial evaluation for hypertensive patients. The urine dipstick is an insensitive test for identification of small amounts of proteinuria.

Retina: Uncontrolled or long-standing hypertension can cause retinopathy and risk for blindness. Patients should have a baseline dilated eye examination at the time of diagnosis.

PAD: As mentioned above, hypertension promotes atherosclerosis in all vascular beds. Patients with symptoms of intermittent claudication should be screened for PAD with an ankle-brachial index. A recent study found that measurement of blood pressure in both arms might help identify patients with PAD. A difference of more than 10 to 20 mm Hg strongly correlated with PAD in this study.

3. Identification of secondary causes of hypertension: See Table 39-4.

A minority of patients (approximately 5%–15%) have an identifiable disease causing hypertension. Thorough history and review of systems along with basic laboratory tests are indicated for all new patients diagnosed with hypertension. The JNC-7 report recommends hematocrit, potassium, creatinine, GFR, and calcium for all patients. In practicality, a CBC and a BMP are inexpensive and include those tests recommended by the JNC-7 providing clues for secondary hypertension. Examples include the association of metabolic alkalosis and hypokalemia with hyperaldosteronism and Cushing, an abnormal creatinine and GFR for chronic kidney

Table 39-4. Identifiable Causes of Hypertension

Sleep apnea
Drug-induced or drug-related
Chronic kidney disease
Primary aldosteronism
Renovascular disease
Chronic steroid therapy and Cushing syndrome
Pheochromocytoma
Coarctation of the aorta
Thyroid or parathyroid disease

Reproduced from Chobanian AV, Bakris GL, Black HR, et al. Joint National Committee on Prevention, Detection, Evaluation, and Treatment of High Blood Pressure. National Heart, Lung, and Blood Institute; National High Blood Pressure Education Program Coordinating Committee. The seventh report of the Joint National Committee on Prevention, Detection, Evaluation and Treatment of High Blood Pressure. *JAMA*. 2003;289:2560–2572.

disease or renovascular disease, an elevated calcium for hyperparathyroid-ism, and polycythemia in patients with chronic hypoxia. Patients who do not achieve blood pressure goals or patients with abnormal initial labora-tory tests should undergo formal screening for secondary causes of hyper-tension. In recent years, obstructive sleep apnea has become one of the most commonly recognized causes of secondary hypertension.

All patients with a diagnosis of HTN should have the following labora-tory tests ordered: CBC, BMP, fasting blood sugar (or HbA1C), lipid pro-file, urinalysis or urine microalbumin, and EKG.

Treatment Considerations

The ultimate goal of identifying and treating hypertension is to decrease the car-diovascular morbidity and mortality associated with it including ischemic heart disease, congestive heart failure, strokes, PAD, hypertensive nephropathy, and retinopathy, among others.

The JNC-7 has established blood pressure goals of <140/90 mm Hg for the gen-eral population and a more strict goal of <130/80 mm Hg for patients with chronic kidney disease and diabetes. Other organizations including the American College of Cardiology/American Heart Association (ACC/AHA) and the American Society of Hypertension (ASH) have issued similar recommendations and have also stated specific goals for other populations, including patients with coronary artery disease, heart failure, or acute coronary syndromes. There are 2 main strategies to achieve blood pressure goals: lifestyle modifications and pharmacologic therapy.

Lifestyle modifications

All patients with HTN or those at risk (prehypertension) including those on phar-macologic therapy should be educated on dietary habits and physical activity that will lower blood pressure. These include the adoption of the DASH diet rich in fruits and vegetables and low in saturated fats. Aerobic exercise for 20 to 30 min-utes most days of the week and sodium restriction to less than 2400 mg of sodium daily, as well as weight loss for those who are overweight, are also recommended (Table 39-5).

Pharmacologic therapy

Multiple drug classes have proven to be effective in controlling blood pressure and decreasing cardiovascular complications. Clinical trials indicate that obtain-ing blood pressure goals are more important than the choice of a specific agent in decreasing morbidity. The selection of medication depends on stage of hyperten-sion, blood pressure goal, the presence of comorbidities for which a specific treat-ment is recommended (so-called *compelling indications*), cost, and side effects, among others. Most patients require at least 2 medications to reach the goal. This is especially true for diabetic patients who often require more than 2 agents to get to a tighter target of <130/80 mm Hg.

Table 39-5. Lifestyle Modifications to Manage Hypertension[a]

Modification	Recommendation	Approximately Systolic BP Reduction, Range
Weight reduction	Maintain normal body weight (BMI, 18.5–24.9)	5–20 mm Hg/10-kg weight loss
Adopt DASH eating plan	Consume a diet rich in fruits and vegetables, and low-fat dairy products with a reduced content of saturated and total fat	8–14 mm Hg
Dietary sodium reduction	Reduce dietary sodium intake to no more than 100 mEq/L (2.4 g sodium or 6 g sodium chloride)	2–8 mm Hg
Physical activity	Engage in regular aerobic physical activity such as brisk walking (at least 30 min per day, most days of the week)	4–9 mm Hg
Moderation of alcohol consumption	Limit consumption to no more than 2 drinks per day (1 oz or 30 mL ethanol [eg, 24 oz beer, 10 oz wine, or 3 oz 80-proof whiskey]) in most men and no more than 1 drink per day in women and lighter-weight persons	2–4 mm Hg

Abbreviations: BMI, body mass index calculated as weight in kilograms divided by the square of height in meters; BP, blood pressure; DASH, Dietary Approaches to Stop Hypertension.

[a]For overall cardiovascular risk reduction, stop smoking. The effects of implementing these modifications are dose and time dependent and could be higher for some individuals.

Reproduced from Chobanian AV, Bakris GL, Black HR, et al. Joint National Committee on Prevention, Detection, Evaluation, and Treatment of High Blood Pressure. National Heart, Lung, and Blood Institute; National High Blood Pressure Education Program Coordinating Committee. The seventh report of the Joint National Committee on Prevention, Detection, Evaluation and Treatment of High Blood Pressure. *JAMA*. 2003;289:2560–2572.

The 2003 JNC-7 report stated that thiazide diuretics should be used as first line for most patients, alone or in combination with other agents. This recommendation was based on multiple outcome trials. The Antihypertensive and Lipid Lowering Treatment to Prevent Heart Attack Trial (ALLHAT) showed that thiazide diuretics were superior to ace inhibitors, alpha-blockers, and calcium channel blockers in reducing cardiovascular and renal risk in patients with hypertension. The report also recommended ace inhibitors, ARB, beta-blockers, and calcium channel blockers as reasonable first-line options. Although these general recommendations are still in place and widely accepted, multiple more recent studies have challenged some of these statements. For example, the ACC/AHA in their 2007 hypertension guidelines did not include beta-blockers as first-line agents for the general population without a compelling indication such as CAD or heart failure as they seem to be weaker antihypertensive agents compared with others.

The following are different populations and the recommended BP targets and first-line medications for them. This includes recommendations based on the JNC-7 report (2003) *and* the ACC/AHA hypertension guidelines (2007):

- General population with hypertension: Goal <140/90 mm Hg. First-line agents include thiazides, ace inhibitors, ARB, and CCB. Beta-blockers are *not* included in ACC/AHA guidelines.

- Diabetic patients: Goal <130/80 mm Hg. Regimen should include an ace inhibitor or ARB based on data showing decreased risk or delay in progression of diabetic nephropathy.

- Chronic kidney disease patients: Goal <130/80 mm Hg. Regimen should include an ace inhibitor or ARB based on data showing delay of progression of nephropathy.

- Stable angina patients: Goal <130/80 mm Hg. Beta-blocker *and* ace inhibitor or ARB-based regimen. If a beta-blocker is contraindicated, it can be substituted with a non-dihydropyridine CCB such as diltiazem or verapamil.

- Acute coronary syndromes: Beta-blockers *and* ace inhibitor or ARB. If a beta-blocker is contraindicated, it may be substituted with a non-dihydropyridine CCB.

- Heart failure patients with ventricular dysfunction: Goal <120/80 mm Hg. First-line agents include beta-blockers *and* ace inhibitors or ARB-based therapy. Additional agents include aldosterone antagonists, loop diuretics, hydralazine, and nitrate combinations.

- Cerebrovascular disease patients: No specific goal. Thiazide diuretics and ace inhibitors might decrease the recurrence of stroke.

- Elderly patients: No specific goal based on age. Use the same general principles as in the general population. More than two thirds of patients older than 65 years have HTN and they have the lowest rates of control. Systolic blood pressure is a better predictor of complications in this group. Thiazide diuretics and ace inhibitors decrease the risk of stroke and overall mortality on the Hypertension in the Very Elderly Trial (HYVET) published in 2008. Elderly patients are more prone to develop side effects, so closer follow-up and careful titration of dosages are warranted. Conflicting evidence suggests that a diastolic BP less than 70 mm Hg might increase the risk of cardiovascular events as it decreases effective coronary perfusion.

- Pregnant women: Ace inhibitors and ARB are contraindicated in pregnancy. Methyldopa, beta-blockers, and vasodilators are preferred agents.

At the time of this publication, the JNC-8 report has not been published. An algorithm for treatment of hypertension from the JNC-7 report is presented in Figure 39-1. The reader is advised to use caution as new information and recommendations are expected to be released within the next year.

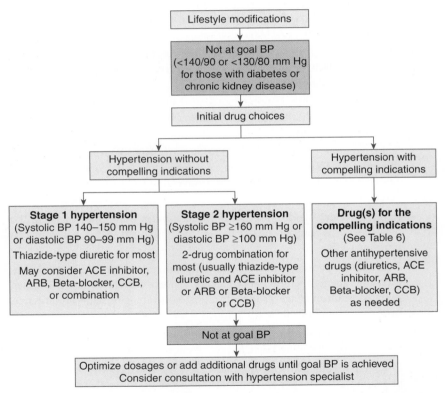

Figure 39-1. Treatment algorithm for hypertension. (Reproduced from Chobanian AV, Bakris GL, Black HR, et al. Joint National Committee on Prevention, Detection, Evaluation, and Treatment of High Blood Pressure. National Heart, Lung, and Blood Institute; National High Blood Pressure Education Program Coordinating Committee. The seventh report of the Joint National Committee on Prevention, Detection, Evaluation and Treatment of High Blood Pressure. *JAMA*. 2003;289:2560–2572.)

Resistant Hypertension

Resistant hypertension is the failure to achieve the blood pressure goal in patients adhering to treatment with optimal doses of 3 medications including a diuretic. Careful evaluation of the patient to exclude "pseudoresistance" caused by improper measurement technique, nonadherence to lifestyle and/or medications, and white-coat effect should be done. Important contributors to resistant hypertension include inadequate diuretic therapy, excess sodium intake, excess alcohol intake, obesity, and OTC or prescription medications that increase blood pressures including NSAIDs, decongestants, and OCP. Patients with resistant hypertension should have an evaluation for secondary causes of hypertension and ideally an ABM study to confirm diagnosis.

The treatment of resistant hypertension should focus on treating secondary causes when present and most importantly on using medications that block different mechanisms of high blood pressure. That includes volume management with diuretics, blockade of the renin–angiotensin–aldosterone system (RAAS), calcium channel blockade, and sympathetic system blockade with vasodilatory beta-blockers (alpha-beta-blockers). Up to 60% of patients will achieve BP control with appropriate diuretic management. For patients with a GFR above 40, thiazides remain the treatment of choice. Chlorthalidone is preferable as it has a longer half-life than hydrochlorothiazide and can be dosed once daily. Loop diuretics should be used once the GFR is below 40. Furosemide has a short half-life and should be dosed twice or 3 times daily. Torsemide has a longer half-life and can be dosed once a day.

Aldosterone antagonists including spironolactone, eplerenone, and amiloride have shown benefits especially in obese patients and those with sleep apnea. Caution with hyperkalemia is warranted.

Secondary Hypertension

Between 5% and 15% of patients with high blood pressure have an identifiable cause. Patients with a history, physical examination, or laboratory tests suggestive of secondary HTN and those with resistant hypertension should have further evaluation to determine etiology.

The most common causes of secondary hypertension include primary hyperaldosteronism, renovascular disease, pheochromocytoma, Cushing syndrome, thyroid disease, and obstructive sleep apnea.

TIPS TO REMEMBER

- Hypertension is the most common cause of ischemic heart disease and strokes in the United States.

- Diagnosis should be confirmed only after multiple readings and using proper technique.
- All patients should have an assessment of end-organ damage and all other CV risk factors.
- Lifestyle modifications include sodium restriction, exercise, and the adoption of the DASH diet.
- Pharmacologic treatment with 2 agents for stage 2 hypertension should be strongly considered.
- Choice of medication should be based on compelling indications, cost, and side effects, among other reasons.
- Thiazide diuretics are a reasonable initial choice for most patients without compelling indications.
- Diabetic and CKD patients should be on an ace inhibitor or an ARB.
- Resistant hypertension is diagnosed after failure to reach goal on 3 medications including a diuretic.

COMPREHENSION QUESTIONS

1. Which of the following is a true statement regarding blood pressure staging?
   A. Normal blood pressure is <120/80 mm Hg.
   B. Prehypertension is a blood pressure between 130 and 139 mm Hg systolic and between 80 and 89 mm Hg diastolic.
   C. Stage 2 HTN is a systolic blood pressure 10 mm Hg above goal.

2. Which of the following is true regarding BP goals?
   A. The BP goal for patients with DM is 140/90 mm Hg.
   B. The BP goal for patients with DM and CKD is <130/80 mm Hg.
   C. The goal for the general population is 130/90 mm Hg.

3. Which of the following is true regarding blood pressure treatment?
   A. Beta-blockers are the medication of choice in the general population.
   B. Ace inhibitors are the treatment of choice for patients with diabetes.
   C. Thiazide diuretics are effective for all patients with chronic kidney disease.

4. Which of the following is true?
   A. Resistant hypertension is the failure to achieve goal after appropriate doses of 2 medications including a diuretic.
   B. A screening test for secondary hypertension should be done in all patients.
   C. Adequate diuretic therapy will improve blood pressures in most patients with resistant hypertension.

Answers

1. **A.** Normal blood pressure is less than 120/80 mm Hg.

2. **B.** Patients with CKD and DM have a more strict goal of BP <130/80 mm Hg.

3. **B.** Ace inhibitors and ARB are the medication of choice for patients with DM and CKD as they help delay onset and progression of nephropathy.

4. **C.** About 60% of patients with resistant hypertension will achieve control after adequate diuretic therapy. Not all patients with HTN should be screened for secondary HTN.

SUGGESTED READINGS

American College of Physicians. *MKSAP 15 Medical Knowledge Self-assessment Program: Nephrology.* Philadelphia, PA: American College of Physicians; 2009.

Beckett NS, Peters R, Fletcher AE, et al. Treatment of hypertension in patients 80 years of age or older. *N Engl J Med.* 2008;358:1887–1898.

Chobanian AV, Bakris GL, Black HR, et al. Joint National Committee on Prevention, Detection, Evaluation, and Treatment of High Blood Pressure. National Heart, Lung, and Blood Institute; National High Blood Pressure Education Program Coordinating Committee. The seventh report of the Joint National Committee on Prevention, Detection, Evaluation and Treatment of High Blood Pressure. *JAMA.* 2003;289:2560–2572.

Clark CE, Taylor RS, Campbell JL. The difference in blood pressure readings between arms and survival: primary care cohort study. *BMJ.* 2012;344:e1327. doi:10.1136/bmj.e1327.

Longo D, Fauci A, Kasper D, Hauser S, Jameson J, Loscalzo J. *Harrison's Principles of Internal Medicine.* 18th ed. New York: The McGraw-Hill Companies; 2012.

Mancia G, De Backer G, Dominiczak A, et al. 2007 guidelines for the management of arterial hypertension: the Task Force for the Management of Arterial Hypertension of the European Society of Hypertension (ESH) and of the European Society of Cardiology (ESC). *J Hypertens.* 2007;25:1105.

Ostchega Y, Dillon CF, Hughes JP, Carroll M, Yoon S. Trends in hypertension prevalence, awareness, treatment, and control in older U.S. adults: data from the National Health and Nutrition Examination Survey 1988 to 2004. *J Am Geriatr Soc.* 2007;55(7):1056–1065.

Pickering T, White W. When and how to use self and ambulatory blood pressure monitoring. *J Am Soc Hypertens.* 2008;2(3):119–124.

Rosendorff C, Black HR, Cannon CP, et al. Treatment of hypertension in the prevention and management of ischemic heart disease: a scientific statement from the American Heart Association Council for High Blood Pressure Research and the Councils on Clinical Cardiology and Epidemiology and Prevention. *Circulation.* 2007;115:2761–2788.

Sarafidis PA, Bakris GL. Resistant hypertension: an overview of evaluation and treatment. *J Am Coll Cardiol.* 2008;52:1749–1757. doi:10.1016/j.jacc.2008.08.036.

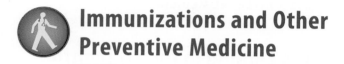

Immunizations and Other Preventive Medicine

Omar A. Vargas, MD, FACP

A 24-year-old Woman Coming for Her Annual Physical Examination

A 24-year-old woman comes for her annual physical examination. She has no pertinent medical history. She takes no medications. She reports no allergies. She is sexually active with a stable partner. She denies a history of STDs. Her last menstrual period was 7 days ago. She denies any symptoms and her physical examination is normal. You review her immunization record and see that she received all the appropriate vaccines during childhood but has not received any immunizations in the last 10 years.

1. Which immunizations should you offer to this patient?

2. What antibody titers (related to immunizations) would it be important to check on this patient?

Answers

1. This patient is a candidate for multiple vaccines. She should be offered the influenza vaccine recommended for all adults. She should start the series of human papillomavirus (HPV) vaccines to prevent cervical cancer and genital warts, as she is within the recommended age group. She should receive the tetanus, diphtheria, and acellular pertussis (Tdap) vaccine that will replace the 10-year tetanus booster.

2. This patient is at risk of becoming pregnant, so it is important to determine immunity against rubella and varicella and vaccinate if appropriate. Women should have rubella titers tested and if negative, should receive the measles, mumps, and rubella (MMR) vaccine.

A 70-year-old Man Coming in for a 6-month Follow-up Appointment

Patient is a 70-year-old man with a history of diabetes mellitus and cirrhosis secondary to hemochromatosis. He comes in for a 6-month follow-up and has no complaints. He takes only metformin for his diabetes. His history and examination are unchanged from previous visits. His immunization record shows a pneumococcal vaccine 7 years ago and a tetanus booster 3 years ago.

1. **Based on his age and comorbidities, which immunizations are indicated for him?**

Answer

1. He is a candidate for several different vaccines, given his age, diabetes, and chronic liver disease. He should receive a 1-time booster of pneumococcal vaccine as more than 5 years have passed since he turned 65. He should receive a dose of Tdap that is recommended for all adults, even those older than 65. Given his chronic liver disease/cirrhosis, he should be immunized against hepatitis A and B if he has not been exposed or does not have protective immunity. He should also receive the zoster vaccine indicated for all adults older than 60 years of age and without contraindications. He should receive an annual influenza vaccine as recommended for all adults regardless of comorbidities or risk factors.

IMMUNIZATIONS AND PREVENTIVE MEDICINE

Preventive medicine includes the routine care of the healthy patient, assessment of lifestyle risk factors, need for immunizations, and screening for prevalent diseases such as hypertension, diabetes, or cancer, among many others.

In regards to lifestyle risk factors, there is evidence that brief primary care–based interventions to modify risk behaviors are effective. This is particularly important in tobacco and alcohol misuse and includes the "5 A's" model for brief counseling: assess (the behavior), advise (clear behavior change advice), agree (mutual collaboration to set goals), assist (aid patient to reach goals), and arrange (schedule follow-up to provide ongoing support). The "5 R's" model can be used for smokers unwilling to quit and includes: relevance (for the smoker to quit), risks (negative consequences of smoking), rewards (benefits of cessation), roadblocks (barriers to quit), and repetition (repeat motivational counseling at future visits).

Screening is defined as an evaluation to detect a disease at an asymptomatic stage. It is appropriate when the population to be screened is accessible and willing to undergo testing, the disease causes burden to patients or society, and the test used is sensitive and specific enough to detect disease without undue false-positives or -negatives. Screening should result in a decrease in mortality. However, screening can also result in significant morbidity to the patient. False-positives tests can generate anxiety, and unnecessary tests and procedures. They can also lead to false-negatives, which gives a false sense of reassurance.

The U.S. Preventive Services Task Force follows rigorous methodology to assess available evidence from clinical trials and issues recommendations for multiple preventive services.

IMMUNIZATIONS FOR ADULTS

The Advisory Committee on Immunization Practices (ACIP) from the CDC annually releases the recommended immunization schedule for children and adults (see Figure 40-1).

In the 2012 schedule, several changes have been made, including new recommendations for Tdap, hepatitis B, and HPV vaccines, among others. Following are some key points about selected vaccines, taken directly from the recommendations:

Pneumococcal polysaccharide (Pneumovax): This 23-valent vaccine is approved for prevention of pneumococcal pneumonia and pneumococcal invasive disease (bacteremia and meningitis). Pneumovax should be given to *all* adults ≥65 years of age. It is also indicated for younger adults with some of the following conditions: chronic cardiovascular or pulmonary disease (eg, CHF, asthma, COPD), chronic liver disease, immunocompromising conditions including HIV, functional or anatomical asplenia including sickle cell disease, and chronic renal failure, and also for all nursing home residents, all smokers, alcoholics, and all diabetics. One-time revaccination 5 years after the first dose is only indicated in patients with renal failure, asplenia, and immunosuppression. Adults who received the vaccine more than 5 years before they turned 65 should also receive a 1-time booster.

Influenza vaccination: Influenza vaccine is indicated for all persons 6 months of age and older. It is available in 3 forms: intranasally administered live attenuated (LAIV), intramuscularly or intradermally administered standard-dose trivalent inactivated vaccine (TIV), and high-dose TIV. LAIV should not be given to patients older than 50, pregnant women, immunocompromised patients, or health care personnel who care for severely immunocompromised persons. The new high-dose TIV is an option for adults older than 65 years. Influenza vaccine is contraindicated if patients have had an anaphylactic reaction to the vaccine or any of its components. Mild allergy to eggs (hives) is not a contraindication for the TIV, but these patients should be observed by health care personnel for 30 minutes after administration.

Recommended Adult Immunization Schedule
UNITED STATES • 2012
Note: These recommendations *must* be read with the footnotes that follow
containing number of doses, intervals between doses, and other important information.

Recommended adult immunization schedule, by vaccine and age group[1]

Vaccine ▼ Age group ▶	19–21 years	22–26 years	27–49 years	50–59 years	60–64 years	≥65 years
Influenza [2,*]	1 dose annually					
Tetanus, diphtheria, pertussis (Td/Tdap) [3,*]	Substitute 1-time dose of Tdap for Td booster; then boost with Td every 10 yrs					Td/Tdap[3/]
Varicella [4,*]	2 doses					
Human papillomavirus (HPV) Female [5,*]	3 doses					
Human papillomavirus (HPV) Male [5,*]	3 doses					
Zoster [6]					1 dose	
Measles, mumps, rubella (MMR) [7,*]	1 or 2 doses			1 dose		
Pneumococcal (polysaccharide) [8,9]	1 or 2 doses					1 dose
Meningococcal [10,*]	1 or more doses					
Hepatitis A [11,*]	2 doses					
Hepatitis B [12,*]	3 doses					

*Covered by the Vaccine Injury Compensation Program.

■ For all persons in this category who meet the age requirements and who lack documentation of vaccination or have no evidence of prior infection

▨ Recommended if some other risk factor is present (eg, on the basis of medical, occupational, lifestyle, or other indications)

▨ Tdap recommended for persons aged ≥65 yrs if contact with <12-month-old child. Either Td or Tdap can be used if no infant contact

☐ No recommendation

Report all clinically significant postvaccination reactions to the Vaccine Adverse Event Reporting System (VAERS). Reporting forms and instructions on filing a VAERS report are available at www.vaers.hhs.gov or by telephone, 800-822-7967.

Information on how to file a Vaccine Injury Compensation Program claim is available at www.hrsa.gov/vaccinecompensation or by telephone, 800-338-2382. To file a claim for vaccine injury, contact the U.S. Court of Federal Claims, 717 Madison Place, N.W., Washington, D.C. 20005; telephone, 202-357-6400.

Additional information about the vaccines in this schedule, extent of available data, and contraindications for vaccination is also available at www.cdc.gov/vaccines or from the CDC-INFO Contact Center at 800-CDC-INFO (800-232-4636) in English and Spanish, 8:00 a.m. – 8:00 p.m. Eastern Time, Monday – Friday, excluding holidays.

Use of trade names and commercial sources is for identification only and does not imply endorsement by the U.S. Department of Health and Human Services.

The recommendations in this schedule were approved by the Centers for Disease Control and Prevention's (CDC) Advisory Committee on Immunization Practices (ACIP), the American Academy of Family Physicians (AAFP), the American College of Obstetricians and Gynecologists (ACOG), the American College of Physicians (ACP), and the American College of Nurse-Midwives (ACNM).

U.S. Department of Health and Human Services
Centers for Disease Control and Prevention

Figure 40-1. Adult immunization schedule. (Centers for Disease Control and Prevention. *Recommended Adult Immunization Schedule, by Vaccine and Age Group.* Atlanta, GA: Centers for Disease Control and Prevention; 2012. <www.cdc.gov>)

Tdap: Pertussis is underdiagnosed and underreported in all age groups. The CDC estimates that the actual burden of pertussis in adults ≥65 years old is at least 100 times greater than reported. There are 2 Tdap vaccines available in the United States, Boostrix and Adacel. ACIP recommends that *all* adults 19 years and older who have not yet received a dose of Tdap should receive a single dose. Tdap should be administered regardless of the interval since the last tetanus-containing vaccine. After Tdap, persons should continue to receive their Td booster every 10 years. Providers should not miss the opportunity to vaccinate all adults older than 65, and either vaccine (Boostrix or Adacel) may be used. Pregnant women should receive Tdap after 20 weeks' gestation or if not received during pregnancy in the immediate postpartum period. It is especially important that all adults in close contact to an infant less than 12 months of age receive the vaccine.

HPV vaccination: HPV infection is the most important risk factor for cervical cancer, genital warts, and anal cancer. Successful vaccination of children is expected to decrease the incidence of these diseases considerably. Two vaccines are available in the United States: bivalent HPV vaccine (HPV2—Cervarix) and quadrivalent HPV vaccine (HPV4—Gardasil). Women should receive either the HPV2 or HPV4 at age 11 to 12 in a 3-dose series or through age 26 if not previously vaccinated. Men should receive the HPV4 at age 11 to 12 or through age 21 if not previously vaccinated. For men who have sex with men, or who are immunocompromised including with an HIV infection, vaccination through age 26 is recommended. HPV vaccine is not a live vaccine and can be safely administered to immunocompromised individuals. It should be administered regardless of a previous history of abnormal PAP, exposure to HPV, or a history of genital warts.

Zoster vaccination: Varicella-zoster virus (shingles) causes significant morbidity in many patients. Postherpetic neuralgia causes severe, chronic, debilitating pain without an effective treatment available. Zoster results from reactivation of past infection with varicella virus (chickenpox). Older age and immunosuppression are clear risk factors. The zoster vaccine has been shown not only to decrease the incidence of shingles but also to decrease the risk of postherpetic neuralgia in affected patients. It is a live vaccine and therefore it is contraindicated in immunocompromised individuals and pregnant patients. Zoster vaccine is currently FDA approved for adults older than 50 years of age, but it is only recommended for adults older than 60 by the CDC-ACIP. A 1-time dose is given regardless of previous history of zoster or chickenpox.

Hepatitis A and B vaccination: Although there are multiple indications for these 2 vaccines, it is important to remember that patients with chronic liver disease should be immunized against both hepatitis A and B and screened for hepatitis C. This is for the purpose of protecting the liver from a second "hit." Hepatitis A and B vaccines are also indicated for drug users, men who have sex with men, and anybody who wants to be protected despite a lack of risk factors. Hepatitis B vaccine is indicated for patients with HIV, those with chronic renal failure on hemodialysis, health care workers, and persons with sexually transmitted diseases or risk factors for them, among others. In the 2012 immunization schedule from the ACIP, there is a new recommendation to vaccinate all diabetic patients younger than 60 years of age as soon as possible after the diagnosis. Diabetics older than 60 years may be vaccinated at the discretion of the health care provider.

Varicella vaccination: All adults without evidence of immunity should be vaccinated. Varicella is a live vaccine; therefore, it is contraindicated in immunocompromised patients and pregnant women. Pregnant women without immunity should receive the vaccine in the postpartum period before hospital discharge.

MMR: Adults born before 1957 are considered immune to measles and mumps. Adults born after 1957 should receive at least 1 dose of MMR if there is no laboratory evidence of immunity or documentation of a dose given on or after the first birthday. For all women of childbearing age immunity against rubella should be determined. If not immune, they should be vaccinated. Pregnant women without immunity should be vaccinated in the postpartum period before discharge from the hospital. MMR is a live vaccine and is thus contraindicated in pregnant women or those who are immunocompromised (except HIV patients with CD-4 above 200 cells/μL).

Meningococcal vaccination: Two vaccines are available for adults, the conjugate quadrivalent (MCV4) and the polysaccharide quadrivalent (MPSV4). The meningococcal vaccine is recommended for patients with anatomical or functional asplenia, those with persistent complement component deficiencies, people who travel to or reside in hyperendemic or epidemic areas (the meningitis belt of sub-Saharan Africa), microbiologists exposed to *N. meningitidis*, and first-year college students through age 21 who live in residence halls. Adults with persistent risk factors should receive a booster every 5 years.

SELECTED PREVENTIVE SERVICES FOR ADULTS

Healthful diet counseling: The USPSTF recommends intensive behavioral dietary counseling for adults with hyperlipidemia or other risk factors for cardiovascular disease and diet-related chronic disease. The USPSTF found only a small benefit for routine counseling about a healthy diet and exercise for adults with no risk factors for cardiovascular disease.

Tobacco use and cessation counseling: The USPSTF recommends screening for all adults and cessation counseling interventions. Use the "5 A's" model for brief counseling and the "5 R's" model for those unwilling to quit.

Alcohol misuse screening: The USPSTF recommends screening and behavioral counseling to reduce alcohol misuse in all adults. (Misuse is defined as >7 drinks per week or >3 drinks/occasion for women and >14 drinks per week or >4/occasion for men or any physical, social, or psychological harm from alcohol use.)

Obesity: The USPSTF recommends screening for all adults and offering intensive counseling and behavioral interventions for weight loss in obese adults (BMI ≥30 kg/m^2).

High blood pressure screening: The USPSTF recommends screening for all adults 18 years of age and older.

Diabetes screening: The USPSTF recommends screening for asymptomatic adults with elevated blood pressure.

Dyslipidemia: The USPSTF recommends screening for all men ≥35 years old and men 20 to 35 years old with risk factors for coronary heart disease (CHD). It also recommends screening for all women ≥45 years old and those 20 to 45 with risk factors for CHD.

Depression screening: The USPSTF recommends screening for adults in clinic practices that have systems in place for adequate diagnosis, treatment, and follow-up of these patients.

Abdominal aortic aneurysm (AAA) screening: The USPSTF recommends screening for all men 65 to 75 years of age who have ever smoked with a 1-time abdominal ultrasound.

Carotid artery stenosis: The USPSTF recommends against screening for asymptomatic adults in the general population.

CHD: The USPSTF recommends against screening for asymptomatic adults at low risk for CHD events. For adults at an increased risk for CHD events, the USPSTF found insufficient evidence to recommend for or against screening.

COPD screening: The ACP recommends against the use of spirometry to diagnose airflow obstruction in asymptomatic patients even in the presence of risk factors. Spirometry should be used to diagnose airflow obstruction in patients with respiratory symptoms.

Osteoporosis screening: The USPSTF recommends screening for all women 65 and older with a 1-time bone density test. Women 50 to 64 years old with a similar risk to that of a Caucasian woman older than 65 should also be screened. This risk can be estimated using the FRAX (fracture risk assessment) tool. This tool can be found at http://www.who-frax.org/. The 10-year fracture risk (FRAX score) of a 65-year-old Caucasian woman is 9.3%. Risk factors for osteoporosis include a mother with osteoporotic fracture, low weight, postmenopausal state, Caucasian race, smoking, alcohol consumption, and chronic steroid use, among others. The National Osteoporosis

Foundation recommends screening for men older than 70 years of age. Men with osteoporosis should be evaluated for hypogonadism.

HIV screening: The CDC recommends routine voluntary HIV screening for adolescents and adults aged 13 to 64 even in the absence of risk factors. The patient should be informed about testing, and the test should not be performed if the patient declines (opt-out screening). HIV screening should be part of routine prenatal testing for pregnant women. Patients with risk factors for HIV should be tested annually. Patients diagnosed with tuberculosis and STDs should also be screened for HIV.

Hepatitis C screening: The current CDC guidelines only recommend screening for patients at risk for hepatitis C. However, in May 2012, the CDC released a draft recommendation to screen all "baby boomers" (those born between 1945 and 1965) 1 single time, since data suggest that 1 in 30 baby boomers can be infected with the virus.

STD screening: USPSTF recommends screening for chlamydia for sexually active women ≤24 years of age and all other asymptomatic women at increased risk for infection. It recommends gonorrhea screening for all sexually active women at increased risk for infection, as well as syphilis screening for all men and women at an increased risk, and all pregnant women regardless of risk factors. Increased risks include: a history of STDs, prostitution, multiple sexual partners, or inconsistent use of condoms.

SPECIAL POPULATIONS

Pregnant women: Pregnant women and their developing babies are especially vulnerable to different infectious diseases, vitamin deficiencies, and metabolic abnormalities that warrant special considerations. All pregnant women should receive the inactivated influenza vaccine during the flu season and the Tdap vaccine after 20 weeks of gestation. Pregnant women who have no immunity against rubella and varicella should receive those vaccines in the postpartum period before hospital discharge. All pregnant women should be screened for HIV, hepatitis B, chlamydia, and syphilis. They should also be screened for asymptomatic bacteriuria with a urine culture between 12 and 16 weeks' gestation, as bacteriuria increases the risk of pyelonephritis and preterm delivery. All pregnant women should be advised to take prenatal vitamins that should include adequate folic acid supplementation (0.4–0.8 mg daily) to prevent neural tube defects. Pregnant women with a history of hypothyroidism need reassessment of their thyroid medication doses as a 25% to 50% increase in requirements should be expected. Although the USPSTF found insufficient evidence to recommend screening for gestational diabetes, the American Congress of Obstetrics and Gynecology (ACOG) recommends that all pregnant women be screened whether by patient history, clinical risk factors, or the 50 g 1-hour tolerance test. The American Diabetes Association (ADA) recommends that women at high risk should be screened with the 50 g glucose test. These include women with at least 1 of the following: >25 years old, BMI >25 kg/m^2, first-degree relative with DM, those from an ethnic group at increased risk for DM, or a previous abnormal glucose tolerance during pregnancy.

Postmenopausal women: In the United States, the average age of menopause is 51 years. The perimenopausal period usually lasts a few years and is heralded by irregularities in the menstrual cycle and hot flashes. Vasomotor symptoms of hot flashes and night sweats are the most common menopause-related complaint. Hot flashes usually last only a few years, but up to 25% to 50% women report a longer duration, up to 10 years in some cases. Estrogens are the most effective treatment with a 50% to 90% response rate. Severe, intolerable hot flashes are probably the only current indication for hormone replacement therapy (HRT). Vaginal atrophy and dryness are common but respond well to estrogen vaginal cream preparations. After menopause, there is a rapid decline in bone mineral density that increases the risk for osteoporosis and fractures. After menopause, women increase their risk for coronary artery disease to that of men. Controversy has surrounded the use of HRT for many years. The results of 3 major studies, Women's Health Initiative (WHI) and the Heart and Estrogen/Progestin Replacement Studies (HERS I and II), have had conflicting results. The WHI study showed an increased risk of cardiovascular events, stroke, thromboembolic disease, and breast cancer for women on the estrogen/progesterone treatment arm. Subgroup analysis suggests that women in the early menopausal period might have in fact had a cardiovascular benefit from HRT. Given the conflicting data and the potential risk for harm, the USPSTF has issued a recommendation against the use of HRT for the prevention of chronic conditions including coronary artery disease and osteoporosis in postmenopausal women. Women older than 65 years of age should be screened for osteoporosis with a DXA scan. Women between 50 and 64 years of age with a similar risk to that of a 65-year-old Caucasian woman should also be screened (FRAX score >9.3%). In 2010, the Institute of Medicine recommended postmenopausal women (up to 70 years of age) take 1000 to 1300 mg of calcium and 600 IU of vitamin D daily. For women older than 70 years, 800 IU of vitamin D was recommended. However, the USPSTF has just issued draft recommendations indicating insufficient evidence to recommend for or against calcium and vitamin D supplementation in postmenopausal women for the prevention of fractures.

Elderly patients: Elderly patients are a susceptible population with significant risks for depression, falls, nutritional deficiencies, polypharmacy, neglect, and abuse, among many others. The USPSTF recommends exercise or physical therapy as well as vitamin D supplementation to prevent falls in community-dwelling adults aged 65 years or older who are at an increased risk for falls. Although the USPSTF has not found enough evidence to recommend for or against screening of all elders for depression, dementia, hearing loss, or visual impairment, the provider should be attentive and perform a detailed history, review of systems, and physical examination. Information should also be obtained from family members and caregivers to assess these issues. The elderly should have their functional status assessed, including their ability to perform activities of daily living (ADLs). Different indices and scales are available to assess ADLs. Elderly patients are more prone to experience side effects from medications and therefore slow titration and low initial doses are recommended. Elderly patients have a blunted sense of thirst and are at a higher risk for dehydration and heat-related illnesses. Home safety evaluations are important for patients especially after hospital discharge or a rehabilitation facility stay.

TIPS TO REMEMBER

● All adults should be screened for obesity, high blood pressure, and lifestyle risk factors such as alcohol and tobacco use.

● Postmenopausal women are at an increased risk for osteoporosis and should be screened at the age of 65. Risk factor assessment should drive the decision to screen before the age of 65.

● Mild egg allergy (hives) is not a contraindication to influenza vaccine.

● Live vaccines are contraindicated in immunocompromised and pregnant patients.

COMPREHENSION QUESTIONS

1. A 40-year-old man comes to your clinic for a routine examination. He has not seen a doctor in many years but feels just fine. He denies any complaints. His review of systems is negative. His social history is positive for a 15 pack year history of smoking. To start counseling for smoking cessation, which of the following interventions are indicated?

    A. Referral to a substance abuse counselor.

    B. The use of the 5 "R's" model for behavioral counseling.

    C. The use of the 5 "A's" model for behavioral counseling.

    D. He is young, asymptomatic, and without other cardiovascular risk factors. Counseling is not indicated at this point.

2. A 20-year-old woman comes to establish care with you. She is sexually active and reports inconsistent use of condoms or other methods of contraception. She

has had 3 sexual partners in the last year. Regarding the HPV vaccine and cervical cancer screening, which of the following statements is true? (Review Chapter 31 for additional information.)

A. She should start the HPV vaccine series if not previously done, and given her risky sexual behavior, a pap smear is also recommended.

B. She has probably been exposed to HPV and vaccination is less likely to be effective; therefore, HPV vaccine is not recommended. She is not 21 years of age yet; therefore, a pap smear is not indicated.

C. She has probably been exposed to HPV and vaccination is less likely to be effective; however, given her age, she should still receive the HPV vaccine. She is not 21 years of age yet; therefore, a pap smear is not indicated.

D. She has probably been exposed to HPV and therefore vaccination is not indicated. She is at higher risk for cervical cancer given her risky behavior; therefore, a pap smear is indicated.

3. A 58-year-old man comes to your office for his annual Medicare visit. He has no complaints. He has a history of diabetes mellitus type 2, dyslipidemia, and hypertension. His social history is positive for a remote 5 pack year history of smoking during his young adult years. His family history is only positive for diabetes and CHD in his father. He has refused immunizations in the past due to a fear of their side effects. He had a normal colonoscopy 5 years ago and a normal PSA 2 years ago. His last HbA1C was 6% 3 months ago. Which of the following statements regarding preventive services for this man is true? (Review Chapter 31 for additional information.)

A. He should be offered a PSA for prostate cancer screening, a repeat colonoscopy for colon cancer screening, and pneumococcal and Tdap vaccines.

B. He should be offered a pneumococcal vaccine, hepatitis B vaccine, Tdap, and zoster vaccine and should be screened for colon cancer with colonoscopy. There is no indication for PSA as he had a normal value before and he is asymptomatic.

C. He should be offered pneumococcal, Tdap, and hepatitis B vaccines. An abdominal ultrasound for AAA screening and a low-dose CT chest for lung cancer screening should also be recommended.

D. He should be offered pneumococcal, Tdap, and hepatitis B vaccines. There is no indication for cancer screening at this time.

4. A healthy 66-year-old Caucasian woman comes to your office asking about osteoporosis screening. She has no family history of osteoporosis, and no personal history of fractures. She takes no medications. She does not drink or smoke. Her review of systems and physical examination are unremarkable. Her BMI is 28 kg/m^2. She takes 600 IU of vitamin D$_3$ and 1000 mg of calcium

carbonate daily. Which of the following statements regarding osteoporosis screening is true?

A. She should be screened for osteoporosis as her BMI is greater than 25 kg/m², putting her at risk for osteoporosis.

B. She has no risk factors for osteoporosis and screening is not indicated.

C. She has a significant risk for an osteoporotic fracture and screening is indicated at this time.

D. Her ethnicity (Caucasian) and age are important risk factors, but given the absence of other risk factors, her overall risk for an osteoporotic fracture is low and screening is not indicated at this time.

Answers

1. **C.** Smoking cessation assessment and counseling are indicated for all adults. The first step is the assessment of the willingness to quit and the understanding of the patient problem. The 5 "A's" model is a useful tool to use initially to counsel patients for alcohol and smoking use. The 5 "R's" model is important in patients who are unwilling to quit after the 5 "A's" model has been applied.

2. **C.** HPV vaccine is indicated in all women between the ages of 11 and 26 regardless of previous sexual history, HPV status, or other risk factors. It is true that this patient probably has been exposed to the HPV and that the vaccine might be less effective than in women never exposed. However, she is likely to benefit because there are different serotypes that can cause cervical cancer. Regarding a pap smear, the current recommendation is to start screening at the age of 21 years regardless of sexual history, so a pap is not indicated at this time.

3. **D.** All diabetic patients should receive the pneumococcal vaccine, and all diabetic patients younger than 60 should start the series of hepatitis B soon after diagnosis. A 1-time Tdap is indicated for all adults. This patient has no symptoms or risk factors for prostate cancer, as well as a previously normal PSA. The USPSTF recommends against PSA-based screening. This patient had a normal colonoscopy 5 years ago and current guidelines recommend colonoscopy every 10 years for average-risk adults with previously normal results.

4. **C.** This patient is a Caucasian postmenopausal woman ≥65 years of age. Her risk for an osteoporotic fracture in the next 10 years is 9.3% even in the absence of other risk factors. The USPSTF recommends screening for all women ≥65 years of age or for younger women with a similar risk to that of a 65-year-old Caucasian woman. Low weight is a risk factor for osteoporosis. The patient is already taking the recommended dose of vitamin D_3 and calcium according to the Institute of Medicine guidelines.

SUGGESTED READINGS

Advisory Committee on Immunization Practices. Recommended adult immunization schedule. United States 2012. *Ann Intern Med.* 2012;156:211–217.

Council for Young Physicians. *Pocket Guide to Selected Preventive Services for Adults.* 10th ed. Philadelphia, PA: American College of Physicians; 2012.

Qaseem A, Snow V, Sherif K, Aronson M, Weiss KB, Owens DK. Screening mammography for women 40 to 49 years of age: a clinical practice guideline from the American College of Physicians. *Ann Intern Med.* 2007;146(7):511–515.

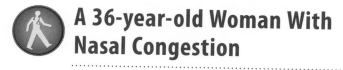

A 36-year-old Woman With Nasal Congestion

Sheryll Mae C. Soriano, MD

A 36-year-old female presents with a 5-day history of clear nasal discharge, nasal congestion, and frontal headaches associated with nonproductive cough. There is no reported fever. On previous similar episodes the patient noted improvement with antibiotics. She has seasonal allergies, and uses loratidine as needed. Vital signs are normal. There is mild bilateral suborbital ridge tenderness present on examination. The nares are patent with a clear mucoid discharge; there is no pharyngeal erythema or exudates, and lungs are clear to auscultation.

1. What is the most appropriate next step?

CASE REVIEW

The patient most likely has acute rhinosinusitis and, thus, symptomatic treatment is recommended. Symptomatic treatments with systemic or local nasal decongestants, saline nasal washes, and NSAIDs have been shown to have some benefit in alleviating symptoms. Antibiotics are unlikely to be effective in most patients who have acute rhinosinusitis as demonstrated by a randomized trial and metanalysis showing no difference in the duration of symptoms between those who were treated with antibiotics and those who were not. Imaging studies such as CT scans and plain films of sinuses with or with out aspiration of sinus/nasal discharge for gram stain and culture are only indicated in cases where a patient is predisposed to atypical infections such as fungal or pseudomonal infections, seen mostly in the immunocompromised. It is recommended to *not* give antibiotics or perform imaging studies in patients with acute rhinosinusitis.

NONSPECIFIC INFECTIONS OF THE UPPER RESPIRATORY TRACT

The common cold, infective rhinitis or nasopharyngitis, encompasses the nonspecific and often uncomplicated upper respiratory tract infections (URIs) without prominent localizing symptoms. They are the major cause of ambulatory visits in the United States, leading to significant direct and indirect costs—accounting for 36 million physician visits per year at an estimated cost of $40 billion annually. They also lead to productivity losses related to lost workdays for adults who get sick and to those whose children get sick. There appears to be a seasonal variation in the United States with increased prevalence from September to March.

Etiology

Viruses are the major pathogens causing URIs. The most common are the rhinoviruses (52%), followed by coronaviruses, influenza A and B viruses, parainfluenza, and adenoviruses. Respiratory syncytial virus (RSV) is a well-recognized cause of URIs in the pediatric population that should also be recognized in the elderly and immunocompromised. Bacterial pathogens are uncommon but those identified are *Chlamydia pneumoniae*, *Haemophilus influenzae*, *Streptococcus pneumoniae*, and *Mycoplasma pneumoniae*. Secondary bacterial infections may complicate viral URIs in 0.05% to 2% of cases and may be manifested as rhinosinusitis, otitis media, or pharyngitis. These often present with recurrent symptoms after an initial improvement, particularly in patients at the extreme of ages and those who are chronically ill.

The mechanism of transmission of viruses and bacteria is via contact with inanimate surfaces and hand-to-hand contact. Hand washing is important to decrease transmission.

Diagnosis

Nonspecific URIs present acutely. Usually they are mild and self-limited. The principal signs and symptoms of nonspecific URIs include rhinorrhea, nasal congestion, cough, and sore throat. Less commonly, fever, malaise, sneezing, myalgia, conjunctivitis, fatigue, lymphadenopathy, and hoarseness may occur. Presentation is variable, which reflects differences in host response as well as in infecting organisms. Physical examination findings are frequently benign, nonspecific, and unimpressive. Although new diagnostic modalities such as PCR of nasopharyngeal swabs are available to identify viral pathogens, the lack of specific effective treatment makes them less useful.

Treatment

Prescribing antibiotics has been a common practice in the outpatient setting for URIs. Antibiotics have no role in uncomplicated URIs as has been consistently demonstrated in clinical trials. Their misuse leads to the emergence of antimicrobial resistance. Symptomatic treatment with over-the-counter decongestants shows consistent benefit in alleviating symptoms. Other symptomatic treatments such as lozenges with topical anesthetics, dextromethorphan, and NSAIDs may be used.

ACUTE SINUSITIS

Acute sinusitis or rhinosinusitis is the inflammation, with or without infection, of the 4-paired sinuses surrounding the nose (maxillary, ethmoid, fontal, and sphenoid sinuses). Acute sinusitis overlaps with URIs in terms of its signs and symptoms. URIs, most often viral, are frequently the precursor of sinusitis. Sinusitis also follows the seasonal pattern seen in common colds—the peak is seen in the winter. When it occurs in children, nearly half will have a coexisting otitis media. The posterior ethmoidal and sphenoid sinuses are more commonly involved in children, and maxillary and anterior ethmoid sinuses are more often affected in adults. Cigarette smoke is a proven risk for the development of bacterial rhinosinusitis due to its effect of reducing the efficiency of the mucociliary clearance of the upper airways. Other risks for sinusitis are allergic rhinitis, cystic fibrosis, asthma, and immunosuppression.

Etiology

Rhinosinusitis can be caused by allergies, or viral, bacterial, and fungal infections. The majority are preceded by URIs, and therefore are often viral in etiology. Viral sinusitis resolves without treatment. Superinfection with bacteria occurs in 0.5% to 1% of URIs. The most common bacterial pathogens implicated are *S. pneumoniae* and nontypable *H. influenzae* (especially in smokers) accounting for 50% to 60% of cases. Methicillin-resistant *Staphylococcus aureus* (MRSA) is an emerging pathogen. Anaerobes rarely cause sinusitis but may gain entry through the premolar teeth adjacent to the maxillary sinuses. *Moraxella catarrhalis* is seen in 20% of children with acute sinusitis. Fungal sinusitis is very rare, but when it occurs, it can be invasive as seen in rhinocerebral mucormycoses and *Aspergillus*. Fungal sinusitis commonly affects the immunosuppressed and patients with diabetes mellitus.

Diagnosis

Acute sinusitis is defined as <4 weeks in duration. It is usually preceded by a URI, hence the overlapping constellation of signs and symptoms of rhinorrhea, nasal congestion, postnasal drip, cough, facial pressure, and headache. Tooth pain and fever may also be seen. Distinguishing viral from bacterial sinusitis is difficult in the ambulatory setting. The purulence of nasal secretion is not sensitive in distinguishing between bacterial and viral sinusitis.

Complicated acute sinusitis is rare and usually presents with painful eye movements, high fever, and periorbital edema/cellulitis with diminished extraocular movements. There may be tenderness over the frontal sinus with soft tissue swelling (Pott puffy tumor), which suggests the presence of a subperiosteal abscess on the frontal bone. Chronic bacterial sinusitis lasts >12 weeks and manifests as constant nasal and sinus congestion with intermittent episodes of increased severity. It may persist for years. Acute fungal sinusitis is seen commonly in immunocompromised hosts. It is usually invasive with proptosis, ptosis, orbital or periorbital swelling, or cellulitis with diminished extraocular movements. These patients appear seriously ill with rapidly progressive deterioration. Acute nosocomial sinusitis manifests atypically, such as with persistent fever, and should be suspected in intubated, hospitalized patients.

Treatment

Discussion in this section mainly focuses on the treatment of acute, uncomplicated sinusitis in the ambulatory setting.

Symptom relief and facilitation of sinus drainage with the use of nasal saline lavage, as well as topical or oral nasal decongestants, are recommended as the initial treatment for mild-to-moderate symptoms of short duration (<7 days). The duration of symptoms has been utilized by experts as a guide, along with diagnostic decision making, to differentiate between likely viral and bacterial sinusitis. Bacterial sinusitis is less common, and especially if symptoms last <7 days, the sinusitis is likely to be viral. Persistent acute sinusitis (symptoms lasting >7 days), along with the presence of purulence, facial pain, and nasal obstruction, was more likely to be bacterial in nature. It is important to note, however, that even in patients who fulfilled these criteria, only 40% to 50% had true bacterial sinusitis.

Penicillin and amoxicillin have shown to be effective in the treatment of bacterial sinusitis. The use of narrow-spectrum antibiotics in persistent and severe community-acquired acute sinusitis is recommended. (Please refer to Table 41-1 for recommended antibiotic treatment.) Broad-spectrum and antibiotic prophylaxis is not recommended and no studies support its use.

Table 41-1. Treatment and Diagnostic Guidelines for Acute Sinusitis

Diagnostic Criteria	Treatment Recommendation
Moderate symptoms (eg, nasal purulence/congestion or cough) for >7 days Or Severe symptoms of any duration, including unilateral/focal facial swelling or tooth pain	**First line** Amoxicillin, 1.5–3.5 g per day divided in 2 or 3 times daily PO for 10 days Penicillin allergy: trimethoprim–sulfamethoxazole 800/160 mg 1 DS tablet PO BID for 10–14 days **Second line** Amoxicillin–clavulanate 500/125 mg BID PO for 10 days Second- or third-generation cephalosporins (eg, cefuroxime 250 or 500 mg BID or cefaclor, 250 or 500 mg TID PO) for 10 days Doxycycline (200 mg day 1, and then 100 mg BID PO for 2–10 days) Macrolides (eg, clarithromycin 500 mg BID or azithromycin 500 mg daily PO for 5 days) Fluoroquinolones (eg, ciprofloxacin 500 mg BID, levofloxacin 500 mg daily PO) for 10 days

In acute disease, CT of the sinuses or sinus radiography is not helpful due to the high prevalence of similar abnormalities among patients with acute viral sinusitis. In the evaluation of persistent and chronic sinusitis, CT of the sinuses is the radiographic study of choice. Sinus aspiration or lavage may be considered in chronic and complicated cases.

PHARYNGITIS

Sore throat is among the top 10 common complaints encountered in the ambulatory setting. It can be an accompanying symptom to URIs when one has postnasal drip causing irritation of the posterior pharynx. Sore throat from pharyngitis can be due to viral or bacterial infection. Sore throat may also be due to gastroesophageal reflux disease (GERD).

Epidemiology

Viral and group A beta-hemolytic streptococcal (GABHS) pharyngitis peaks in the winter and early spring. It has peak occurrences at 5 and 15 years of age, with diminishing risk above 20 years of age, and is frequently recognized in an epidemic pattern. Acute pharyngitis accounts for 1% to 2% ambulatory visits, about 10 million visits per year in the United States.

Diagnosis

Respiratory viruses are the most common cause of pharyngitis. Adenovirus and rhinoviruses account for 80% of cases. Herpes viruses, coxsackievirus, Epstein-Barr virus, and HIV are less common causes. Exudative tonsillitis can be seen in adenovirus (more commonly than in GABHS pharyngitis), and also in coxsackievirus and Epstein-Barr virus pharyngitis.

GABHS, group G or C streptococcus, *Chlamydia, Mycoplasma, Neisseria gonorrhea,* and *Corynebacterium diphtheriae* are the bacterial causes of acute pharyngitis.

Associated symptoms are not reliable predictors of the etiologic agent. The presence of conjunctivitis, coryza, stomatitis, viral exanthem, diarrhea, and ulcerative lesions or sores may point to a viral cause. Exudative pharyngitis with fever, fatigue, posterior cervical lymphadenopathy, and splenomegaly is seen in infectious mononucleosis. In GABHS and non-GABHS pharyngitis, there is an absence of coryzal symptoms such as cough.

Fusobacterium necrophorum causes a life-threatening infection (Lemierre disease) in about 10% of adolescents and young adults 15 to 24 years of age. It is manifested as worsening pharyngitis with neck swelling from suppurative thrombophlebitis of the internal jugular vein. Bacteremia with metastatic infection such as lung abscesses may occur. This disease requires intensive care, including anaerobic coverage with antibiotics and surgical drainage.

Treatment

The primary task of the physician is to distinguish between non-GABHS and GABHS pharyngitis. The reason for this is to adequately treat GABHS pharyngitis to improve symptoms, reduce spread, and reduce the complications such as peritonsillar abscess, poststreptococcal glomerulonephritis, and rheumatic fever. The necessity of this task led to the development of the 4-point Centor criteria. One point is given for each of the following: subjective or documented fever (temperature >38.1°C/100.5°F), absence of cough, tonsillar exudates, and tender anterior cervical lymphadenopathy. Each score corresponds to recommended testing and treatment (Table 41-2). Fulfillment of 3 or 4 criteria has a positive predictive value of 40% to 60%, whereas the absence of 3 or 4 criteria has a negative predictive value of about 80% for GABHS infection.

The rapid streptococcal antigen detection test has a high degree of specificity (90%–95%) but a sensitivity range of 65% to 95% when compared with standard blood agar throat culture. (However, the latter will also identify patients who are colonized but may not be infected.) The rapid antigen test is more cost-effective, and thus recommended. Other available tests for other pathogens such as the heterophile agglutination assay in suspected infectious mononucleosis, and gonorrhea cultures are available.

Treatment failure occurs in 11% to 45% of penicillin V–treated patients. Alternative antibiotics such as amoxicillin appear to be effective with lower rates of treatment failure (5%–10%). Other antibiotics such as azithromycin and clarithromycin have not shown better results than penicillin and amoxicillin. They are used as alternatives for patients with a penicillin allergy. Other second-line agents are first-generation cephalosporins (eg, cephalexin 50 mg/kg per day PO in 4 divided doses for 10 days and clindamycin 20 mg/kg per day PO in 3 divided doses for 10 days).

Table 41-2. Clinical Predictors for GABHS Infection by Centor Criteria

Centor Score	Recommended Testing	Treatment
0	No test	Symptomatic
1	No test	Symptomatic
2	Rapid streptococcal antigen detection test	If positive, penicillin V[a] or amoxicillin[b]
3	Rapid streptococcal antigen detection test	If positive, penicillin V[a] or amoxicillin[b]
	No test	Empiric penicillin V[a] or amoxicillin[b]
4	No test	Empiric penicillin V[a] or amoxicillin[b]

[a]Penicillin V 500 mg BID for 10 days.
[b]Amoxicillin 40 mg/kg per day for 10 days.

The carrier state does not require treatment. Antibiotic use in non-GABHS pharyngitis, *Mycoplasma* and *Chlamydia* in particular, may offer symptomatic improvement, but indiscriminate antibiotic therapy for these infections should be avoided until a specific test for them is developed. Testing for cure in GABHS pharyngitis is unnecessary. *N. gonorrhea* pharyngitis requires antibiotic treatment with ceftriaxone or fluoroquinolones.

Of note, the feared complications from GABHS pharyngitis, poststreptococcal glomerulonephritis and rheumatic fever, are rare and antibiotics have not been shown to prevent these complications.

Tonsillectomy may benefit children with repeated episodes of GABHS pharyngitis (3 or more episodes in 6 months or 4 episodes in 12 months), as well as in adults where it may lessen the incidence of further recurrence.

TIPS TO REMEMBER

- The common cold and acute sinusitis are commonly of viral etiology; particular attention to hand washing is important in decreasing transmission.
- Antibiotic use in uncomplicated URIs and acute sinusitis of <7 days' duration has no proven benefit, and instead may facilitate emergence of antibiotic resistance. Therefore, its routine use is not recommended.
- Narrow-spectrum antibiotics are used in acute sinusitis with moderate-to-severe symptoms of >7 days' duration.
- CT of the sinuses is the preferred imaging modality in persistent, chronic, or complicated sinusitis.
- Antibiotics are not recommended for patients presenting with acute pharyngitis with none or only 1 of the following features (Centor criteria): fever, tender cervical lymphadenopathy, tonsillar exudate, and absence of cough.
- Rapid streptococcal antigen testing is a cost-effective diagnostic test when used with Centor criteria, but throat culture remains the gold standard diagnostic test for GABHS pharyngitis.
- The first-line antibiotic of choice in patients with GABHS is penicillin V 500 mg BID or amoxicillin 40 mg/kg per day for 10 days.

COMPREHENSION QUESTIONS

1. A 46-year-old man with well-controlled hypertension is seen in the clinic due to a 5-day history of nasal congestion, rhinorrhea, sore throat, and nonproductive cough. He denies fever, history of allergic rhinitis, or sick contacts. His current medications include hydrochlorothiazide and ibuprofen for occasional body aches. He says antibiotics have helped in his past episodes. On physical examination, his temperature is 37.4°C (99.4°F). There is clear nasal discharge, mildly congested turbinates, and no pharyngeal exudate or cervical lymphadenopathy, and he has clear lungs.

What treatment has shown symptomatic benefit in patients with the above complaints?

2. A 28-year-old woman presents with a 2-week history of sinus congestion. It started initially with sneezing, rhinorrhea, and nasal congestion. She self-treated with over-the-counter oral pseudoephedrine and diphenhydramine, and initially felt better. However, her nasal congestion returned with yellowish nasal secretions, which have increased, and she started to have low-grade fevers, headache, and facial fullness. On physical examination, her temperature is 37.3°C (99.2°F). Her turbinates are swollen and erythematous with a thick yellow nasal discharge and she has left maxillary tenderness. What is the most appropriate next step in managing this patient?

3. A 23-year-old female day care teacher presents with a 2-day history of a sore throat associated with pain on swallowing, rhinorrhea, nonproductive cough, and generalized body aches. There is no associated rash or fever. She has no past medical history or allergies. Her vital signs are normal. There is no cervical lymphadenopathy. There are bilateral white tonsillar exudates present. What is the best next step?

4. A 34-year-old woman is evaluated for a 4-day history of sore throat, malaise, and low-grade fever. She denies nasal discharge or cough. She has not had any contact with persons who are ill. She has no drug allergies. On physical examination, temperature is 38.1°C (100.5°F). She has clear lungs. The oropharynx is erythematous with minimal whitish exudates, but tonsils are not enlarged. She has tender anterior cervical lymphadenopathy. What is the most appropriate management?

5. A 19-year-old male has a 3-day history of a sore throat, malaise, increasing fatigue, low-grade fever, and nonproductive cough. He has no known drug allergies and takes no medications. His girlfriend had these same symptoms 2 weeks ago but has now recovered. On physical examination, temperature is 38.1°C (100.5°F). The patient has clear lungs, and there is a faint macular rash on his torso. He has no tonsillopharyngeal exudates but has bilateral posterior nontender cervical lymphadenopathy. Rapid streptococcal antigen test is negative. What should be done next?

Answers

1. The patient has a URI, most likely viral in etiology. Treatment for URIs is mainly supportive with nasal decongestants such as pseudoephedrine, which has been shown to lessen the severity of symptoms, although it does not shorten the duration of the illness. Antihistamines, ascorbic acid, zinc, and echinacea have all shown mixed results, and therefore there is insufficient evidence to support their use. Pseudoephedrine is safe in patients with adequately controlled hypertension.

2. This patient meets the criteria for acute rhinosinusitis. She has had symptoms of more than 1 week. Her illness started as a common cold and improved with nasal decongestants. However, her symptoms subsequently worsened ("double sickening phenomenon"). Since her symptoms are more severe (fever and facial pain) and have exceeded 7 to 10 days, she will likely benefit from narrow-spectrum antibiotics (amoxicillin, trimethoprim–sulfamethoxazole, or doxycycline for 10 days) that cover *S. pneumoniae* and *H. influenzae* to reduce the duration of symptoms. Of note, the character of the nasal discharge or presence of facial pain is not a reliable sign of acute sinusitis.

3. This patient is at very low risk for GABHS because her Centor score is 1 (based on the presence of tonsillar exudates). Conservative management to reduce her symptoms is sufficient. The 4-point Centor criteria were developed to guide the management of acute pharyngitis in distinguishing GABHS infection from other causes. It assigns 1 point for each of the following: fever, absence of cough, presence of tender cervical lymphadenopathy, and tonsillar exudates (see Table 41-2).

4. Her Centor score is 4; therefore, empiric treatment without testing is warranted. Amoxicillin for 10 days should be started.

5. The patient meets 2 of the Centor criteria (fever, cervical lymphadenopathy); therefore, doing a rapid streptococcal antigen test is warranted. The test was however negative. The diagnosis of infectious mononucleosis should be considered in patients presenting with pharyngitis associated with fever and lymphadenopathy, most often involving the posterior cervical lymph nodes. A heterophile antibody (monospot) test to diagnose infectious mononucleosis is indicated in this patient. He also has a rash and his girlfriend was recently sick. He has had possible exposure to Epstein-Barr virus, which is the etiologic agent for infectious mononucleosis (also known as the "kissing disease").

SUGGESTED READINGS

Alguire P, Kroenke K, Ende J, et al. *MKSAP 15 General Internal Medicine*. Philadelphia, PA: American College of Physicians; 2010.

Centor R, Allison J, Cohen S. Pharyngitis management: defining the controversy. *J Gen Intern Med*. 2007;22:127–130.

Longo D, Fauci A, Kasper D, Hauser S, Jameson J, Loscalzo J. *Harrison's Principle of Internal Medicine*. 18th ed. New York, NY: McGraw-Hill; 2011.

Mainous A III, Pomeroy C. *Management of Antimicrobials in Infectious Diseases: Impact of Antibiotic Resistance*. 2nd ed. New York, NY: Humana Press; 2010.

Turner B, Williams S, Taichman D. In the clinic. Acute sinusitis. *Ann Intern Med*. 2010;153: ITC3-3–ITC3-16. American College of Physicians; 2010.

Wong D, Blumberg D, Lowe L. Guidelines for the use of antibiotics in acute upper respiratory tract infections. *Am Fam Physician*. 2006;74(6):956–966.

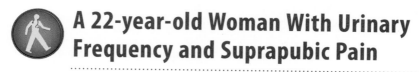

A 22-year-old Woman With Urinary Frequency and Suprapubic Pain

Muralidhar Papireddy, MD and Susan Thompson Hingle, MD

A 22-year-old female presents to the ED with 3 days of increased urinary frequency and suprapubic pain after micturition. She has no fevers, chills, or flank pain, nausea or vomiting, and urethral discharge. There have been no similar complaints in the past. She is sexually active and uses a barrier mode of contraception. She has no history of sexually transmitted diseases. She has no allergies to medications or food. Physical examination is unremarkable. Spot urinary pregnancy test is negative. Urinalysis is significant for 12 white blood cells (WBCs) and 3 red blood cells (RBCs), and the urine is nitrite positive. She has no primary care physician.

1. What is the diagnosis and the next step of action?

Answer

1. Simple or uncomplicated urinary tract infection. Prescribing short course (3 days) of Bactrim or ciprofloxacin is the next step as she has an uncomplicated lower urinary tract infection that can be managed as an outpatient. She does not need admission to the hospital or need imaging as she has a simple UTI.

CASE REVIEW

Urinary tract infection is one of the commonest infections encountered by a physician. Clinical presentation could range from annoying urinary symptoms to severe sepsis and death. Further management depends on the severity of the infection. In the above case, the patient is a sexually active young female with no systemic symptoms or comorbid conditions. Lower urinary tract infections are common among sexually active women due to the anatomy of the female urinary tract. Short antibiotic therapy without further imaging is the best course of management for this patient.

URINARY TRACT INFECTIONS

Simple or uncomplicated UTIs are urinary tract infections occurring in healthy premenopausal women without structural or neurological abnormalities. Rest of the UTIs are classified as complicated (males, pregnancy, immunosuppression, diabetes, structural abnormalities including stones, strictures, neurogenic bladder, tumors, etc).

Urinary tract infections are classified on an anatomical basis into lower and upper UTIs. Lower urinary tract infections include urethritis, cystitis, prostatitis, and epididymitis. Upper urinary tract infections include pyelonephritis. We will discuss topics related to cystitis and pyelonephritis in this section.

Common Organisms Causing UTIs

E. coli, Proteus, Klebsiella, Pseudomonas, Staphylococcus saprophyticus, Chlamydia (suspect in patients with history of STDs), and *Candida* (in patients with indwelling Foley catheter or immunosuppression).

Cystitis

Cystitis is the infection/inflammation of the urinary bladder and patients present with urinary frequency, urgency, dysuria, suprapubic discomfort/pain, and hematuria. Physical examination may be positive for suprapubic tenderness.

Cystitis is a clinical diagnosis, and routine urinalysis or reflex cultures are not required unless there is a recurrence. Urinalysis is considered positive if any of the following are present; nitrite positive or LE positive or >10 WBC/hpf. Men are treated for longer duration due to the concern of prostatitis. Empiric treatment is as per Tables 42-1 and 42-2.

Pyelonephritis

Pyelonephritis is the infection of the kidney and patients present with fevers, chills, rigors, nausea/vomiting, and flank pain along with symptoms of cystitis. Elderly patients may present with confusion and vague abdominal pain with or without symptoms of cystitis. Costovertebral angle tenderness is a common physical finding in pyelonephritis. Urinalysis, urine cultures, and blood cultures should be done prior to starting antibiotics.

Table 42-1. Empiric Treatment of Simple Cystitis

Empiric antibiotics for women
Trimethoprim–sulfamethoxazole double strength PO bid × 3 days *or* nitrofurantoin 100 mg PO bid × 5–7 days
Trimethoprim 100 mg PO bid × 7 days *or* fosfomycin 3 g × 1 dose (less efficacy compared with Bactrim or quinolones)
Ciprofloxacin 250 mg PO bid × 3 days *or* levofloxacin 250 mg daily for 3 days
Beta-lactams 3–7 days

Table 42-2. Empiric Treatment of Pyelonephritis and Complicated Cystitis

Empiric antibiotics for outpatient treatment

Ciprofloxacin 500 mg PO bid or levofloxacin 500 mg PO daily × 7 days

Trimethoprim–sulfamethoxazole double strength PO bid for 14 days

If presenting to the ED, may use 1 dose of ceftriaxone 1 g IV and discharge on quinolones or trimethoprim–sulfamethoxazole

Empiric antibiotics for inpatient treatment

Intravenous ciprofloxacin 400 mg Q 12 h, or levofloxacin 500 mg daily

Intravenous ceftriaxone 1 g daily

Aminoglycosides with or without ampicillin

Patients presenting with sepsis should receive carbapenems to cover for extended-spectrum beta-lactamases (ESBL) until the culture sensitivities are available

Treat complicated pyelonephritis for 10–14 days.

Pyelonephritis is a clinical diagnosis. There is no need for imaging on presentation. CT of the abdomen and pelvis in the image of choice. Do imaging if the patient remains febrile for more than 48 hours after being on appropriate antibiotic therapy. Consider early imaging in patients with diabetes or immunosuppression to look for complications of pyelonephritis including perinephric abscess, gangrenous pyelonephritis, and emphysematous pyelonephritis. Consider cyst abscess in patients with underlying cystic kidney disease.

UA shows pyuria (WBC >10/hpf) or is positive for leukocyte esterase or nitrites with or without positive urine cultures. Complete occlusion of the ureter may give a normal UA or negative cultures, as the infected part is compartmentalized. Blood cultures are positive in up to 20% of patients, but it has no prognostic significance.

Criteria for admission to the hospital depend on clinical condition. If the patient is in sepsis or dehydrated from poor oral intake due to severe nausea/vomiting and not able to take oral medication, then he or she should be admitted for intravenous antibiotics, hydration, and close monitoring. Otherwise, he or she can be managed in the outpatient setting with close-monitoring. Start empiric antibiotics as in Table 42-2. De-escalate to appropriate antibiotics on availability of sensitivities. The patient may need urgent urological intervention if there are signs of ureteral obstruction or perinephric fluid collections. Young women often present with much severe flank pain and systemic symptoms that last longer than the other groups of patients due to degree of inflammation. Patients may be discharged if they are afebrile for more than 24 hours and are able to tolerate PO antibiotics.

Asymptomatic Bacteriuria (ASB)

Urine culture growing more than 100,000 colony-forming units (cfu) without symptoms of UTI. ASB increases with age and is more common in women. Screen for ASB only in pregnant women and patients going for urological procedures that cause mucosal bleeding. These are the patients who benefit from treatment. Some data suggest screening might help in patients going for hip surgery. If someone else did the culture and you have the results, stick to the same principle. Do not treat culture results, except for those special populations as listed above.

Patients With Indwelling Bladder Catheter

There is no need for routine screening for UTI. Patients may not have typical symptoms. Screen for UTI if the patient has fevers, flank pain, suprapubic pain, hematuria, or sepsis. In these cases, remove the indwelling catheter and repeat the cultures via a new catheter or midstream urine sample for UA and urine cultures. Treat for 7 to 14 days if criteria for catheter-associated UTI are met. Candiduria is common with indwelling catheters, especially if patients are on antibiotics or are diabetic. Replace the Foley catheter and repeat the cultures. If still positive, treat with fluconazole 100 mg PO for 5 days. Avoid the use of a long-term catheter if not indicated. Intermittent catheterization is better than an indwelling catheter, if feasible.

Recurrent Cystitis and Prophylaxis

If the symptoms do not resolve or recur within 2 weeks, problem could be due to resistant organisms or rarely reinfection. Obtain urine cultures and treat with a more broad-spectrum antibiotic such as quinolones. If the symptoms recur after a month, use short course of the first-line agents but a different antibiotic.

Prophylactic antibiotics (Table 42-3) may be considered if the patient is willing and in cases of 3 or more episodes of cystitis in 1 year, or 2 or more episodes in 6 months of which at least 1 is culture proven.

Other behavioral and biologic agents for prophylaxis are mentioned in Table 42-3.

TIPS TO REMEMBER

- Significant bacteriuria:
  - For clean catheter sample in men and women: 100 cfu/mL
  - For clean catheter sample or midstream urine for catheter-associated UTI: 1000 cfu/mL; catheter removed within last 48 hours
  - For midstream urine in men for UTI: 10,000 cfu/mL

Table 42-3. Prophylactic Measures for Recurrent Urinary Tract Infections

Antibiotics for prophylaxis postcoital or daily
Nitrofurantoin 50–100 mg
TMP-SMX, 40–200 mg (3 times weekly is also effective) (Category C medication, may cause adverse events to the fetus)
Cephalexin 250 mg (125 mg is also effective if taken daily)
Fosfomycin 3 g every 10 days
Nonantimicrobial prophylaxis
Reduction in frequency or abstinence of intercourse (not a feasible strategy)
Avoid spermicide or spermicide-coated barrier method of contraception
Urinate after intercourse
Cranberry juice or tablets (recent RCT showed no benefit)
Topical estrogens in postmenopausal women (not systemic)

- ▪ For midstream urine in women for UTI: 100,000 cfu/mL
- ▪ For midstream urine in both men and women for ASB: 100,000 cfu/mL
- ● Pyuria: WBC >10 in unspun midstream urine. LE positivity suggests WBCs are present in the urine. May repeat UA if WBCs are not seen but LE is positive, but it is a good enough indicator for pyuria if the patient has symptoms of UTI.
- ● Nitrites: Enterobacteriaceae reduce nitrate to nitrite. Suggest bacteriuria >100,000 cfu/mL. There can be false-positives with beet consumption or with use of phenazopyridine.
- ● Treat simple UTI with short course of trimethoprim–sulfamethoxazole or nitrofurantoin or fosfomycin as first-line agents. Quinolones and beta-lactams are second-line agents.
- ● If there is a complicated UTI, treat for 7 to 14 days. Drugs of choice—quinolones or trimethoprim–sulfamethoxazole as an outpatient. Longer duration of antibiotics in men, due to the concern of prostatitis.
- ● Severe pyelonephritis needs admission to the hospital and treatment with IV antibiotics such as ceftriaxone or quinolones. If septic from UTI, use carbapenems until the sensitivities are available to cover for extended-spectrum beta-lactamase (ESBL)–producing *E. coli*.
- ● Use ampicillin, cephalosporins, or trimethoprim–sulfamethoxazole in pregnant women. Do not use trimethoprim–sulfamethoxazole in late pregnancy and early nursing mothers to prevent neonatal jaundice. Do not use quinolones or tetracyclines.

- Imaging of the GU tract is not necessary unless the patient is critically ill on presentation or if there is no improvement of symptoms in 48 hours despite appropriate antibiotic therapy.

- Men do not need imaging with their first UTI, but will need further evaluation to rule out structural abnormalities if the treatment fails or the patient has a repeat infection.

- Think about chronic prostatitis in a man with ASB or in one who has had recurrent UTIs with no other structural abnormalities.

- Do not treat candiduria in a patient with an indwelling Foley catheter. First, remove the catheter and repeat the midstream urine cultures before or after insertion of a new Foley catheter.

- Routine UA and cultures should be ordered only if the patient is a pregnant woman or for any patient about to undergo urological procedures. Only these patients should be treated for bacteriuria without symptoms.

- Do not order routine UA. Most diagnoses are clinical, and the labs should be ordered only to confirm or refute your diagnosis.

COMPREHENSION QUESTION

1. A 57-year-old man presents with nausea, vomiting, and fevers for 1 day. He also complains of dark urine. He had burning micturition for 1 day a few days ago, along with colicky abdominal pain radiating to the groin. He had a similar episode 2 weeks ago that improved with levofloxacin 500 mg PO daily for 7 days. Urine culture was done at that time, but the results are not available. Physical examination is significant for a temperature of 102.6°F, heart rate of 116 bpm, BP 112/70 mm Hg, saturating 98% on room air, and respiratory rate of 20/min. There is costovertebral angle tenderness on the right. CBC is significant for elevated WBCs at 15,000 cells/mm^3 with a left shift. Urine is dark with increased specific gravity, otherwise unremarkable. Urine and blood cultures are sent. What is the best next step of action?

        A. Admit to medicine floor, start fluids and IV meropenem, and obtain a CT of the abdomen and pelvis with renal protocol.

        B. Switch to PO ciprofloxacin and discharge home.

        C. Do a rectal examination, and if the prostate examination is unremarkable, discharge with PO Bactrim.

        D. Admit; call Urology and Infectious Disease consults for the management of pyelonephritis.

Answer

1. **A.** Patient probably has a renal calculus that is acting as a nidus for recurrent infection. If the calculus is completely occluding the ureter, the UA can be

normal. The patient in this case has sepsis and needs to be admitted to the hospital for IV antibiotics, hydration, and closer monitoring. He needs imaging to look for complications of pyelonephritis and hydronephrosis that may need surgical intervention, as there is a concern of stone impaction. Patients in sepsis should be covered for ESBLs until the sensitivities are available. Carbapenems are the preferred agents. Antibiotics should be switched as per the sensitivities available from urine or blood cultures.

SUGGESTED READINGS

Barbosa-Cesnik C, Brown MB, Buxton M, et al. Cranberry juice fails to prevent recurrent urinary tract infection: results from a randomized placebo-controlled trial. *Clin Infect Dis*. 2011 1;52(1):23–30.

Gupta K, Hooton TM, Naber KG, et al. International clinical practice guidelines for the treatment of acute uncomplicated cystitis and pyelonephritis in women: a 2010 update by the Infectious Diseases Society of America and the European Society for Microbiology and Infectious Diseases. *Clin Infect Dis*. 2011;52:e103–e120.

Hooton TM. Clinical practice. Uncomplicated urinary tract infection. *N Engl J Med*. 2012;366(11): 1028–1037.

Hooton TM, Bradley SF, Cardenas DD, et al. Diagnosis, prevention, and treatment of catheter-associated urinary tract infection in adults: 2009 international clinical practice guidelines from the Infectious Diseases Society of America. *Clin Infect Dis*; 2010;50:625–663.

McMurray BR, Wrenn KD, Wright SW. Usefulness of blood cultures in pyelonephritis. *Am J Emerg Med*. 1997;15(2):137–140.

Nicolle LE, Bradley S, Colgan R, et al. Infectious Diseases Society of America guidelines for the diagnosis and treatment of asymptomatic bacteriuria in adults. *Clin Infect Dis*. 2005;40:643–654.

Section III.
Transitions of Care

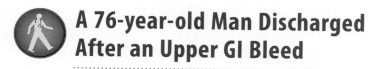

A 76-year-old Man Discharged After an Upper GI Bleed

Christine I. Todd, MD, FACP, FHM

A 76-year-old man with an eighth-grade education who is chronically antico-agulated on warfarin for a history of paroxysmal atrial fibrillation, is admitted to the hospital with an upper GI bleed. His warfarin is reversed with vitamin K, and upper endoscopy reveals an actively bleeding duodenal ulcer. A CLO test confirms the ulcer was caused by *H. pylori*, and the patient is then placed on a proton pump inhibitor and appropriate antibiotics. After discussion with the GI consultants, the hospitalists advise the patient as he is being discharged to follow up with his primary care physician (PCP) and that he can restart his warfarin in 6 weeks.

When the patient arrives for his outpatient follow-up visit, his PCP is sur-prised to hear that her patient was in the hospital. No discharge summary is avail-able, so his doctor relies on the patient to tell her what happened. Unfortunately the patient does not remember all the details. He does remember something about the problem being caused by an "infection in my stomach," and he also notes that he was taken off his warfarin. Worried that her patient might have a stroke if he remains off his anticoagulant and thinking her patient had a viral gas-tritis, the PCP restarts his warfarin. One week later, the patient develops melena and is readmitted to the hospital with a recurrent GI bleed.

1. **What barriers might have prevented the patient from accurately remember-ing the details of his hospital stay?**

2. **What practices could prevent this type of medical error?**

Answers

1. In the above scenario, there are several potential barriers. First and foremost, the patient was told vital information about his warfarin at the time of his dis-charge—a time during which his mind may have been on many other things: how he was going to arrange for transportation home, how he was going to pay for his new prescriptions, when the nurse would be along to take out his IV, etc. His advanced age and the fact that he was recovering from a significant acute illness also play a role in his ability to remember information—elderly patients can be significantly cognitively impaired when ill and this impairment can be very hard to detect in the normal course of a conversation. Finally, this patient's educational status should alert us to the fact that he might have basic or below-basic health literacy status. Patients with low health literacy find it particularly difficult to understand and retain information given to them in a 1-time, verbal format.

2. One way doctors can be sure they have communicated effectively to patients is through the process of "teach-back." Teach-back involves discussing an issue with a patient, and then asking the patient to share with you what was understood about the concept being discussed. The process is then repeated until the patient demonstrates full understanding of the concept. Use of printed documents, drawings, and pictures can enhance the process. Engaging patients in this method of education over several days is often necessary when the issues are myriad or complex, so it is a part of the discharge process that cannot be done effectively at the last minute.

Aside from empowering patients through effective education, it is important that physicians working in the hospital master the skill of effective transfer-of-care communication. Prompt, accurate, and succinct communication with a patient's PCP is of paramount importance in preventing the type of miscommunication illustrated in the example above. Strong ties between the electronic health records used in hospitals and the systems used at outpatient referral sites can also help health care practitioners receive adequate and up-to-date information about their patients.

CASE REVIEW: TRANSITIONS OF CARE
COMMON PITFALLS AT DISCHARGE

Physicians are often surprised at the paucity of information that patients retain, even after they "have been told" the details of their medical condition. It is important to remember that simply telling a patient something does not mean the patient will understand it or can remember it. As physicians, it is important to make sure we communicate effectively. Being aware of the barriers our patients have to retaining information can help doctors be more effective communicators.

Shift work, duty hour limitations, and the increasing disconnect between hospital-based and clinic-based physicians have conspired to make the time during and immediately after discharge from the hospital fraught with opportunities for medical error. Thus, the ability to discharge a patient according to the best practices outlined in the medical literature is a necessary skill for all medical residents. In the next paragraphs, we discuss common areas for poor practice and propose a checklist at discharge to help avoid these pitfalls.

Availability of discharge documentation: Although it seems obvious that a patient discharge from the hospital would work best as a collaborative effort between the discharging hospitalist team and the receiving ambulist team, a true collaboration rarely happens. Only 3% of PCPs report that they are routinely involved in discussions about the discharge of 1 of their patients. Fewer than 20% feel that they are routinely informed in any way about 1 of their patients being admitted to or discharged from the hospital. Twenty-five percent of dictated discharge summaries never reach the intended PCP and, not surprisingly, 66% of patients who arrive for a follow-up visit are seen without a discharge summary available to the PCP. A clear and ordered discharge process would improve these statistics.

First, discharging physicians must complete discharge documentation immediately on a patient's discharge. Forward-looking hospital systems often require that a discharge summary be dictated, and status transcribed and signed before a patient is allowed to leave the hospital. The second step is to make sure the PCP receives the information as soon as possible. Remember that although the patient may not see the PCP for 1 or 2 weeks, questions directed to the PCP may begin mere minutes after the patient leaves the hospital (ie, from a pharmacy questioning a drug dosage or interaction). PCPs find personal letters (as opposed to a copy of the discharge summary) and phone calls to be the most helpful way to communicate issues at discharge. While this may not be possible for all discharges, it is important to consider making personal contact with the PCP on complex or sensitive patient cases. Phone calls between providers at discharge can be immensely helpful, as it permits a 2-way conversation about the patient. In our opening scenario, it is clear that the absence of a discharge summary when the patient presented for a follow-up began the chain of events that led to a poor patient outcome.

High-quality documentation: The data related to the quality of the discharge information that does reach the PCP suggest that there are many opportunities for better practice. Written paperwork is illegible at least 10% of the time, the main diagnosis is missing from the documentation 17.5% of the time, reasons for medication changes are clearly explained only 21% of the time, and the name of the main doctor caring for the patient during the hospitalization is missing in 1 quarter of all discharge summaries. Recalling the opening scenario in this chapter, a legible discharge summary explaining why warfarin was being held would have eliminated the need for the PCP to make an educated guess about her patient's pathology (which, in this case, turned out to be wrong).

Pending laboratory tests: Tests that have been ordered and performed but not resulted by the time of discharge deserve special attention by the discharging physician. A full 3 quarters of patients leaving the hospital have pending lab tests, 15% of which turn out to be abnormal. Most of these abnormal tests are seen by neither the hospitalist team after discharge nor the PCP's team, which is unaware that any testing has been done. The medical and legal liability of letting a patient "fall through the cracks" at discharge in this way is of significant concern. Few hospital systems have a foolproof way of making sure these results are seen by a physician who can take responsibility for acting on the results.

In order to avoid these common errors at discharge, it is important that physicians get into the habit of following a checklist of tasks when discharging a patient.

1. Make sure the patient and/or his or her caregivers understand the important diagnoses or issues that necessitated the admission to the hospital. Use the teach-back method to make sure the patient understands, and supply brochures, handouts, or illustrations to help reinforce the concepts. Make sure to dictate these diagnoses into the discharge document.

2. Summarize the pertinent medical history and the key physical findings in discharge documentation. For instance, for a patient with CHF and pulmonary fibrosis, it would be important to note that even when the patient was clinically no longer in a CHF exacerbation, there were still crackles on the lung examination due to fibrosis.

3. Include the dates of hospital admission and discharge with a brief narrative of the hospitalization. Novice doctors often spend most of their time on this part of their discharge summary, when in reality it is the least read section. Be brief and problem oriented.

4. List the procedures done and key lab results in the discharge summary. Do not create an unreadable "data dump" by including all available information—make a decision about what to include based on the patient's active problems. For instance, that a patient's creatinine remained normal for 10 days only needs to be mentioned once, but the evolving INR and changing warfarin doses for new-onset atrial fibrillation should be mentioned in detail.

5. Include a medication list, broken down into previous medications and current medications. Call attention to medications that have been stopped, had their doses changed, or have been added. List not only the medications but their indications as well. Finally, make sure to "de-autosubstitute" medications. For instance, if your hospital automatically changes your patient's omeprazole to an equivalent dose of esomeprazole, make sure his or her medication list at discharge lists his or her home medication, omeprazole, as his or her PPI. Failure to do so can result in harmful (and expensive) medication class duplication.

6. If your patient was seen by specialists, include a list of them in the discharge summary. Make sure to list the names of the attending physicians and the problem for which they saw the patient. "Patient was seen by Dr. Friend of GI for peptic ulcer disease" is much more informative than "Patient was seen by GI."

7. If you spent time educating a patient or family on a medical issue, indicate that in the discharge documentation. "Since patient was new to warfarin,

we discussed eating a vitamin K–consistent diet and supplied a handout" can help the PCP know education needs remain for the patient.

8. Describe the patient's functional and mental status at discharge, so that the PCP knows if the patient's "baseline" has changed. If changes have been made in the DNR status or advanced directives, make sure to describe them. If the patient is being sent to an extended care facility (ECF) or home with assistance, note that in the summary.

9. List all the follow-up appointments and recommendations in the discharge document so that both the PCP and the patient (who may receive this information by way of written prescription or a printed list at discharge) know future plans. By doing this, you make it easy for the PCP to be on the lookout for follow-up information, and make it easier to help the patient comply with follow-up recommendations.

10. Call special attention to the patient's critical follow-up needs. The last section of the discharge document should be a bulleted list of important follow-up issues. Using the patient from our opening scenario as an example, it is clear that a summary statement in a discharge summary that said "Important Follow-up Issue: Per Dr. Friend of GI, this patient can restart his warfarin therapy in 6 weeks barring further issues" would have prevented the medical error that was made.

11. Include the name of the attending physician in the hospital and contact information. Patients meet many new people during their hospital stays, and few can name their attending physicians. Providing this information is crucial to facilitating good communication between the hospital team and the patient's outpatient team.

12. Give or send the patient a copy of the discharge summary. This is vitally important for patients who have yet to establish with a PCP or who are from out of town. On a very literal level, the only way to ensure that a patient arrives at an outpatient appointment with all pertinent information is to place the information in the patient's hands.

TIPS TO REMEMBER

- Issues at discharge are myriad and complex. Work as a team to accomplish the tasks and remember that the patient's outpatient team (PCP, caregivers, family) should be included in the process.

- Prompt discharge documentation that lists pending labs and important follow-up issues is the most important piece of a successful transition from the hospital to home.

- Use a checklist approach to make sure your discharge work is complete and that your discharge summary gives important information to the patient's PCP.

COMPREHENSION QUESTIONS

1. Use the checklist of items to consider at discharge and turn them into workable "section headings" you can use in a discharge document.

2. List 5 problems that patients could have immediately following discharge that could result in a readmission to the hospital.

Answers

1. Although the hospital at which you work may suggest a template for discharge summaries, they can insufficiently address the complex discharges doctors in internal medicine must manage. In general, you can use a template of your own devising when dictating discharge summaries. Using the checklist discussed above, a template for discharge summaries could be:

> Primary and secondary diagnosis
> Pertinent history and physical findings
> Dates of hospitalization and hospital course
> Previous (home) medications
> Medication list at discharge
> Results of procedures and labs
> Subspecialists involved in care
> Educational issues addressed
> Patient's functional status/advanced directive at discharge
> Follow-up arrangements made
> Specific follow-up needs
> Name and contact information of discharging team

2. It is important to put yourself in the patient's shoes and think about the problems that might occur after discharge. These issues can be as likely as exacerbations of acute illness to result in a readmission. Common issues include:

- Medications:
  Inability to afford new prescription medication
  Interactions or severe side effects from new medications
  Mixing up old and new doses of medications
  Continuing to take medications that have been stopped

- Home environment:
  Not having the keys to get back into the house
  Being unable to climb the stairs to enter the house
  Being alone with no access to food/telephone/toileting/heat/air conditioning

Family/caregivers who are unprepared for patient's needs
Needing equipment that has not been arranged/delivered (home oxygen, hospital bed)

- Follow-up:
Losing the papers listing follow-up appointments
Finding out about a scheduling conflict with 1 of the follow-up appointments
Not being able to arrange transport to a follow-up appointment

SUGGESTED READINGS

Halasyamani L, Kripalani S, Coleman EA, et al. Transition of care for hospitalized elderly patients—development of a discharge checklist for hospitalists. *J Hosp Med.* 2006;1:354–360.

Kripalani S, Jackson A, Schnipper J, Coleman EA. Promoting effective transitions of care at hospital discharge: a review of key issues for hospitalists. *J Hosp Med.* 2007;2:314–323.

Kripalani S, LeFevre F, Phillips CO, Williams NC, Basaviah P, Baker DW. Deficits in communications and information transfer between hospital-based and primary care physicians: implications for patient safety and continuity of care. *JAMA.* 2007;297:831–841.

Moore C, Wisnivesky J, Williams S, McGinn T. Medical errors related to discontinuity of care from an inpatient to an outpatient setting. *J Gen Intern Med.* 2003;18:646–651.

A Woman With Mild Dementia and a CHF Exacerbation

Christine I. Todd, MD, FACP, FHM

You are an intern on the General Ward Service. Ms Brown, one of your patients, is a woman with mild baseline dementia who was admitted 2 days ago with a CHF exacerbation. For the last 2 nights in the hospital she has had agitation and confusion at night, which your team has attributed to "sundowning." She received quetiapine for these symptoms by the night resident, which worked well.

On hospital day 3, your team sees Ms Brown on rounds and decides, based on persistent crackles in her lung bases, elevated JVD, and continued shortness of breath that continued diuresis is needed before discharge can be contemplated. Forty milligrams of IV furosemide is prescribed as a 1-time dose that morning, and when you check back on Ms Brown later in the day, she seems to feel better.

When handing your patients off to the night residents before your shift is over, you go over Ms Brown's case, explaining that her diagnoses are dementia and CHF and letting your teammates know that she is stable and hopefully will be discharged soon.

When you arrive to the hospital the next day, you see Ms Brown and find that she is not doing well. She complains of shortness of breath, has prominent JVD, and has bilateral lower lobe crackles. You see by her intake and output tally that she had quite a bit to drink the night before, and even though she had 1 L of urine after her morning dose of furosemide, she had 3 L of intake to only 2 L of output for the last 24-hour period. She is still in a CHF exacerbation, and will not be able to be discharged today.

In addition, the night residents tell you that she was very agitated last night, and became even more agitated after they gave her a dose of benzodiazepines to calm her down. In fact, they had to restrain her arms in order to keep her from pulling out her IV line, which was very upsetting to her family, who had to be notified about the restraint order.

1. **What unintended consequences did Ms Brown suffer during her hospital course? What was the root cause of these errors?**

Answer

1. This case illustrates a few of the many mishaps that can occur when patients receive care from shifting teams of providers, as opposed to one provider who is responsible for them throughout a hospital stays. There are many good reasons why doctors and other health care providers must transfer the responsibility for a patient's care among each other during a patient's hospital

stay, but these transition points are also fraught with the opportunity for serious error. In this case, Ms Brown fell victim to 2 errors, both traceable to handoff issues.

Although Ms Brown was identified as a patient with CHF during the hand-off, she was not classified as a patient in a CHF *exacerbation*. Thus, the night team did not know that the primary team intended for the patient to be in a negative fluid balance during their shift. Second, the information that Ms Brown's "sundowning" responded well to quetiapine was not relayed to the night team. Without this knowledge, they chose a medication to which the patient had unintended side effects when a superior medication for the patient was available. The combination of these 2 preventable unintended outcomes, or medical errors, will likely prolong Ms Brown's hospital stay.

CASE REVIEW: HAND-OFFS WITH ANTICIPATED COMMUNICATION

A high-functioning health care team puts best practices into effect in managing handoffs. The medical literature suggests a number of ways to insure handoffs happen seamlessly, (discussed in detail below). In the scenario above, a handoff that made acute issues explicit by specifying that Ms Brown had a CHF *exacerbation and needed further diuresis* would have made it more clear to the night team that they needed to watch her I's and O's and possibly give her additional doses of furosemide.

Besides offering specific information about acute issues, good-quality handoffs also give recommendations about anticipated complications. In Ms Brown's case, her dementia makes her prone to nighttime delirium or "sundowning," and since it has happened on the first 2 nights of her hospitalization, it is very likely to happen again. Since there was a treatment that worked for her, a handoff to the night team should have included not only the warning that she might get delirious but also a specific recommendation for the medication that helped her.

Anticipated Problems

Poor-quality handoffs have been implicated in the medical literature as one of the most common sources of medical errors in the hospital. Even though everyone on a health care team feels responsible for the patients in the hospital, it remains difficult to "know" the patients you did not admit or for whom you do not have primary responsibility. Teams that aim to give excellent care to their patients work hard on avoiding the "voltage drop" of information at handoff by effecting succinct, accurate, and helpful communication at the point of transition. Chief among the skills it takes to do this is the ability to

give specific tasks on active issues and specific recommendations about anticipated problems.

When asked to hand off a patient to a covering physician, many novice physicians will begin by relating the patient's narrative, starting with the events that led
to the patient's illness and working in chronological order through the events of
the hospitalization. Although this type of handoff can impressively demonstrate
how thoroughly you know your patient, it usually does not help the receiving
doctor manage the patient's needs. More helpful is a non-narrative bulleted presentation of the patient's acute or active issues along with specific recommendations for anticipated problems. In this way, you can most efficiently pass your
knowledge of the patient to your colleague. It is important to be as specific as
possible—not just "give furosemide," but relay *how much* furosemide has worked
in the past for the patient. Don't advise giving a patient blood "if he or she needs
it" rather, give specifics for the hemoglobin level at which you feel a transfusion is
warranted, and why.

For novices, a good way to organize a bulleted list of acute issues is to work
from the problem list you've generated as part of your SOAP note on the patient.
You do not need to mention every issue on your problem list during your handoff,
but you should mention the ones you feel are likely to need intervention. Your
senior resident can help you develop your list of acute issues for handoff. The
senior can also help you think of specific recommendations for actions on these
acute issues until you are comfortable coming up with these on your own.

Table 44-1 lists common inpatient issues and suggests specific recommendations that may be needed to help covering residents take care of your patient when
you are not on shift.

When handing off your patients to a colleague, accurate, to the point, and
specific about the issues facing your patient. It is equally important that you be
engaged in the handoff process when you are the resident who will be covering a group of patients for a shift. Pay close attention to the information you are
being given, and write notes to yourself so that you can remember the specific
actions recommended to you by your peers. Be assertive in asking questions so
that you get the type of information you need in order to take care of the patient.
For instance, if you are told a patient may "need extra insulin," be sure to ask what
kind of insulin is indicated and in what doses it is likely to work.

The course of a patient in the hospital is not always predictable, and sur-
prises, emergencies, and generally unforeseen events occur frequently. It is
impossible to account for every issue that may arise for your patient—covering
residents will always have to keep an open mind, be flexible, and see the patient
for themselves to decide on the best course of action for every situation. However, a succinct summary of active issues along with specific recommendations
for action can help everyone on the health care team work together to create
good outcomes for the patient.

Table 44-1. Common Inpatient Issues and Recommendations for Covering

Symptom or Diagnosis	Anticipated Issues
Chest pain	Do you suspect cardiac or noncardiac pain?
	What should be ordered if the pain recurs—EKG, chest X-ray, antacid, antianxiety medicine?
Dyspnea	What would be the most likely cause in this patient?
	What are the patient's baseline oxygen needs?
Oliguria	If this occurs, is it likely that the patient needs a diuretic, or a fluid bolus?
GI bleed	Is the bleeding active, or has it clinically stopped?
	How likely is the patient to rebleed?
	When will the next hemoglobin be checked? What value is likely to represent further bleeding?
	What should be done if further bleeding is suspected—bleeding scan? Notify GI team?
CHF	What is your goal for diuresis in the next 24 h?
Infection	What should be done for a fever? Reculture or change in antibiotics?
Pain	What additional steps should be taken if the patient's pain is not controlled? Should the current analgesic be increased in dose or frequency? Should there be an additional workup as to the source of the pain?
IV access	How important are the IV medications the patient is on? If the patient loses IV access, can his or her medications be changed to oral equivalents, or should a central line be placed?
Advanced directives	If this patient's status worsens, what steps should be taken? Should a transfer to ICU be contemplated, or does the patient wish to de-escalate care at that point?
	Who is the power of attorney, and what is the contact information?

TIPS TO REMEMBER

- The handoff is one of the few places in medicine in which a narrative approach to communication will not benefit the patient.

- Put work and thought into making a complete and prioritized problem list for your patient. This cannot be done "on the fly" and is the most important step toward a high-quality handoff.

- Think of patient care in terms of a 24-hours-a-day, 7-days-a-week cycle. What can you communicate at the point of handoff that will make sure that your patient's care will be advanced during the shifts in which you are absent?

- Incorporate unexpected events into updated action steps you include in the next handoff on the patient.

- If you are receiving a handoff that does not include specific tasks and delineates active issues, be assertive! Clarify vague recommendations, and make sure you clearly understand the active patient issues.

COMPREHENSION QUESTIONS

1. Your patient, Mr Brown, has end-stage COPD, and is hospitalized with a COPD exacerbation. After a day of hospitalization, the IV steroids, antibiotics, and breathing treatments seem to be improving his symptoms. However, your senior warns you on rounds that he is "not out of the woods yet." You note that he is a full code, but wonder if resuscitation would be much of a benefit to him should his condition suddenly worsen. What is the best way to hand off this patient to your colleagues at the end of your shift?

2. Your co-intern is finished with her work and is ready to go home. During the handoff, she mentions that one of her patients has become more dyspneic this afternoon, and a CT angiogram of the chest to look for pulmonary embolism has been ordered, but hasn't been done yet. She asks you to follow up on this test and start anticoagulation if it is positive. What kinds of questions would give you more specific information to help you take care of this patient?

Answers

1. It is important to discuss unresolved issues, such as goals of care in patients with serious illnesses, before handing off a patient's case to your colleagues. The time you have spent with your patient and his or her family establishes an important rapport and allows your patient the chance to have an informed conversation about the condition and make a clear-headed choice about care should the condition worsen. Without the benefit of this relationship, conversations between covering residents and patients done during a time of medical crisis can lead to

decisions that all parties regret. By discussing end-of-life issues with your patient in preparation for handoff, you can offer your peers specific information and action steps in case your patient's condition deteriorates.

2. Although your co-intern has supplied you with a specific request—to follow up on her patient's CT scan—there are a few issues that bear further questioning so that the patient can get high-quality care. First, it would be a good idea to ask how strongly a PE is suspected—if the clinical suspicion is high, starting anticoagulation before getting the CT results back is warranted. Next, it would be helpful to know what other diagnoses the patient's primary team is contemplating for the patient's dyspnea. That way, you can continue a workup for the problem if the CT scan is negative for PE. Finally, asking if there are any relative contraindications or concerns for anticoagulation can help you be alert for concerning symptoms while you are caring for the patient.

SUGGESTED READINGS

Arora VM, Manjarrez E, Dressler DD, Basaviah P, Halasyamani L, Kripalani S. Hospitalist handoffs: a systematic review and task force recommendations. *J Hosp Med*. 2009;4(7):433–440 [review].

Burton MC, Kashiwagi DT, Kirkland LL, Manning D, Varkey P. Gaining efficiency and satisfaction in the handoff process. *J Hosp Med*. 2010;5(9):547–552 [Epub August 17, 2010]. doi:10.1002/jhm.808.

Riesenberg LA, Leitzsch J, Massucci JL, et al. Residents' and attending physicians' handoffs: a systematic review of the literature. *Acad Med*. 2009;84(12):1775–1787 [review].

A Patient in Respiratory Distress

Christine I. Todd, MD, FACP, FHM

You are on call for the General Wards service, and it's late in the afternoon. One of your co-interns, Dr George, went home a few hours ago. He sent you a text page telling you that a list of his patients is taped to the door of the resident's lounge and that "every one is stable." As you were busy admitting a sick patient when you got his text, you did not have time to call Dr George back and ask for more detailed information.

Just as you are getting ready to eat supper, you get a page from a nurse. He tells you that one of Dr George's patients is in respiratory distress and needs to be assessed. This patient is not on the list that Dr George printed out for you, but when you check the patient's chart, you see that he has been seeing and writing notes on the patient daily. Unfortunately, his note in her chart from today is largely illegible. When you go to the patient's room to assess her and begin asking questions, the patient becomes irritated. "I already answered these questions a million times! Don't you people talk to each other?"

1. What are the communication challenges present in this scenario?

2. How can a handoff process be structured in order to mitigate the communication breakdowns present in the above case?

Answers

1. In the above scenario, there are many opportunities for improvement in communication of handoff information. First, and perhaps most importantly, the handoff does not occur in a face-to-face fashion. Since the giving and the receiving interns do not meet and discuss the patients, the only information shared is a list of names and the vague panacea that all patients are "stable." Because there is not an appointed time and place for the handoff to occur, the list ends up being posted in a potentially public area, and the receiving intern is too distracted by a new patient to be able to take the time to ask Dr George important questions about the patients on his service. Lastly, the list of patients to cover is incorrect, leading to additional time spent by the covering intern gathering facts from the patient and chart, which is illegible. The patient's perception that this is a poor way to approach patient care is correct.

2. Although the focus on skills for successful transfers of care is relatively new, there are best practices advocated for and supported by a growing body of medical literature. It is important that your residency program provides a consistent structure for handoffs. A specific time and place for handoff, consistent written and verbal formats, content guidelines, and an insistence on legible, accurate charting should be strong elements of the resident culture around transfers of patient information and care. These items should be perceived as mandatory by

house staff and done as a matter of routine in order to create a safe environment for patients.

TRANSITIONS OF CARE—HANDOFFS

Handoffs, an ever more frequent occurrence in the course of hospitalized patient care, are a time when significant patient safety issues can occur. Residents working in today's compressed, shift-work-oriented environment must develop the ability to competently give and receive handoff information.

Novice house staff may think that poor-quality handoff communication occurs in a somewhat random fashion due to lack of experience. They may assume that as they gain confidence and general know-how, they will naturally produce high-quality transfers of care. In fact, errors in handoff communication are very predictable, and can be largely avoided, even by novices, by adhering to a consistent structure for handoff. The Joint Commission, the national association that accredits health care organizations, lists a standardized approach to handoff communication as a mandatory National Patient Safety Goal.

There is no substitute for face-to-face handoffs. When you personally meet to transfer patient care, the quality of the information shared is higher. In addition, the person receiving the handoff has the opportunity to ask questions. For instance, in a patient with a complex illness and an involved family, a face-to-face handoff makes it more likely that ongoing treatment decisions and the vocabulary used to explain them will be consistent across caregivers. This leads to care that advances despite changes in staff and higher patient and family satisfaction.

There should be a consistent time and place for handoff communication. Handoffs that take place as each team finishes work and leaves for the day are inefficient as they occur at random and unplanned times. Although the residents giving the handoff information may have tied up all loose ends and are ready to focus on the handoff, the receiving resident is frequently in the middle of a task. A distracted resident will not be able to listen and participate in the handoff process. A routine, specific time for handoff should be established so that both teams of caretakers can be ready to participate in the process. It's also important to choose a place for handoff that is quiet, private, and HIPPA compliant.

Participants should use a standard template for written and verbal handoffs. There are many popular templates to guide information transfer, such as SBAR and I PASS THE BATON. You should use the one endorsed by your institution, as it can be very helpful when both nurses and doctors use the same handoff template. Verbal handoffs that are accompanied by written prompts result in better-quality handoffs than verbal handoffs by themselves. Recent studies suggest that computer-generated printouts that autopopulate important fields can make handoffs more accurate. They also lead to fewer patients being forgotten and left off the list at handoff. These types of lists are increasingly available for use at hospitals that have instituted electronic health records with computerized physician order entry. In any case, when composing a written list or cards to pass along at handoff, remember the "garbage in, garbage out" rule. Written handoffs are only as good as the information they display, so it is important to update information such as code status, active problems, and medication lists.

It is important to create an environment during handoff that minimizes distractions. Participants should be seated so that they can take notes and focus on their task. The room should be quiet, with no side conversations taking place among house staff waiting their turn to sign out patients. Supervising residents should relieve the resident taking over patient care of the pager, so that the resident is not rushed and the handoff process is not fractured by frequent pauses while the on-call intern returns a page.

Lastly, remember that no matter how good a handoff is, it is impossible for all information to be transferred and all issues to be anticipated. In many cases, an issue evolving on a patient will require some time spent with the chart in order to make good clinical decisions. It is thus very important to maintain high standards of quality in written charting. Legible handwriting is mandatory. Legible signatures (or legible written names appended to signatures) are of utmost importance in terms of helping others know who to contact for patient issues. For institutions that use a computerized record, remember that overuse of cut and paste in composing notes can lead to the perpetuation of outdated and incorrect information in a patient's chart. Original content, particularly in the assessment and plan area of your SOAP note, is a hallmark of quality care.

TIPS TO REMEMBER

- There is no substitute for a standardized approach to patient handoffs that includes a face-to-face conversation at a preestablished place and time and with a standardized informational template.

- Verbal handoffs that are accompanied by a written document lead to better outcomes.

- Prepopulated computer-generated sign-out documents can lead to more efficient handoffs and fewer missed patients.

- Handoffs are 2-way conversations. The resident handing off patients must be accurate and efficient, and the resident receiving the handoff should actively participate by asking questions clarifying complex issues.

COMPREHENSION QUESTIONS

1. Although handoffs are often discussed in the context of inpatient care, what are some scenarios where good handoff skills could be used to augment ambulatory care?

2. You are on call and realize that one of your co-interns has gone home without signing out her patients to you. You have handled a few straightforward calls on her patients, but will be responsible for her patients until the end of your shift. What should you do?

Answers

1. The overall acuity of an outpatient panel is lower than that of a group of inpatients, but at any given point in time, there are patients in an outpatient practice who have important evolving issues. Outpatient practitioners should consider a formal handoff of this group of patients to one of their partners when they will be away from their practice for a substantial period of time—that is, vacation, educational leave, or medical leave. Residents might consider an inpatient handoff during training months during which their clinic time will be limited, as it may be during a month in the ICU or working night shifts. A short session where a verbal and written sign-out of patients with acute issues is discussed between colleagues (and potentially other staff, such as clinic nurses) would further patient continuity.

2. A handoff must occur so that patient care can be rendered safely, and it is your duty to purse the information you need to take care of patients for whom you are responsible. Unfortunately, due to work duty hour restrictions, you may not be able to page your co-intern to obtain handoff information. In this case, contacting either your co-intern's senior resident or attending for handoff information would be the advised course of action. Asking your program to establish a routine time and place where all teams gather for handoff (and the process does not start without all participants present) would alleviate this problem in the future.

SUGGESTED READINGS

Arora VM, Manjarrez E, Dressler DD, Basaviah P, Halasyamani L, Kripalani S. Hospitalist handoffs: a systematic review and task force recommendations. *J Hosp Med*. 2009;4(7):433–440.

Joint Commission. *2006 Critical Access Hospital and Hospital National Patient Safety Goals*. Oakbrook Terrace, IL. <www.jointcommission.org/PatientSafety/NationalPatientSafetyGoals/06_npsg_cah.htm>; 2006.

Kripalani S, Jackson AT, Schnipper JL, Coleman EA. Promoting effective transitions of care at hospital discharge: a review of key issues for hospitalists. *J Hosp Med*. 2007;2(5):314–323.

Solet DJ, Norvell JM, Rutan GH, Frankel RM. Lost in translation: challenges and opportunities during physician-to-physician communication during patient handoffs. *Acad Med*. 2005;80:1094–1099.

Williams MV, Flanders SA, Whitcomb W, et al. *Comprehensive Hospital Medicine*. Philadelphia, PA: Saunders; 2007.

A 78-year-old Woman Taking Multiple Medications

Tiffany Leung, MD, MPH and
J. Mark Ruscin, PharmD

A 78-year-old woman with hypertension, diabetes mellitus, and osteoporosis presents to the emergency room with her son with unilateral weakness and garbled speech. She was found on the floor of her home after an unknown period of time. She takes hydrochlorothiazide, candesartan, a baby aspirin, metformin, and alendronate. On examination, she appears lethargic but respirations are unlabored. Her blood pressure is 98/65 mm Hg with a heart rate of 128 bpm. Oxygen saturation is 97% on room air. Her speech is slurred. She is oriented to self but not to place or time. Cardiac examination demonstrates an irregularly irregular rhythm. A thorough neurologic examination reveals a right-sided facial droop, and she is unable to lift her right arm or leg off the bed. A CT brain shows a left middle cerebral artery ischemic stroke. An EKG shows atrial fibrillation. A pelvic x-ray shows a left pubic ramus fracture. Her laboratory data show a blood glucose of 360 mg/dL, and findings consistent with acute kidney injury and mild rhabdomyolysis. During hospitalization, she develops a right lower extremity deep vein thrombus and is started on therapeutic anticoagulation.

She will be discharged to home in the next 24 hours, with assistance from her son and a hired caregiver. She now needs assistance with taking her medications. You review her medication list and find the following:

- Hydrochlorothiazide and metformin were discontinued.
- Alendronate was not given during hospitalization.
- Aspirin was continued during hospitalization.
- Candesartan was originally substituted with losartan, but then changed to ramipril.
- New medications include insulin glargine, insulin lispro, metoprolol tartrate, diltiazem, warfarin, atorvastatin, pantoprazole, hydrocodone–acetaminophen, and calcium with vitamin D_3.

1. **What are important next steps in managing her medication list as you prepare her discharge?**

2. **What counseling should you provide to this patient and her caregivers while preparing for discharge?**

Answers

1. A thorough and detailed medication reconciliation (see definition in Table 46-1) must occur at every transition of care between health care settings. It is important

Table 46-1. Definitions

Medication reconciliation	The process of verifying that a patient's current list of medications (including dose, route, and frequency) is correct and that the medications are currently medically necessary and safe
Medical error	Failure of a planned action to be completed as intended. Errors during the transition from discharge to post-acute or outpatient care include medication errors and potential adverse drug events, test follow-up errors, and workup errors
Medication discrepancy	Lack of agreement (or incompatibility) between different medication regimens, which may be recorded (eg, in the medical record) or reported (eg, provided by the patient verbally or with medication bottles)

to recognize that medication errors can compromise patient safety and contribute to increased rates of rehospitalization within 30 days after discharge. Reconciliation helps to reduce these errors. Medication changes must be clearly identified and appropriate counseling provided to the patient and caregiver in a patient-centered manner that is sensitive to both health literacy level and cultural background. Additionally, preparing for this transition of care should include direct communication of the recommended medication changes to the patient's primary care provider.

2. Medication-specific counseling must be provided in order to insure safe medication administration outside of the closely monitored setting of the hospital. For example, this patient has been started on warfarin to reduce her personal risk of recurrent cardioembolic stroke and also to prevent additional deep vein thrombosis. Warfarin administration necessitates detailed counseling on the effects of variable vitamin K intake in the diet, education on symptoms and signs of potentially life-threatening bleeding, and emphasis on scheduled follow-up to check INR in order to continue this medication safely. Similarly, skill-focused education is important to ensure that the patient and family understand how to safely administer the right insulin doses and types of insulin at the right times, check blood sugars with a glucometer, and monitor for signs of hypoglycemia. Additional counseling on possible adverse effects of all medications must be provided.

CASE REVIEW

Throughout this patient's hospital course, multiple medication changes were required to address her new and prior medical problems. Additionally, she now has an increased need for assistance in performing activities of daily living, has impaired mobility, and is at risk for additional functional, cognitive, and communication impairments that would increase the complexity of her post-acute care and long-term recovery.

This patient's medication regimen has become increasingly complex but clinically indicated in order to manage her multiple medical problems. Each new medication has a side effect profile that must be recognized in order to maximize safe prescribing by the physician and safe administration for the patient by her caregivers. Medications discontinued during the hospitalization must be acknowledged to ensure that appropriate medication adjustments have been made to match the patient's current clinical condition.

Medication reconciliation can require a significant amount of time and effort, but there are clear care, quality, and patient safety benefits of a detailed medication review. An inaccurate or incomplete medication list obtained at admission will likely result in an inaccurate and incomplete list at discharge. Additionally, when the initial reconciliation is performed, medication adherence should be addressed. In other words, it is also important to determine if the patient was using medications as prescribed prior to admission. It may not be necessary to add medications or change dosing regimens on discharge. It is possible that counseling on the appropriate use of existing medications is all that is necessary to manage existing or new medical conditions.

Anticipating potential medication-related complications prior to discharge can help to prevent problems with medications after discharge from hospital to home. If potential errors are identified, then specific counseling to address these potential errors can help minimize their impact on the patient's health outcome. For example, it is important to recognize that when the patient returns home, medications reconciled on admission may still be available at home for the patient to use. Without adequate medication counseling, significant errors and poorer outcomes may occur if the patient continues to take home medications in addition to medications added or changed on discharge from the hospital. In the case presented, hydrochlorothiazide and metformin have been discontinued in the hospital and, in the setting of insufficient counseling, the patient may inappropriately continue to take these medications.

Another common source of errors and miscommunication about medications is the use of brand names and generic names interchangeably. Therapeutic substitution of similar medications within a medication class is also common during hospitalization, for example, candesartan and losartan are in the class of angiotensin II receptor blockers, and ramipril is an angiotensin-converting enzyme inhibitor, as was done in this case. It is important to remember to resume use of the admission medication on discharge to avoid therapeutic duplication, unless an alternative is indicated based on the clinical scenario.

The risks and benefits of each new or modified medication or dosing regimen must be considered at each transition of care. Warfarin in this patient provides an evidence-based benefit of secondary stroke prevention, given the presumed etiology was a cardioembolic thrombus related to undiagnosed atrial fibrillation, and also protection against a recurrent venous thromboembolic event. However, the patient is on both aspirin and warfarin, which increases the risk of significant bleeding complications. Such risk–benefit considerations must be carefully weighed before making the final decision to adjust the medication regimen on discharge from the hospital. The clinical scenario and diagnoses should always guide decision making about appropriate use of medications.

GENERAL APPROACH

Epidemiology

Discharge from the inpatient hospital to a continuing care facility or to home is a time of increased patient vulnerability to medical errors and adverse clinical outcomes. Transitions of care become increasingly complex when additional factors are considered, including multiple chronic diseases, polypharmacy, vulnerable populations including geriatric patients, increased demands for patient self-management, complex follow-up care plans, and multiple medication and treatment changes. All transition of care processes also depend heavily on clear patient–provider communication and communication between providers during handoffs, particularly between the discharging hospitalist and primary care physician.

Nearly half (49%) of patients experience a medical error after discharge, and an estimated 19% to 23% of patients experience an adverse event after discharge, most commonly attributable to an adverse drug event. Chart reviews of hospital discharge instructions demonstrate that at least 1 medication discrepancy occurs in approximately 14% of patients. Medication discrepancies are variable in type and sometimes can occur without immediate awareness of the discrepancy at the point of care (Table 46-2). About half of medication discrepancies are related to patient-associated factors and half related to system-associated factors. Additionally, rehospitalization rates within 30 days after discharge are significantly higher (14.3%) among patients who have at least 1 medication discrepancy identified compared with patients who do not have any medication discrepancies (6.1%). The 4 most commonly implicated drugs leading to rehospitalization, especially in the elderly, are warfarin, insulin, oral antiplatelet agents, and oral hypoglycemic agents.

The 2001 Institute of Medicine report *Crossing the Quality Chasm* was a mission statement to improve the safety of the nation's health care system. In 2005,

Table 46-2. Factors Contributing to Medication Discrepancies After Hospital Discharge

Patient-associated factors

Nonadherence (nonintentional or intentional)

Financial barriers

Did not fill prescription

Did not need prescription

Performance deficit

Adverse drug effect or intolerance

System-associated factors

Incomplete, inaccurate, or illegible discharge instructions

Conflicting information from different informational sources

Duplication

Prescribed with known allergies/intolerances

Confusion between brand and generic names

Incorrect label, quantity, or dosage

Cognitive impairment, sight/dexterity limitations, or need for assistance not recognized

the Joint Commission incorporated medication reconciliation into the National Patient Safety Goals program, promoting medication reconciliation at care transitions in order to minimize adverse patient events. In 2006, the Institute for Healthcare Improvement implemented the 100,000 Lives campaign, and then subsequently the 5 Million Lives campaign, to reduce adverse patient outcomes systemwide. Medication reconciliation as a key component of each of these initiatives seeks to improve patient safety across the continuum of care.

Treatment

Accurate medication reconciliation can increase patient safety and quality of care in each health care setting *and* across transitions of care between health care settings. When managing the care of a hospitalized patient, the medication reconciliation begins on admission. This includes assessment of each medication's dose, frequency, and route of administration. Medications should include prescriptions from different providers, nonoral medications, over-the-counter products, and supplements. Possible sources of medication information include the patient, the

Table 46-3. Types of Medication Discrepancies

Omission	The patient was receiving, before admission, medication that was not prescribed at discharge, with no clinical explanation for the omission
Substitution	Prescription, at discharge, of a medication using different dosage, route of administration, or frequency from that which the patient received before admission, when this difference was not justified by a change in the patient's clinical condition
Commission (or addition)	A medication was ordered at discharge that the patient did not take before hospitalization. There was no clinical explanation for adding the medication to the patient's therapy
Incomplete prescription	The dosage, frequency, or duration of treatment was not included for 1 medicine on the discharge medication list
Duplicate medication	More than 1 drug of the same class was prescribed

patient's caregiver or family members, nursing home personnel, a primary care provider or other providers, and pharmacies. During the course of the hospitalization, medications may be stopped or substituted and new medications begun, with clinical justifications supporting each change ideally occurring during the course of the patient's hospitalization.

Discharge medication reconciliation must be reviewed and finalized, incorporating the same components noted on admission: dose, frequency, and route of administration. Each discrepancy identified when comparing the admission medication list and discharge medication must be justified or intended based on the patient's clinical status and diagnoses (Table 46-3). A clearly written document that summarizes the complete and reconciled medication list should be provided to the patient and his or her caregiver, along with appropriate counseling on the changes. When preparing a patient for discharge from the hospital, attention to potential barriers to taking medications as recommended must also be considered and addressed proactively (Table 46-2). Involving the assistance of a pharmacist can promote a robust and effective medication reconciliation and discharge process. Clear communication between the discharging hospitalist and the patient's primary care provider or the continuing care facility receiving the patient is essential to ensure that a detailed medication reconciliation performed at a post-acute care follow-up appointment can be performed as well.

Counseling

Medication counseling is an important element of the hospital discharge that must be provided in a sensitive manner. One of the most common methods used is a teach-back technique, which is an iterative technique in which the physician assesses patient comprehension, tailors important learning points in response to the patient's level of comprehension, and then reassesses patient comprehension until the patient has mastered the knowledge or skill taught. In essence, the physician is "closing the loop" of communication to ensure that the intended message was received by the patient. In the case of learning about appropriate medication administration, a physician might assess patient comprehension in a nonjudgmental manner by stating, "I want to make sure I explained your medicines well. Please tell me how you plan to take each one." Other general rules to follow for clear patient communication include speaking slowly and in plain, nonmedical language, limiting the amount of information conveyed, and repeating or summarizing the information for clarity.

Closing the Loop of Communication

Step 1: Clinician explains new information or advice to patient.

Step 2: Clinician assesses patient recall and comprehension of new information shared.

Step 3: Clinician clarifies and tailors explanation, based on patient's response in Step 2.

Step 4: Steps 2 and 3 are repeated iteratively until patient expresses comprehension of new information.

TIPS TO REMEMBER

- Medication reconciliation must be performed carefully at every care transition, including hospital admission and discharge, noting medication dosage, frequency, and route of administration.
- Discharge medication discrepancies include omissions, substitutions, commissions, incomplete prescriptions, and duplicate prescriptions.
- Clinical justification must be present to explain each medication change identified when performing the discharge medication reconciliation.
- Discharge medication changes must be communicated clearly to the patient, the patient's caregiver, and post-acute care provider, including the continuing care facility and the patient's primary care physician.
- Medication-specific counseling on hospital discharge can help to improve patient understanding, safety, and outcomes.

● Anticipate potential problems with medications and consider potential sources of error, including where and when errors might occur.

COMPREHENSION QUESTIONS

1. In addition to identifying the name of each medication, what are the 3 most important elements of each medication that must be collected in a detailed and accurate medication reconciliation?
> A. Dose, prescribing physician, and dispensing pharmacy
> B. Dose, route, and frequency
> C. Brand name, dose, and route
> D. Indication, dose, and frequency

2. On admission, a patient reports taking famotidine daily. When she is discharged from the hospital, she is given discharge instructions and a prescription for ranitidine. At her follow-up visit with her primary care physician, she is found to be taking both famotidine and ranitidine. What type of medication discrepancy best describes this scenario?
> A. Omission
> B. Commission
> C. Substitution
> D. Duplication

3. What communication techniques should be utilized in counseling patients about their discharge medications?
> A. Use nonmedical language.
> B. Speak slowly.
> C. Use teach-back.
> D. Summarize information.
> E. All of the above.

Answers

1. **B.** It is important to identify the dose, route, and frequency of administration of each medication when reconciling a patient's medications at each care transition. Care transitions include admission, interhospital or intrahospital transfers, and discharge.

2. **D.** This patient is taking 2 H2-receptor antagonists. Duplication, which is the administration of 2 medications of the same class, is the correct answer. If famotidine was omitted from and no antireflux medication was provided on the discharge medication list when it was intended, then this would be an error of omission. If the intent was to discontinue antireflux medications, but famotidine

was included on the discharge medication list, then this would be an error of commission. If the intent was to continue the patient's home antireflux medication but instead ranitidine was prescribed, then this would be an error of substitution.

3. E. All of the options are important communication techniques to use when counseling patients about new medications and potential adverse effects. Communication should also be nonjudgmental, culturally sensitive, and ideally performed in an environment where the patient and his or her caregivers can feel at ease asking questions and engaging in conversation with the physician about medical recommendations.

SUGGESTED READINGS

Bedell SE, Jabbour S, Goldberg R, et al. Discrepancies in the use of medications: their extent and predictors in an outpatient practice. *Arch Intern Med.* 2000;160:2129–2134.

Budnitz DS, Lovegrove MC, Shehab N, Richards CL. Emergency hospitalizations for adverse drug events in older Americans. *N Engl J Med.* 2011;365:2002–2012.

Coleman EA, Smith JD, Raha D, Min SJ. Posthospital medication discrepancies: prevalence and contributing factors. *Arch Intern Med.* 2005;165:1842–1847.

Council NR. *Crossing the Quality Chasm: A New Health System for the 21st Century.* Washington, DC: The National Academies Press; 2001.

Council NR. *To Err Is Human: Building a Safer Health System.* Washington, DC: The National Academies Press; 2000.

Greenwald JL, Halasyamani L, Greene J, et al. Making inpatient medication reconciliation patient centered, clinically relevant and implementable: a consensus statement on key principles and necessary first steps. *J Hosp Med.* 2010;5:477–485.

Herrero-Herrero JI, García-Aparicio J. Medication discrepancies at discharge from an internal medicine service. *Eur J Intern Med.* 2011;22:43–48.

Kripalani S, Jackson AT, Schnipper JL, Coleman EA. Promoting effective transitions of care at hospital discharge: a review of key issues for hospitalists. *J Hosp Med.* 2007;2:314–323.

Moore C, Wisnivesky J, Williams S, McGinn T. Medical errors related to discontinuity of care from an inpatient to an outpatient setting. *J Gen Intern Med.* 2003;18:646–651.

Paasche-Orlow M. Caring for patients with limited health literacy: a 76-year-old man with multiple medical problems. *JAMA.* 2011;306:1122–1129.

Schillinger D, Piette J, Grumbach K, et al. Closing the loop: physician communication with diabetic patients who have low health literacy. *Arch Intern Med.* 2003;163:83–90.

The Care Transitions Program: Health Care Services for Improving Quality and Safety During Care Hand-offs. <http://www.caretransitions.org/>; 2012. Accessed 05.03.12.

A 63-year-old Man With Urosepsis

Tiffany Leung, MD, MPH

A 63-year-old man with benign prostatic hypertrophy and diabetes mellitus presents to the emergency department with gradual decrease in urine output for the past 1 week, and inability to urinate today. Over this time, he has developed abdominal pain and fullness. His medical history is otherwise unremarkable. His only medications are finasteride, terazosin, metformin, and a baby aspirin daily. On examination, his temperature is 99.8°F, blood pressure is 138/86 mm Hg, heart rate is 97 bpm, respiratory rate is 14/min, and pulse oximetry is 99% on room air. He appears uncomfortable but in no acute distress. His cardiopulmonary examination is unremarkable. He has suprapubic pain to palpation and dullness to percussion in the same region. He does not have costovertebral angle tenderness. Laboratory evaluation demonstrates WBCs of 13,000 cells/mm^3. After repeated attempts to place a straight urinary catheter, a Coudé catheter is finally placed successfully with resultant 1 L of urine output. Urinalysis shows large hematuria, leukocyte esterase, and nitrites, with 10 to 50 WBCs/hpf. Serum chemistry is normal. Urine and blood cultures are drawn, and empiric ciprofloxacin is started intravenously.

He is admitted for observation and discharged in less than 24 hours with an indwelling urinary catheter, a prescription for oral ciprofloxacin, and instructions to follow up with his primary care provider (PCP) in 24 to 48 hours. He is lost to follow-up and presents to the ED 1 week later with fever, hypotension, and acute kidney injury. His urinary catheter is no longer draining, but he cannot recall when it stopped doing so. Review of his chart shows that the urine and blood cultures drawn 1 week ago grew *E. coli* that were resistant to ciprofloxacin. He is admitted to the hospital and started on piperacillin–tazobactam intravenously for urosepsis.

1. What type of medical error occurred?

2. How could this error have been prevented? What could the inpatient physician (emergency department physician, PCP, hospital, patient) have done differently to prevent rehospitalization?

Answers

1. Test follow-up error occurred, in which a test result that was pending at the time of discharge was not followed up. The patient had urine and blood cultures ordered and in process, which usually take at least 24 to 48 hours for a preliminary result, and up to 5 days for a final result. This patient stayed in the hospital for observation only, and thus was discharged in less than 24 hours. The case does not provide enough information to determine if an adequate handoff regarding the pending test result occurred and who would be responsible for

following up on the final result with the patient. The positive blood and urine cultures indicated that the oral antibiotic prescribed at discharge would not provide adequate antimicrobial coverage. The result was potentially actionable in this case, meaning that the result would have changed the plan of management or, more specifically, the choice of antibiotic.

2. Many interventions are possible to prevent medical errors and promote patient safety during the transition from the inpatient setting to the outpatient setting. One commonly recognized intervention is transmission of a discharge summary to the PCP. The goal is to use the discharge summary to communicate pending tests, in addition to other key discharge information, to the PCP for postdischarge follow-up. This method provides, at a minimum, the passive transmission of information via a discharge summary to indicate issues that need to be addressed during the postdischarge follow-up period. A direct verbal provider-to-provider handoff is also highly recommended.

   The summary should also include other important information about the discharge care plan, such as diagnoses, medication changes, pending diagnostic tests or laboratory results needing follow-up, and recommended outpatient workup such as additional diagnostic or laboratory testing, or specialty referrals. Stakeholders in the transmission of patient discharge information include the inpatient or emergent department physician, both of whom are the providers of new information obtained during an emergency room visit or hospitalization, respectively, and the PCP, who is the receiver of this information. Pending issues must be adequately handed off at each transition of care from 1 provider to each subsequent care provider.

   It is important to recognize that the patient is clearly the primary stakeholder, but the patient should not be solely relied on to be the courier or the retainer of important information regarding the care transition. In an accountable care arrangement, it is not acceptable to rely on the patient as courier of such important information. The hospital, postdischarge care facility, and/or primary care physician may be accountable for the transmission of discharge information by establishing standards of service, developing a culture of patient safety, and providing supportive information technology systems. Effective methods of minimizing medical errors during this important transition should address the potential outcomes of poorly managed care transitions. Outcomes may include increased rehospitalization rates, adverse clinical outcomes, and patient and provider dissatisfaction with discharge care planning.

TRANSITIONS OF CARE: PENDING ISSUES AT DISCHARGE

After medication errors, the next most common errors in the postdischarge period include test follow-up errors and workup errors (Table 47-1). Adequate and timely communication between care providers during the transition from the

Table 47-1. Types of Error Related to Discontinuity of Care From the Inpatient to Outpatient Setting

Medication continuity errors	Medication was documented in the hospital chart, but not in the medication list of the first postdischarge PCP visit
Test follow-up errors	A test result was pending at discharge, but was not acknowledged in the outpatient chart
Workup error	An outpatient test or procedure suggested or scheduled by the inpatient provider was not adequately followed up by the outpatient provider

inpatient setting to the outpatient setting is an important target in high-quality, safe patient care. In a health care system where PCPs are increasingly less likely to be a patient's hospital physician, the transition of care from the inpatient setting to the outpatient setting becomes a time of increased patient vulnerability to medical errors and adverse clinical outcomes. From a patient-centered perspective, the transition between care settings should occur as a smooth continuum of patient care, rather than discrete, punctuated care settings. Transition-of-care processes must be executed efficiently through clear communication between the inpatient providers and outpatient PCP during the patient handoff. Accurate, timely information exchange during this transition is recognized as the benchmark for a successful care transition.

The primary goal of all discharge planning processes is to ensure a patient-centered, well-coordinated care transition that minimizes readmission, medical errors, and adverse events, and promotes the timely execution of appropriate patient care (Figure 47-1). The Joint Commission's National Patient Safety Goals program recognizes the importance of care transitions in managing patient care and safety.

Epidemiology

Three main categories of medical errors exist that are unique to the inpatient-to-outpatient care transition (Table 47-1). Medication continuity errors are the most common of the 3 categories to occur during this care transition. Medication changes at discharge are a topic discussed in detail in another case and thus will not be addressed further here. In a study examining test follow-up errors, a retrospective review of charts of patients discharged over a 5-month period revealed that half of patients had pending tests at discharge. Of these test follow-up errors, 9% were considered potentially actionable, of which more than

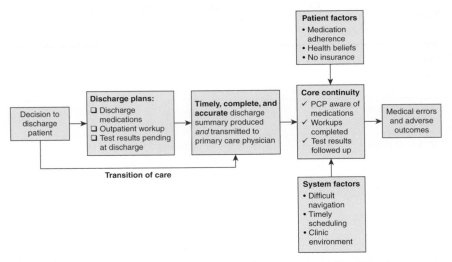

Figure 47-1. Conceptual framework for the discharge transition from inpatient to outpatient care.

one third would change the diagnostic or therapeutic plan, and 12.6% required urgent action.

Workup errors occur when an inpatient provider recommends outpatient tests or referrals but the recommended workup is inadvertently not completed (Figure 47-2). Approximately 27.6% of inpatients are recommended to have outpatient workups, of which only 35.9% are completed. In an observational study at an academic general internal medicine clinic, patients with at least 1 workup error were more than 6 times as likely to be rehospitalized within 3 months after the first postdischarge PCP visit compared with patients without workup errors. In the same study, medication continuity errors and test follow-up errors were less likely to lead to rehospitalization.

General practitioners surveyed about the care transition from the inpatient to outpatient setting described hospitalization of their patients as a "black box," in which inadequate communication led to lack of knowledge of the patient's clinical status and important continuity of care issues. The method of communication was far less important than the expectation that communication occurred at all. In an observational study, direct communication between hospital physicians and PCPs occurred only 3% to 20% of the time, and a discharge summary at the first postdischarge visit was available in only 12% to 34% of cases. Direct communication is arguably the most effective means to ensure adequate discharge communication between inpatient provider and primary care physician because it is more than simply a transfer of information—it provides an opportunity for 2-way dialogue.

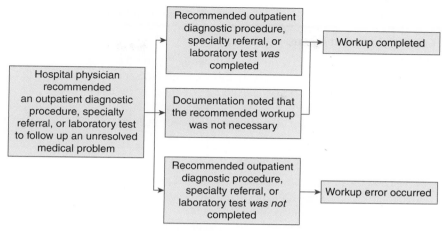

Figure 47-2. Assessment of workup completion.

Treatment

Various methods to achieve safe and efficient care transitions from the inpatient to outpatient setting have been studied. The foundation of the majority of proposed interventions depends on clear communication between providers in each of these settings. Clear communication skills about the care transition and appropriately detailed content of the transition should guide handoff etiquette (Table 47-2).

Another common method of ensuring appropriate content of a discharge summary is a checklist (Table 47-3). Implementation of a discharge checklist may be integrated into the hospital care process at various levels or may be the responsibility of different individuals. Multidisciplinary discharge teams are increasingly recognized as an important part of a well-coordinated discharge. Additionally, teams that continue care remotely in the postdischarge period prior to primary care follow-up are increasingly common. The impact of these and other interventions on medical errors and adverse outcomes is an active area of continuing research. Integration of information technology tools also has the potential to greatly enhance the discharge process, including production of an effective discharge summary that includes pending test results, recommended further workups, and medication changes. For example, many inpatient electronic health records have the capability to customize hospital discharge summary templates designed to ensure that all the discharge checklist items have been completed and effectively communicated to the patient, family, PCP, and other important postdischarge care providers, including home health care services and nursing homes.

Table 47-2. Six Principles of the Inpatient-to-outpatient Handoff

Communicate, but do not irritate

The primary care physician should be sufficiently informed so that a question from a patient or family member can elicit an appropriate response. The hospitalist should select a communication method based on local primary care physician preference and patient population served, and can be by telephone, fax, or, increasingly, electronically

Consult the primary care physician

The PCP can be an invaluable source of information about the patient, particularly when difficult circumstances arise, for example, discussions about code status. More importantly, the patient should not receive conflicting messages and the patient may be comforted to know that the primary care physician is in agreement with the plan of care

Timeliness is next to godliness

Timeliness of primary care physician notification of patient admission to the hospital, involvement of the primary care physician at important decision points in care, and transmission of discharge summaries before the postdischarge follow-up visit are essential

Partner with the patient

The patient should be empowered to be involved in his or her care, and the primary care physician can provide some insight into the patient's preferences regarding this process. The hospitalist's role is to develop rapport with the patient during a challenging time in the patient's continuum of care

Make it clear that you are the patient's advocate

A hospitalist's institutional role in designing and implementing critical pathways, guidelines, and cost control measures cannot interfere with the hospitalist's role as a patient's doctor. The hospitalist should be the patient's advocate without conflicts of interest with his or her institutional roles

Pass the baton as graciously as you received it (or even better, more graciously)

Ensure appropriate follow-up care is arranged and the patient is aware of whom to contact and how regarding problems in the postdischarge period

Table 47-3. Checklist for a Discharge Summary

Minimum Elements of a Transition Record	Ideal Additional Elements of a Transition Record
Main diagnosis, or problem that led to hospitalization	Anticipated problems and suggested interventions, and contact number and person
Discharge medications, with reasons for any changes to the previous medication regimen	Proposed treatment and diagnostic plan
Name and contact information of transferring physician	Recommendations of subspecialty consultations
Discharge destination	Brief hospital course
Details of follow-up arrangements made	Pertinent physical findings and key findings, including results of procedures and laboratory tests
Pending laboratory work and tests	
Patient's cognitive status	Information given to the patient and family, and documentation of patient education
	Specific follow-up needs, including wound care, durable medical equipment, etc
	Advance directives, power of attorney, consent
	Assessment of caregiver status

TIPS TO REMEMBER

- Medication continuity errors, workup errors, and test follow-up errors are the 3 most common errors that occur during the discharge transition.
- Timely communication with the PCP, including transmission of a complete and accurate discharge summary, improves the coordination of care during a patient's discharge transition.

COMPREHENSION QUESTIONS

1. What is the most important foundational principle of an effective care transition?

      A. Providing a detailed discharge summary to the patient and family

      B. Communicating with the patient's PCP in a timely manner

C. Electronically transmitting a discharge summary to the patient's PCP

D. Calling the patient within 48 hours after discharge

E. Using teach-back to ensure patient understanding about the discharge

2. What information should be clearly communicated in a discharge summary or handoff to the patient's primary care physician to ensure pending issues are addressed after discharge?

A. Pending test results and procedure or radiology reports

B. Recommended outpatient workup, including tests and referrals

C. Medication reconciliation, changes, and timeline (eg, for antibiotics course)

D. All of the above

Answers

1. **B.** Communication with the PCP regarding pending issues is essential to a well-coordinated care transition from the inpatient to the outpatient setting. The discharge checklist helps to guide the discharge planner and/or hospitalist to ensure that all important clinical and follow-up information is provided in an efficient discharge summary.

2. **D.** Medication continuity errors, workup errors, and test follow-up errors are the 3 most common errors that occur during the discharge transition. Special attention to these components of the discharge summary will ensure that the handoff to the primary care physician is as well informed as possible. Scheduling and completing a follow-up appointment with the primary care physician for a postdischarge hospital follow-up visit within 30 days may be able to reduce readmission for certain high-risk conditions, and is one of the important drivers of the anticipated Medicare reimbursement penalty for hospitals that have higher-than-expected rates of readmissions.

SUGGESTED READINGS

American College of Physicians. *Creating a Better Discharge Summary: Is Standardization the Answer?* <http://www.acphospitalist.org/archives/2009/03/discharge.htm#sb1>; 2009. Accessed May 2012.

Coleman EA, Williams MV. Executing high-quality care transitions: a call to do it right. *J Hosp Med.* 2007;2:287–290.

Goldman L, Pantilat SZ, Whitcomb WF. Passing the clinical baton: 6 principles to guide the hospitalist. *Am J Med.* 2001;111:S36–S39.

Hansen LO, Young RS, Hinami K, Leung A, Williams MV. Interventions to reduce 30-day rehospitalization: a systematic review. *Ann Intern Med.* 2011;155:520–528.

Kripalani S, Jackson AT, Schnipper JL, Coleman EA. Promoting effective transitions of care at hospital discharge: a review of key issues for hospitalists. *J Hosp Med.* 2007;2:314–323.

Kripalani S, LeFevre F, Phillips CO, Williams MV, Basaviah P, Baker DW. Deficits in communication and information transfer between hospital-based and primary care physicians: implications for patient safety and continuity of care. *JAMA*. 2007;297:831–841.

Moore C, McGinn T, Halm E. Tying up loose ends: discharging patients with unresolved medical issues. *Arch Intern Med*. 2007;167:1305–1311.

Moore C, Wisnivesky J, Williams S, McGinn T. Medical errors related to discontinuity of care from an inpatient to an outpatient setting. *J Gen Intern Med*. 2003;18:646–651.

Roy CL, Poon EG, Karson AS, et al. Patient safety concerns arising from test results that return after hospital discharge. *Ann Intern Med*. 2005;143:121–128.

Snow V, Beck D, Budnitz T, et al. Transitions of Care Consensus policy statement: American College of Physicians, Society of General Internal Medicine, Society of Hospital Medicine, American Geriatrics Society, American College of Emergency Physicians, and Society for Academic Emergency Medicine. *J Hosp Med*. 2009;4:364–370.

Tandjung R, Rosemann T, Badertscher N. Gaps in continuity of care at the interface between primary care and specialized care: general practitioners' experiences and expectations. *Int J Gen Med*. 2011;4:773–778.

The Joint Commission. *National Patient Safety Goals*. <http://www.jointcommission.org/standards_information/npsgs.aspx>; 2012. Accessed May 2012.

van Walraven C, Mamdani M, Fang J, Austin PC. Continuity of care and patient outcomes after hospital discharge. *J Gen Intern Med*. 2004;19:624–631.

WEB SITES

AHRQ Discharge Process Information for Clinicians and Consumers: http://www.ahrq.gov/qual/impptdis.htm.

Project RED (Re-engineered Discharge): https://www.bu.edu/fammed/projectred/.

Society of Hospital Medicine's Project BOOST (Better Outcomes for Older adults through Safe Transitions): http://www.hospitalmedicine.org/ResourceRoomRedesign/RR_CareTransitions/CT_Home.cfm.

The Care Transitions Program: http://www.caretransitions.org/.

A 72-year-old Man With Social Issues

Stacy Sattovia, MD, FACP

The patient is a 72-year-old man with a past medical history significant for congestive heart failure with an ejection fraction of 25%. Your inpatient team is called by the emergency room to admit the patient who has presented with decompensated congestive heart failure. Review of his records reveals 6 admissions in the past 4 months. Each time he is admitted he rapidly improves, and your team wonders why the patient requires so many hospitalizations.

1. What social issues may be contributing to the patient's frequent hospitalizations?

Answer

1. Readmissions often signal a failure to address aspects of a patient's social situation that might limit the patient's ability to comply with a complex medical regimen and thus hinder a successful recovery. Numerous social issues may exist for any patient.

CASE REVIEW

With this case, you further discover that while the patient's condition, medication regimen, and dietary restrictions seem standard to you, he doesn't understand it. His wife previously took care of him—she ensured that he took his medications correctly and prepared nutritious low-sodium meals for him; however, she passed away 8 months ago. In addition, the patient doesn't read very well and finds the small print on the bottles difficult to decipher. Even if he can read them, he doesn't always understand the directions. His meals consist mostly of frozen dinners and cans of soup, both of which tend to have a high sodium content. In general, the patient is very frustrated and beginning to feel hopeless about his medical condition, and he misses his wife terribly.

TRANSITIONS OF CARE: PATIENTS WITH SOCIAL ISSUES

Discharge is a complex transition of care that leaves a patient highly vulnerable to adverse events. The key to a successful transition from the inpatient to the outpatient setting begins at the time of admission. Numerous social issues might exist that can complicate patients' hospital stays and compromise their success during this critical transition of care.

The literature cites that up to 20% of US hospitalizations result in readmission within 30 days. The Medicare Payment Advisory Committee found that up to 76% of 30-day readmissions in Medicare beneficiaries are potentially avoidable. Similar literature states that unplanned rehospitalizations may signal a failure in hospital discharge processes, patients' ability to manage self-care, and/or the quality of care in the next community setting. Patients' ability to manage self-care is, in part, closely related to their social context.

Eliciting these social issues in the setting of medical illness requires the physician to think broadly—to move beyond symptoms, diagnosis, and treatment to inquire about aspects of the patient's life that may be quite personal. The physician may also need to obtain collateral information from family or other persons close to the patient.

Important factors to consider include:

1. Living situation:

   Where does the patient live?

   Does the patient live alone?

   Does the patient have family support?

   Is the support that exists healthy enough to care for the patient?

   Will the patient be able to return to independent living?

   Who does the patient support? Will the patient still be able to do so?

   What are the physical attributes of the home, specifically related to the patient's functional status? For example, how many steps are required to move from the bedroom to bathroom?

   What durable medical equipment might help the patient remain as functional and independent as possible?

2. Finances:

   Does the patient have insurance coverage?

   Can the patient afford medications and follow-up care?

   Can the patient afford rent, house payments, and food?

3. Transportation:

   How will the patient get home from the hospital?

   Can the patient get to follow-up appointments?

   If the patient used public transportation prior to hospitalization, is the patient still able to physically do this?

4. Health literacy:

   What is the patient's literacy level?

   Can the patient understand discharge instructions and medications?

5. Other issues:

   Does the patient have a primary care physician?

   Does the patient know how to contact his or her primary care physician?

   Are there substance abuse issues confounding the patient's health?

How to Assess

Eliciting this information needs to begin at admission. Begin with asking the patient about these issues—for example, "tell me about your life at home." Starting with an open-ended question can elicit factors that you may not consider asking about, particularly when you remember that everyone's social situation is unique. You may then move into specific questions to develop a more complete understanding of the patient's social context and the needs the patient might have.

There are typically resources that can be of tremendous benefit to the patient and the provider. Social workers possess the expertise to counsel patients and identify resources that might provide social and financial support. For example, there may be commercial or community programs that can help a patient afford medications. Some patients may qualify for help at home in the form of home health or senior support services, thereby allowing the patient to remain more independent. Obtaining physical therapy and occupational therapy evaluations are particularly helpful in assessing a patient's functional status. These experts can then lend recommendations to provide a physically safe discharge plan for the patient.

The ultimate goal is to be able to formulate a plan at discharge that provides maximal support to the patient—this requires understanding not only the disease process and therapy but also the impact the social context has on each particular patient's overall health.

TIPS TO REMEMBER

- Patients' social situations are often quite complex. Asking about their lives at home can be very helpful to elicit barriers to adherence with the plan of care.
- Social service experts are typically available in the inpatient setting and their expertise should be leveraged to help patients at the time of discharge.

COMPREHENSION QUESTIONS

1. The patient is an 89-year-old female who lives alone. She has had 6 admissions in the last 9 months, each for a different reason. At the time of the current discharge, she declines a short stay in a nursing home for continued rehabilitation, stating that her family will stay with her and provide 24-hour assistance. The family is in the room with her and they confirm this. However, the situation and solution do not seem that simple to you. What is a reasonable next step?

    A. Discharge the patient to the care of her family—you cannot force her to accept assistance.

    B. Ask social services to see the patient—perhaps she will qualify for some further assistance in her home.

C. Ask the patient if you can speak with her alone to obtain further social history.
D. Obtain a psychiatry consultation to assess decision-making capacity.

2. The patient is a 34-year-old male with a past medical history significant for schizophrenia that is well compensated. He has been admitted twice in the past 1 week for a lower extremity cellulitis. Each time he responded very well to IV antibiotics but worsened after discharge. You discover that he did not obtain his antibiotics at discharge and did not follow up with his primary care provider.
　He is again ready for discharge. How can you ensure his medical success?
　　A. Consult psychiatry—they might be effective at helping him take his medications.
　　B. Discharge him to an extended care facility to finish his intravenous antibiotics—this may represent oral antibiotic failure.
　　C. Provide oral antibiotics at the time of discharge.
　　D. Ask the patient what he needs to be able to comply with the recommended plan of care.

Answers

1. C. If something about the social situation seems unworkable to you, it is worth further exploration. On further discussion, alone with the patient, you discover that while she loves her family, she financially supports 2 of her adult children and there is concern that if she enters a nursing home, even for a short stay, she will not be able to provide this assistance to her children. Additionally, in the past, despite the recommendations of her providers, her children have not provided 24-hour care. She is scared she will not be able to meet her own medical needs.
　This is a delicate, but not uncommon, social situation. At this point, enlisting the assistance of the social services experts will be helpful as you begin an important discussion with the family—the key is to place the patient's needs first.

2. D. Asking the patient what his needs are is an excellent way to help ensure his success. In this situation you would discover that he was unable to obtain his antibiotics because he was discharged over a holiday weekend and the pharmacy that he typically uses was closed and thus unable to deliver his medications. In addition, he did not attend his outpatient follow-up because the appointment was scheduled in the morning and the bus he takes to his appointments only runs in the afternoons. With attention to these 2 issues, you find that over the next few days, the patient did indeed obtain and take his medications appropriately and did attend his afternoon follow-up appointment with his primary care provider, with resolution of his cellulitis.

SUGGESTED READINGS

Berenson RA, Paulus RA, Kalman NS. Medicare's readmissions-reduction program—a positive alternative. *N Engl J Med.* 2012;366:1364–1366.

Cain CH, Neuwirth E, Bellows J, Zuber C, Green J. Patient experiences of transitioning from hospital to home: an ethnographic quality improvement project. *J Hosp Med.* 2012;7:382–387.

Mudge AM, Kasper K, Clair A, et al. Recurrent readmissions in medical patients: a prospective study. *J Hosp Med.* 2011;6(2):61–67.

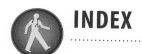

INDEX

Page numbers followed by *f* or *t* indicate figures or tables, respectively.